edited by H Hinzen and V H Hundsdörfer

The TANZANIAN Experience

Education for LIBERATION and DEVELOPMENT

Published by
Unesco Institute for Education, Hamburg
and
Evans Brothers Limited

Published by Evans Brothers Limited
Montague House, Russell Square
London WC1B 5BX

Evans Brothers (Nigeria Publishers) Limited
PMB 5164, Jericho Road
Ibadan

First published 1979

Set in 10 on 11 point Baskerville
Printed by BAS Printers Limited,
Over Wallop, Hants.
ISBN 0 237 50405 1   PRA 6864

Contents

Foreword

The current research programme of the Unesco Institute for Education includes in its various avenues of research two series of analytic-descriptive studies dealing with selected educational experiences. From the case studies centring on national reforms of a comprehensive nature, insight is expected into the many-sided aspects of 'total' or 'global' systems of lifelong education as well as into the preconditions for and the various phases of their implementation. The studies on practices with a restricted scope in terms of objectives, target groups, programmes, resources and implications, on the other hand, should contribute to the understanding of the meaning and implications of lifelong education at the institutional or classroom level.

Both series share a common interpretation of lifelong education which influences the focus of the studies. Both aim at contributing to a comprehensive, consistent and reliable theory of lifelong education, through the validation of its assumptions and through identification of its practical consequences when it is applied to a specific educational area.

Thus, while the individual case studies are self-contained and consistent in terms of immediate objectives, specific scope and research methodology, they are not ends in themselves but form part of a cumulative process intended to provide an empirical basis for the development of a comprehensive theory of lifelong education.

The methodological controversies surrounding case studies are common knowledge. They seem to derive from the characteristics of the various fields of knowledge in which they are used, from the purpose for which they are undertaken as well as from the varying emphasis placed on the successive phases of the research process. The present study adds to these controversial features some of its own. Eighteen educators (most of them Tanzanian) closely connected with the implementation of the national reform were requested to describe, assess and forecast its development in the areas with which they are particularly familiar. The authors measure the achievements and the outcomes of a quinquennium of work against the original intentions guiding the reform and the national expectations vested in it. Their involvement guarantees a reliable interpretation of the preconditions, the purposes and the pattern of the changes introduced.

The Tanzanian educational developments are regarded in lifelong education literature as an example of the reorganisation of the whole range of educational activities (formal, non-formal and informal) into a global system characterized by flexibility, articulation, adaptation and universalization. Thus, although the term 'lifelong education' rarely appears in the Tanzanian Reform, the principles guiding this Reform for Liberation and Development and the practices introduced coincide closely with the ideas usually stated and the practices recommended in connection with lifelong education.

The descriptions and analyses made by the contributors to this report, while centring on those aspects of the reform which are considered significant for the clarification of the idea and for the implementation of the principles of lifelong education, have not been influenced by this intention. They simply describe the reform as conceived and viewed by educators in Tanzania.

The linking of the features of the reform with the characteristics of lifelong education is tentatively carried out in a brief concluding chapter, which indicates, in general terms, the main areas of similarity. In addition, a subject index setting the various aspects of the reform against the key concepts of lifelong education, provides an instrument for a detailed understanding of what is meant by the coincidence between the principles of the Tanzanian Reform and those of lifelong education. The study also offers a comprehensive, up-to-date and selected bibliography on the Tanzanian Educational Reform, substantially complementing those already in existence.

The Unesco Institute for Education has been singularly fortunate in receiving the generous support of Julius Nyerere, President of the United Republic of Tanzania, with whose permission the articles in Chapter 2 are reproduced. The Ministry of Education and the Tanzanian Unesco National Commission have also greatly facilitated the various stages of the work. Nor could the book have reached its satisfactory conclusion without the interest and help of the many Tanzanian educators contributing to the study. We are indebted to them for devoting so much of their valuable and limited free time towards the making of this book. Finally we must gratefully acknowledge the whole-hearted dedication and enthusiasm of the editors V H Hunsdörfer and H Hinzen whose familiarity with the Tanzanian Educational Reform and links with a large number of educators in the country made this study possible.

M Dino Carelli
Director
Unesco Institute for Education

Introduction

The idea of starting to work on a case study of the Tanzanian educational reform in the perspective of lifelong education was conceived at a meeting in the UIE early in 1975. It arose from the realization that the conceptual framework of this reform, as set out, for instance, in *Education for Self-Reliance*, is in many aspects closely linked to the general conception of lifelong education.

The project started on a modest scale by collecting relevant published documents from Tanzania. Later, the need was felt to produce a consistent study that would take the most recent developments into consideration. It was, therefore, agreed to request Tanzanian educationists to contribute original sections based on the research and development work in which each of them had been engaged in connection with the current educational reform. Thus the editors approached several scholars they already knew, either personally from past joint work or from their research reports and publications, and asked them to propose other colleagues who had the necessary competence and were willing to co-operate. All participants invited were given an outline of the whole proposed study and suggestions on the desired content and form of presentation of its individual parts. The team created in this manner expanded both the topics and the methods of the initial study plan. From a mere collection of relevant articles already published the project thus became an original study on the Tanzanian education for liberation and development.

The rationale for the structure of the report derives from the innovations introduced by the reform and the overall conception of education in Tanzania. As both are guided by the content of writings and speeches by President Nyerere, the most important of these are presented in Chapter 2 as an introduction to the detailed description of the Tanzanian educational reform. Next the pattern of integration of formal and non-formal education, which seems to be one of the characteristics of a system of lifelong education, is analyzed. It is followed by a chapter on schooling, covering different aspects of the history and present situation in primary and secondary education and teacher training. Problems such as curriculum development, evaluation procedures, expansion of education from very restricted access to universal primary education and diversification of secondary education, are discussed at length in that chapter. The wide range of learning opportunities for adults that are provided on different levels and with diverse purposes could, it was felt, be best covered under the broad heading *The Non-formal and Formal Sector in Education and Training of Adults*. The chapter is subdivided into basic and manpower-oriented sectors to reflect the diversification and integration of adult education. The chapter on research shows different modes and methods of applied research in Tanzania, and provides an insight into selected problems existing in formal and non-formal education. That chapter also presents a research project which involves participation in research by the people themselves. The structured and selected bibliography at the end suggests a number of titles on each of the topics dealt with to those interested in further reading or research.

Chapter 7 finally attempts to point out the principles of lifelong education which would seem to be supported by the Tanzanian educational reform.

This organization of the report has been chosen because it was thought that it would best serve the reading public for which it is mainly intended, i.e. educationists in Third World countries, professionals interested in lifelong education and specialists in the fields of development planning and policy.

It is hoped that this book will help the reader to understand the Tanzanian educational concept, the changes it has undergone in this decade, the reasons for them, and the deficiencies from which it is still suffering, and so provide an opportunity for profiting from the Tanzanians' experiences, good and bad ones alike.

We, as editors, would like to thank the Unesco Institute for Education for incorporating our proposal in its research programme, and all its staff for the contributions they have made to this study. Our special thanks go to the Director, Dr Dino Carelli, and our ever-present co-ordinating officer, Miss Hede Menke, for their valuable comments and help throughout the course of the project, and to Mrs J Kesavan for her untiring co-operation in the later editing.

Finally we want to express our deep appreciation of the willingness with which so many Tanzanians have participated in the study, thus permitting people in different parts of the world to share their valuable experiences. To all of them we are sincerely grateful for their excellent co-operation. May the study be looked upon as a committed contribution to the tenth anniversary of the declaration of 'Education for Self-Reliance'.

Roisdorf/Wiesbaden   Heribert Hinzen
January 1977   V Harry Hundsdörfer

List of Abbreviations

AE	Adult Education
AI	Ardhi Institute, Dar es Salaam
BRALUP	Bureau of Resource Assessment and Land Use Planning, UDSM
CC	Cooperative College
CEC	Cooperative Education Centre, Moshi
CESO	Centre for the Study of Education in Changing Societies, The Hague, Holland
CNE	College of National Education
CUT	Cooperative Union of Tanganyika
CWM	College of Wild Life Management, Mweka, Moshi
DE	Diploma in Engineering
DEO (AE)	District Education Officer for Adult Education
DO	District Officer
DSM	Dar es Salaam
DTC	Dar es Salaam Technical College
EALB	East African Literature Bureau
EAPH	East African Publishing House
ERB	Economic Research Bureau, UDSM
FTC	Full Technician Certificate Course
IAE	Institute of Adult Education, DSM
IDM	Institute of Development Management, Mzumbe, Morogoro
IE	Institute of Education, DSM

KFI	Kunduchi Fisheries Institute, DSM
MTUU	(Kiswahili abbreviation for) Tanzania/Unicef/Unesco Primary Education Reform Project
NACE	National Advisory Committee on Education
NAEAT	National Adult Education Association of Tanzania
NCI	National Correspondence Institution, IAE, DSM
NDC	National Development Corporation
NEC	National Executive Committee of TANU
NIP	National Institute of Productivity, DSM
NUTA	National Union of Tanzania's Workers
NVTC	National Vocational Training Centre
NVTP	National Vocational Training Programme
OL	Olmotonyi Forestry Institute, Arusha
OS	Overseas
OUP	Oxford University Press
REO (AE)	Regional Education Officer for Adult Education
RTD	Radio Tanzania Dar es Salaam
SIDA	Swedish International Development Authority
SIDO	Small Scale Industries Development Organisation
TANU	Tanzania or Tanganyika African National Union
TAPA	Tanzania or Tanganyika African Parents' Association
TPDF	Tanzania or Tanganyika Peoples' Defence Forces
TLS	Tanzania or Tanganyika Library Service
Tsh	Tanzanian Shilling (rate in March 1977 Tsh 8 = US \$1)
TYL	TANU Youth League
UDSM	University of Dar es Salaam
UMak	Makerere College, Kampala, Uganda
UNai	University of Nairobi, Kenya
UNDP	United Nations Development Programme
UNECA	United Nations Economic Commission for Africa
UNESCO	United Nations Educational, Scientific and Cultural Organization
UPE	Universal Primary Education
UWT	United Women of Tanganyika
WOALPP	Work-Oriented Adult Literacy Pilot Project, Lake Regions, Tanzania

Notes on Contributors

Bwatwa, Y D M
Currently Lecturer in Adult Education and Research in the Department of Education, University of Dar es Salaam.

Chale, E M
Resident Tutor in the National Correspondence Institution, Institute of Adult Education, Dar es Salaam.

Cropley, A J
Professor of Psychology at the University of Regina, Saskatchewan, Canada. Presently spending two years' leave as Principal Research Specialist at the Unesco Institute for Education, Hamburg.

von Freyhold, Michaela
Formerly in the Department of Sociology, University of Dar es Salaam, now in the Institute of Finance Management, Dar es Salaam.

Hinzen, H
Research Scholarship Holder at Institute of Education, University of Heidelberg, at the time this study was made. Now Programme Officer, German Adult Education Association, Bonn.

Hundsdörfer, V H
Assistant Professor at the Institute of Ethnology and African Studies, Mainz University.

Ishumi, A G M
Senior Lecturer in the Department of Education, University of Dar es Salaam.

Joachim, A K
Organizer in the Research and Planning Department, Institute of Adult Education, Dar es Salaam.

Kassam, Y O
Senior Lecturer in Adult Education in the Department of Education, University of Dar es Salaam.

Mahai, B A P
Head of the Research and Planning Department, Institute of Adult Education, Dar es Salaam.

Maliyamkono, T L
Lecturer in Economics of Education, Department of Education, University of Dar es Salaam.

Malya, S
Principal Tutor Academic, Institute of Adult Education, Dar es Salaam.

Mbilinyi, Marjorie
Senior Lecturer in the Department of Education, University of Dar es Salaam.

Mbunda, F L
Senior Lecturer in Education in the Department of Education, University of Dar es Salaam.

Meena, A S
Senior Lecturer in Science Education in the Department of Education, University of Dar es Salaam.

Menke, Hede
Associate Expert in Educational Research and Development, Unesco Institute for Education, Hamburg.

von Mitschke-Collande, P
Lecturer in the Department of Mechanical Engineering, University of Dar es Salaam.

Mlekwa, V M
Resident Tutor in the Training and Personnel Department, Institute of Adult Education, Dar es Salaam.

Mmari, G R V
Head of the Department of Education, University of Dar es Salaam.

Muze, M S
Lecturer in the Department of Education, University of Dar es Salaam.

Shengena, J J
Formerly Head of Workers' Education Section in the Ministry of National Education, now Head of the Functional Literacy Section in the Ministry of National Education, Dar es Salaam.

Swantz, Marja Liisa
Formerly Senior Fellow in the Bureau of Resource Assessment and Land Use Planning, University of Dar es Salaam, now in the Institute of Ethnology, University of Helsinki.

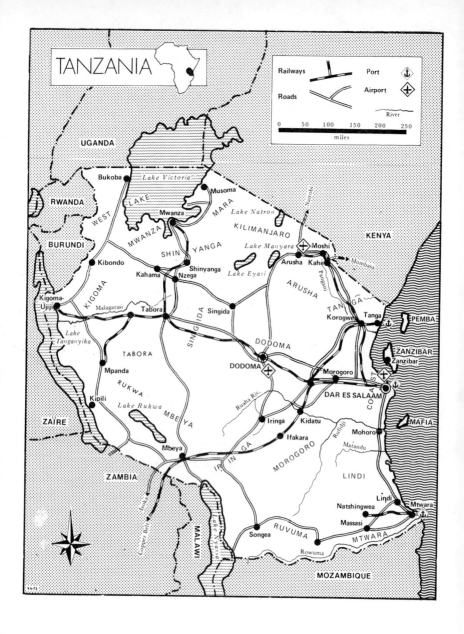

Chapter 1 Education in Tanzania

1.1 Historical Outline
V H Hundsdörfer

To write about 'The Tanzanians' is somewhat difficult. The 15 million inhabitants of Tanzania comprise many different communities and groups which in the past constituted more than 120 differing societies, each with a number of unequal strata. In modern times there was little or no political or social communication between them.

This constellation was the result of geographical, ecological and political circumstances that had conditioned the process of societal development for the last two centuries. Tanzania, a tropical country with a very humid coastal strip and temperate highlands consisting of different vegetative zones—stretches of very fertile land with lush vegetation within semi-arid woodland—had seen constant population movements as far back as human history in that part of the world is known. The pressure on areas with good soil and sufficient regular rainfall led to the separation and splitting of tribal groups and the scattered structure of indigenous societies.

Intensive communication and cultural exchange between the inhabitants of East Africa and other peoples living at the edges of the Indian Ocean can be traced back to the seventh century A.D. Even earlier there had been trade relations with countries such as China, and contacts of an unknown nature with other foreign peoples, such as the inhabitants of legendary 'Azania'—as the Greeks called the interior behind the East African coast.

The history of armed struggle by the local inhabitants of this part of East Africa against foreign invaders dates back to the early sixteenth century, when the Portuguese were trying to conquer the coast. Although the Portuguese managed to rule these people for about two centuries, they never succeeded in subjugating them completely, not even after they had destroyed most of their cities and towns. The Portuguese were defeated by Arabs from Oman, who in

1846 moved their capital to Zanzibar. In the interior of the country there had been constant moves by Nilo-Hamitic groups from the north invading the highlands between Mount Meru, Mount Kilimanjaro, the Pare Mountains, Lake Victoria and the Central Plains around Dodoma. They are reported to have settled down at the beginning of the nineteenth century—just in time for the next invasion. Zulu groups, called Ngoni, who had been defeated by the British and the Boers in South Africa, fled to the north fighting the peoples who had been living on fertile ground in eastern Africa. They finally settled to the east of Lake Nyasa, with their centre at Songea. Some of their groups or families moved up to the forests of Ifakara waging wars against other societies in that region. Slave raiders and traders profited from this so called 'tribal' warfare. Some of them may even have partially financed it. At any rate they encouraged it and bought the captives, though they also engaged in slave hunting of the kind known in West Africa.

From the beginning of the nineteenth century at least half the population of this area was thus taken as slaves to the islands of Zanzibar, Pemba, Mauritius and the Seychelles or killed during the slave raids, or perished on their way to the slave market. Slaves carrying ivory from the interior to the coast provided big business in the decades up to 1873, when the slave market of Zanzibar was closed.

The German colonizers arrived on the shores of East Africa in the early 1880s. A few years later, the area between the Indian Ocean and Lake Tanganyika, between Ruvuma River and Lake Victoria, which was then called Tanganyika and is now mainland Tanzania, became a German protectorate. Germans fought for nearly three decades to pacify the country. At least two fifths of it was, for instance, involved in the supratribal Maji Maji rebellion against German colonization (1905–1907). Very harsh methods were applied to put down this insurrection. The colonizers destroyed not only the villages they suspected of harbouring guerillas, but also the fields and entire harvests, in order to make it impossible for the population to offer further resistance. Thus they depopulated formerly flourishing regions and let fertile cultivated areas revert to bushland or deserted plains. The resulting famine was the most serious in the history of the people.

The Germans tried to prepare the country for colonial development. But before they had reached their goal, World War I put an end to their efforts. Nearly all of the newly created infrastructure was destroyed by the war.

Two other factors contributed to the decline of the legendary high civilization of the olden days. The first is an implicit one. When all of the small surplus gained by communities living mostly in a subsistence economy is needed for defence purposes, little if anything is left in terms of capital or unused labour to promote social progress. Moreover, when defence is the main occupation of a population of peasant farmers, as it was in the East African hinterland in the late eighteenth century, agricultural output is bound to be minimized.

The second reason for the decay of East African agriculture in those areas was a change in the climate and the sudden occurrence in the last decades of the nineteenth century of cattle diseases such as rinderpest. This is reported to have almost annihilated Tanganyikan livestock so that even rich families who had owned thousands of head of cattle found themselves on the verge of starvation.

Thus, at the end of World War I the population of Tanganyika was really underdeveloped in several respects. The surviving human beings lived in scattered homesteads hidden in the bush. Most of them had accepted apathy and political indifference as their way of life in order to avoid trouble with the rulers—a lesson their long history of surrender had taught them.

During the mandate period (1919–1961) the British had little interest in any development activity that did not bring them profits in simple economic terms. They continued to pursue the policy of exploitation to which the inhabitants of Tanganyika had been subjected by all their invaders for the last four and a half centuries. Since Tanganyika was rather poor, all colonial activities concentrated on agriculture. But, as John Iliffe observed, after a period of growing prosperity just after World War II, 'by the 1950s, Tanganyika's farmers were more ready to resist than they had been since 1905'.

Owing to increasing demand for their products on the world market, Tanganyika's farmers tended to oppose obvious economic exploitation by British and Asian traders and the governmental marketing boards. They formed co-operative unions in order to profit as much as possible from their own surplus. When their natural rights were seriously violated, as they had been, for instance, in the Maru land case where the mandatory power expelled local inhabitants from their own grounds to sell their land to European settlers, they organized themselves in political groups together with young African entrepreneurs. And the educated elite, previously organized in debating clubs, demanded for themselves and all African inhabitants of this territory the rights which, as they had learnt from the missionaries, were human rights. These three roots of the independence movement combined in 1954 into one central political organization, the Tanganyika African National Union (TANU), under the leadership of Julius Kamberege Nyerere.

Unlike independence movements in other African countries, TANU was able to take its complaints against the British Mandatory Power to the UNO Trusteeship Council and the General Assembly and thus draw the world's attention to events in Tanganyika. TANU's president Nyerere did so several times in those years. Step by step TANU won more constitutional rights for Tanganyika and international support at the UN level. It proved to be a mass movement when it won all the elections that were gradually permitted by the British administrators. At the first general election in 1960, victory seemed to be complete: TANU got all but one of the seats in Parliament—and this remaining seat was won by an old TANU member who had been standing for election independently for local reasons but later rejoined the party.

On 9th December 1962 Tanganyika finally became a sovereign state, after only seven years of struggle for independence: a battle without violence, a very diplomatic fight, fought mainly on the international scene and led by the representatives of TANU, a true mass movement that had united all the different political streams under the banner of independence.

Nyerere became Prime Minister, but after two months he resigned: once national independence had been achieved, the unifying political factor had gone. He preferred to tour the country, to work and talk with the peasants about their problems, and so to reorganize TANU as a government party instead of an independence movement. He was elected President of the Republic by 97 per cent of the votes, and has since been re-elected in 1966, 1970 and 1974.

The road to independence had been so short and the colonial administrators' policy of keeping the African population down so effective, that there were not enough qualified Tanganyikan citizens to take over the posts held by foreign managers and administrators immediately after independence. Africanization of the government machinery thus created problems. As the people had suffered too much from the discrimination practised by their European governors to accept the old staff in the posts of the new state for any length of time, a long-range manpower programme was designed to speed up the Africanization of senior positions. But, since there was a discrepancy between the technical and administrative competence of the new civil servants and their political mandate, many of them had initial difficulties in decision-making. They needed advice and they obtained it from international experts who, although they tried their best, also lacked the political competence needed in Tanganyika in those days.

Some of the new Tanganyikan civil servants had inherited from their colonial predecessors not only their posts but also their attitudes. A few years after independence TANU's officials recognized that the principles of an egalitarian social structure were not becoming effective and that the social development tended to create a class structure divorcing the peasants and workers from the managers, administrators, government employees and politicans, with a few big landowners on their side. In the mid-sixties there was a real danger that a national 'parasitic bourgeoisie' with neo-colonial attitudes might establish itself. The gap between the five per cent town dwellers and the mass of the tax-paying rural population had grown so wide that it became obvious even to an uninformed peasant in the remotest area that officials and managers, landowners and employees were living at the expense of the poor masses.

The turning point was reached when Dar es Salaam students organized a protest demonstration against a planned government regulation that every student was to do a period of National Service at the beginning and after the end of his or her university education. On seeing this demonstration the President was struck by the students' elitist attitude and expelled all of them from the university, had them sent back to their respective places of origin and ordered them to spend their time working hard in the fields together with their relatives. However, their uneducated fathers applied for their re-enrolment at the university, and after one year nearly all of them were readmitted. On the very day on which the students had been expelled the President decided to cut all higher salaries in the country, including his own, by 20 per cent. Together with his party colleagues he then worked out the principles embodied in the 'Arusha Declaration' and the subsequent policy statement 'Education for Self-Reliance'. The first of these documents was adopted by the National Committee of TANU at their annual meeting in February 1967 at Arusha, and the second was published only one month later.

In these papers TANU had drafted a concept of political development towards socialism. It was the signal for the beginning of a new era: after the epoch of decolonization and Africanization these documents marked a positive approach to development, with the main emphases on land, the people, good policies, and good leadership (Nyerere. See Chapter 2.)

It is within the context of such major political changes that the educational reform of Tanzania was conceived, discussed and gradually implemented.

1.2 Aspects of Conception and Implementation
H Hinzen

1. The conception of education

If one looks at some aspects of education in Tanzania within the overall developmental process, one will find that education and society are seen as being dialectically related to each other. On the one hand, the structure and content of the education system depend on the stage of socio-economic development the society has reached: '. . . education cannot be considered apart from society. The formal school system cannot educate a child in isolation from the social and economic system in which it operates . . . the truth is that education is unavoidably part of society'.[1] On the other hand, education is looked upon as one of the key variables in the growth of the human potential to influence the process of development of a society in accordance with the needs and aspirations of the people living and working within it. 'We must change our conditions of life ourselves; and we can learn how to do this by educating ourselves.'[2] This again relates education to a concept of development in which 'development means the development of people',[3] a process which is meaningless without an educational element.

The general purpose of education is seen to be 'to transmit from one generation to the next the accumulated wisdom and knowledge of the society, and to prepare the young people for their future membership of the society and their active participation in its maintenance or development'.[4] In view of the present situation of Tanzania and most African countries, their colonial past and the many new kinds of international dependency, Nyerere adds to his definition: 'the primary purpose of education is the liberation of man'.[5]

Thus, education in Tanzania is purpose-oriented. Nyerere describes and profoundly analyzes what education for self-reliance, for liberation, and for development means in the Tanzanian context. But in his overall educational conception he adds another dimension that stems from the lifelong process of development, the struggle for liberation and self-reliance, from human life itself: '. . . education is something that all of us should continue to acquire from the time we are born until the time we die. This is important both for individuals and for our country as a whole.'[6] His conception thus includes all forms and all stages of education covering virtually the entire life-span of the individual—more informal ones when the child is very young, predominantly formal ones during the time of schooling or training, and all the different kinds of learning in adulthood, be they informal, formal or non-formal. The following figure showing some aspects of the relationships of formal and non-formal education and training for youths and adults in Tanzania may give an impression of the potential role all kinds of adult education play within a conception favouring lifelong education for all, whether on a basic or on higher levels.

The need for integrating education with living and working is another cornerstone for innovations in the Tanzanian system of education. But in contrast to a 'one after the other' or 'from time to time' approach Nyerere stresses the need for lifelong integration of education, working and living. Taking adult education as an example he said: 'If we are to make real progress in "adult education", it is essential that we should stop trying to divide up life into sections,

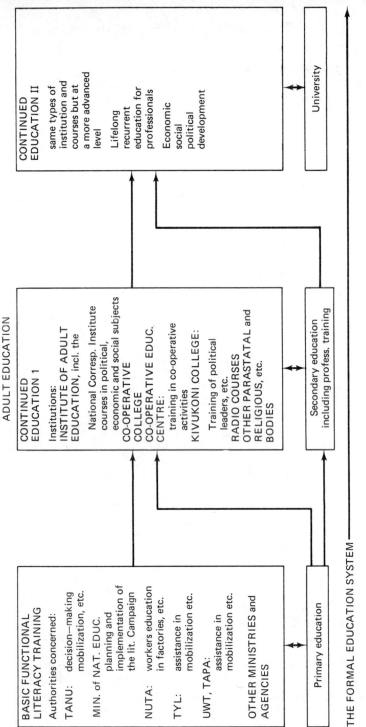

Figure 1.1

Structure of Adult Education in Relation to Formal Education

Source: Kibira, E *Adult Education in Tanzania*, p. 11 Bibl. 137.

one of which is for education and another, longer one which is for work—with occasional time off for "courses". In a country dedicated to change we must accept that education and working are both parts of living and should continue from birth until we die.'[7] Integration of work with education and of education with work or, better, with all aspects of life, is seen to be both a prerequisite for and a fruit of education for self-reliance and for liberation.

2. Educational resolutions and laws within the conceptual framework

The Tanzanian conception of education evolved within, and as a part of, the overall national policy of socialism and self-reliance. Hence its various aspects were not elaborated nor introduced into the educational system simultaneously by means of a new and comprehensive educational law, but gradually. Over a number of years several laws, resolutions and recommendations, mostly dealing with specific parts of the whole and catering for diverse modes of implementation, were issued by the government and its representatives, by TANU, or by President Nyerere. The following brief overview may be useful to the reader.

In 1967 'Education for Self-Reliance' was published. It aimed at making the education provided more relevant to Tanzania by merging the educational needs and aspirations of the individual with those of the community, thus integrating education and society. Primary schooling was to become a complete basic cycle of learning, instead of being regarded, as it used to be, as mainly a preparatory stage and an instrument for selecting the lucky few who would go on to secondary education. At the same time, those receiving secondary school education would be expected to render more service to the communities financing their education. The school curriculum was to be changed so as to make the content of all subjects more relevant to Tanzanian children, to introduce productive activities such as work on farms and in workshops, to relate the lessons very closely to the daily life and work of the pupils, and to merge theory and practice. The parents were to take part in the school activities, and farmers and agricultural extension workers could act as teachers.[8] Education would thus become supportive of the overall development of the country.'

The Second Five-Year Plan (1969–1974), envisaged changing the primary schools into 'community educational centres'[9] which, in addition to providing education by functioning as primary schools, would take care of the educational needs of out-of-school-youths and of adults. In this way formal and non-formal education would be integrated at the village level.

In 1969 the Education Act was passed. It provided, with immediate effect, 'for the development of a system of education in conformity with the political, social and cultural ideals of the United Republic'.[10] The government took over the responsibility for all schools, employing all teachers as government servants. The Ministry of Education was renamed Ministry of National Education and had henceforth to co-ordinate all educational matters on a national level.

In 1971 the 15th Biannual TANU Conference passed two major resolutions concerning education. The first called for an extensive functional literacy campaign so as to make everybody in the country literate; this was seen as an important part of basic education for those who had received no education under colonialism or thereafter. The second stressed the necessity of merging work with education in adult life, so that 'education should be an integral part of any work programme throughout the nation'.[11]

In 1973 the Prime Minister took up again the aim of the second resolution. He demanded that 'Workers' Education must involve ALL WORKERS, starting with the illiterate worker up to the university graduate worker or those holding high posts in leadership, and that this education and training must take place 'during normal working hours for a duration of not less than one hour every day'.[12] This circular has opened wide perspectives for the development of general and professional education on all levels. It provides for continued education after completion of the basic cycle of learning and perhaps some more formal education throughout life covering the whole life-span of the individual in accordance with the needs of the society.

Another 1973 event was the establishment of the National Examinations Council of Tanzania. One of its major objectives is 'to formulate examinations policy in accordance with the principles of education for self-reliance accepted by the people of Tanzania'.[13]

In 1974 the TANU National Executive Council reviewed the progress that had been made in transforming the educational system. On the basis of the findings it passed further resolutions, generally called the 'Musoma Resolutions', [14] to the effect that universal primary education should be realized by 1977. To make this possible, very flexible methods should be employed. For instance, older pupils should teach younger ones; there should be shift lessons in the morning and afternoon; and parents, teachers, and pupils should construct classrooms in self-help activities. In respect to secondary education the TANU resolutions stated that it should be regarded as another cycle of education complete in itself and not as an instrument of preparation and selection for university education. All secondary school leavers should start to work or to be trained for work; this would be facilitated by diversified secondary education in the fields of technical education, agriculture, commerce, and home economics. These provisions resulted in the abolition of direct entry to university education. In future, candidates would be selected from people who were already working, and their work performance as well as their academic ability would be taken into consideration in the selection. The existing examination system was criticized for being incompatible with the guiding principles of education for self-reliance. For instance, primary school leaving examinations were still not conducted in the perspective of assessing the pupils' competence to live and work in their communities and to contribute to the development of socialism and self-reliance; the criteria used were still those suitable for selecting a small number of students for secondary education, the others being regarded by society and themselves as failures. To correct this mistake, primary schooling should either finish without any final examination or the old mode should be replaced by one assessing pupils' capacities for life, education and work, i.e. their academic progress, productive work, and social responsibility shown during school years.

The purpose of the foregoing outline of the Tanzanian conception of education as expressed in some important official statements has been to sketch the framework for the transformation of the education system. Some aspects of implementing educational innovations in Tanzania will be discussed in section 4.

3. Organizing the integration of all education
Today the Ministry of National Education, working in close co-operation with many institutions and bodies, such as the National Advisory Committee on Education, Kivukoni College, and the Ministry of Manpower Development, is the organizing force of educational development and planning. The following figure shows the organizational structure of the Ministry, which by integrating all matters related to education, is concerned with the whole cycle of life and learning. Its four divisions (primary, secondary/technical, teacher, and adult education) indicate that equal recognition is given to all types of education.

Among the 'parastatals', i.e. independent institutions closely linked to the Ministry, are the Institute of Education, and the Institute of Adult Education. Along with other duties, the former is heavily involved in curriculum development and in writing and testing of materials mostly for primary, secondary, and teacher education.[15] The latter is engaged in planning and research on adult education, training of adult educators, administration of mass radio study group campaigns and, through its different regional centres, in conducting courses and evening classes and providing correspondence education for participants in all parts of the country.[16] The Ministry also has close working relationships with, e.g. the University of Dar es Salaam, the Tanzania Library Service which, in co-operation with the Ministry, is endeavouring to establish in the near future libraries everywhere in the country from the national down to the ward level, and Tanzania Elimu Supplies, which is concerned with providing stationery and educational materials of all kinds.

The Ministry of National Education is represented on the regional, district, divisional and ward levels through its officers and co-ordinators. Integration and co-operation are further supported on all those levels by advisory committees representing different institutions and agencies concerned with education and training.

4. Aspects of the implementation of educational innovations
Tanzania has now had only about 15 years for transforming the colonial, and even less for the early post-colonial, structure and content of education. 1977 will be the tenth anniversary of the adoption of 'Education for Self-Reliance' as a guiding principle for the future. It seems, therefore, an opportune moment to investigate to what extent the intensive efforts Tanzania has made in these ten years have succeeded in implementing the intended educational innovations and reaching the desired objectives. Many of the achievements and shortcomings in primary, secondary, and teacher education, and in the various kinds of training and

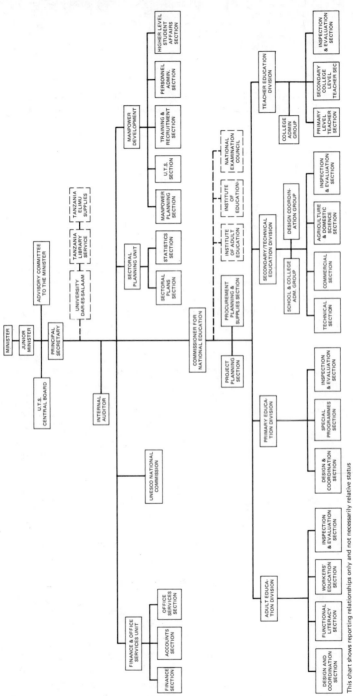

This chart shows reporting relationships only and not necessarily relative status

Figure 1.2

Ministry of National Education—New Structure

Source: Hall, B L, *The Structure of Adult Education and Rural Development in Tanzania.* (IDS Discussion Paper No. 67), Brighton: University of Sussex, Institute of Development Studies (January 1975), App. II.

education of adults, are discussed in detail in the subsequent chapters; some additional general information and problems are presented below.

It was one of the chief designers of the educational concept described above, President Nyerere himself, who said two years ago: '. . . I am becoming increasingly convinced that we in Tanzania either have not yet found the right educational policy, or have not yet succeeded in implementing it—or some combination of these two alternatives'.[17] In the following brief discussion of three priorities in educational development in Tanzania, this critical approach will be adopted, in that an attempt will be made to identify problems and pose questions rather than give ready-made answers.

If Figure 1.3 showing the more formal sector of education, including schooling, is taken as a starting point, the hierarchical nature of the educational structure, rising from the many at the base to the very few at the top, becomes immediately evident. Up to 1975 only about 50 per cent of all school age children entered Standard I in primary school. Of those who finished Standard VII only a small number were selected for secondary schools and an even smaller number for higher education and training after passing some examinations. A look at Figure 1.4 suggests a very close relationship between education and occupation. In this regard, a working group of Tanzanian educationists stated: 'The relationship between the formal educational system and the formal occupational structure is the basis for the people's expectations for education. The major determinant of getting work is the amount of formal education an individual has acquired. The more education someone has, the "bigger" the job he will get (which relates to more income, more fringe benefits, a bigger house, better health services, and greater prestige).'[18]

Education thus seems to be one of the chief factors furthering social stratification of the Tanzanian society through promoting an interest in further education and training mainly in those who have already benefited up to a certain level and can thus benefit again by getting a certificate which will enable them to obtain better employment or a higher salary, most probably in the urban sector. The objectives and content of education for self-reliance and for liberation (see, for example, the curriculum for primary and secondary schools), and hence all the principles deriving from this policy, are trying to educate children against the given reality which has been and is still socializing the students, often enough through the expectations of their parents. The question is whether such 'counter-education' and 'counter-action' are at all possible under present conditions, or whether some further thinking and action are required on the lines suggested by the hypothesis: 'In order for complete transformation of the educational structure to take place, the occupational structure must be transformed.'[19]

In the light of these observations, the following three priorities deserve further comment:

(a) Universal Primary Education (UPE) by 1977
(b) Eradication of illiteracy by 1980
(c) Self-sufficiency in manpower requirements by 1980

(a) UPE by 1977
Giving basic schooling to every Tanzanian child will fulfil a basic right. Though

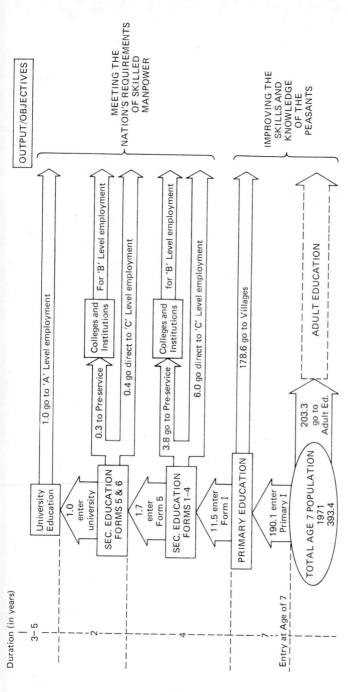

Figure 1.3

Education and Training Prospects of the Age Seven Population in 1971 (in thousands)
*'Adult Education' here refers to literacy and other forms of basic education.

Source: Mwobahe, B L and Mbilinyi, M J (eds.), *Challenge of Education for Self-Reliance in Tanzania*, p. 11, (slightly altered by addition of 'Duration in Years')

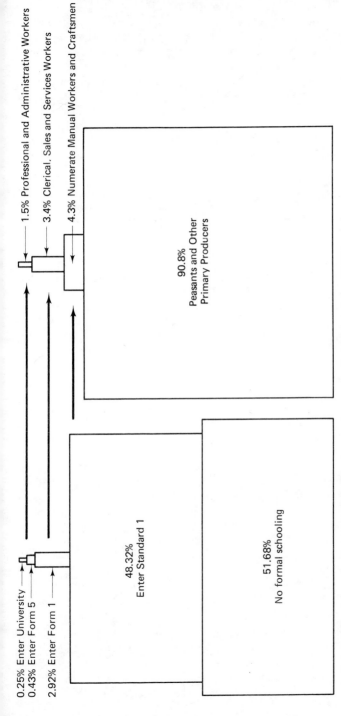

Figure 1.4

Educational and Occupational Structure in Tanzania in 1971

1.5% Professional and Administrative Workers

3.4% Clerical. Sales and Services Workers

4.3% Numerate Manual Workers and Craftsmen

90.8% Peasants and Other Primary Producers

0.25% Enter University
0.43% Enter Form 5

2.92% Enter Form 1

48.32% Enter Standard 1

51.68% No formal schooling

Total age seven population—1971 (393 400) Major occupation groups, Tanzania mainland (1967)

13

realization of the target will certainly generate a lot of problems and difficulties for pupils, parents, teachers, and administrators, they can be solved if all the experience gained since 1967 in transforming the education system is utilized right from the beginning of implementation. In particular this means the need for complete integration of UPE classes with all other primary education, for permanent training and re-training of teachers, and for integration of education with the community by gaining the interest and participation of parents. On the other hand, even when UPE has been achieved, primary education will remain part of the existing education pyramid and lead to some definite place within the given occupation structure. It may thus be influenced more by some 'hidden curriculum' than by aims and objectives in accordance with a lifelong education for self-reliance and liberation.

(b) Eradication of illiteracy
In the fight for nationwide literacy Tanzania seems to be on the winning side. The results of the national campaign launched in 1970 have shown that 'with extra effort added to the present pace of the campaign and also by checking that relapse into illiteracy does not take place, it should be possible for the nation to reduce the illiteracy rate to 10 per cent–15 per cent by 1980 . . .'.[20] But despite this success, the discussion on: 'After literacy, what?' seems to reveal a somewhat defensive attitude. This tendency is articulated in phrases like: 'How can we avoid relapse into illiteracy?' instead of asking: 'How can we use literacy to enhance the skills we already have?' Literacy can, for instance, contribute to wider political participation at the grassroots level and on higher levels, in that plans and reports could be written and read by the masses, and representation in all kinds of development committees and councils would no longer be predominantly reserved for those with formal schooling. It can improve productivity because the masses would be able to read, discuss and write about what, how much, and when to produce, and to go in for further training and upgrading of skills. Literacy can be useful to the masses for transforming society, for the wide range of activities in social life, leisure time, and self-improvement of the individual. Whilst the writing, printing, and distribution of books and newspapers does present considerable difficulties, they are technical ones that can be overcome with overall rural development and should not prevent the masses and leaders from solving their problems. There still seems to be a tendency in the bureaucracy to 'do something for' the masses, instead of encouraging them to take their own decisions and actions. 'But people cannot be developed; they can only develop themselves. . . . He develops himself by what he does; he develops himself by making his own decisions, by increasing his understanding of what he is doing, and why; by increasing his own knowledge and ability, and by his own full participation—as an equal—in the life of the community he lives in.'[21]

(c) Self-sufficiency in manpower requirements
The Daily News headline: 'Manpower policy needs retouching' points to another contradictory process of education and development. While Tanzania has changed its overall development policy to one of intensified rural development, this shift does not seem to be reflected in the manpower development policy. The statement still applies today that the rural sector 'had been denied the vital

middle and lower level skilled workers. Whereas we have declared that our villages will form the nucleus of development, plans for manpower needs have not been made to accommodate this reality.'[22] If rural development is considered to be the way to overcome underdevelopment, then specifically educated and trained manpower is required to improve the agricultural sector, promote small-scale factories, and provide social services. Why has Tanzania not taken the necessary steps in that direction by improving first of all the productive manpower at the lower levels, instead of sticking to a manpower development policy designed mainly to fill middle and higher level administrative posts in the bureaucracy? The dismissal of a number of civil servants in 1976 was somehow related to this problem—but it only scratched the surface. The new Ministry of Manpower Development in conjunction with the Ministry of National Education still has to seek for long-term solutions for manpower development and allocation in accordance with rural development within the national policy of socialism and self-reliance.

5. Future prospects

For the future it will be of the highest importance that the integrated institutions for education at the grassroots level, namely the community education centres, really become institutions of the masses, where the people will identify their educational needs, organize and evaluate their progress, and thereby create their lifelong education for a self-reliant and liberated development. Major problems confronting the political, economic and social development of Tanzania may have further repercussions on her educational plans, since past and present history show that education in Tanzania is inevitably affected by the objectives and realities of overall national and international development. It remains to be seen whether lifelong education for liberation and development can dialectically influence the national realities by supporting the transformation of the political and economic sectors of the society that is necessary to bring about the human and social development demanded by the masses and committed leaders for the benefit of all. It can certainly not be a substitute for such transformation, which has to be realized by the masses and leaders themselves. What contribution it can make will be a matter for future research.

Notes

1 Nyerere, J K 'Our Education Must Be for Liberation' *The Tanzania Education Journal* 3 (1974), No. 8, p. 6
2 Nyerere, J K 'Education Never Ends' in *Adult Education and Development in Tanzania*, edited by National Adult Education Association of Tanzania, p. 7 Bibl. 145
3 Nyerere, J K *Freedom and Development* p. 59 Bibl. 12
4 Nyerere, J K 'Education for Self-Reliance' in *Freedom and Socialism* by J K Nyerere p. 268 Bibl. 11
5 Nyerere, J K 'Our Education Must Be for Liberation' p. 4 (See Note 1)
6 Nyerere, J K 'Education Never Ends' p. 6 (See Note 2) Bibl. 145
7 Nyerere, J K 'Ten Years After Independence' in *Freedom and Development* by J K Nyerere p. 301 (see Note 3) Bibl. 12
8 Nyerere, J K 'Education for Self-Reliance' pp. 279–290 (See Note 4) Bibl. 11
9 The United Republic of Tanzania. *Tanzania Second Five-Year Plan for Economic and Social Development* Vol. I p. 156 Bibl. 18
10 The United Republic of Tanzania. 'The Education Act, 1969.' *Bill Supplement of the Gazette of the United Republic of Tanzania* L (November, 1969) No. 51 p. 3 Bibl. 70

11 Mbunda, D 'Adult Education and Socialist Development' in *Adult Education and Development*, edited by National Adult Education Association of Tanzania, p. 40 (See Notes 2 and 6) Bibl. 145
12 Kawawa, R M 'Circular Concerning Adult Education: Workers' Education' in *Case Studies in Workers' Education No. 1: Tanzania and Somalia*, edited by G Mkunduge, pp. 12 and 13 (stress given in the text) Bibl. 173
13 The United Republic of Tanzania 'National Examinations Council of Tanzania Act, 1973 (No. 8 of 1973)' *Bill Supplement to the Gazette of the United Republic of Tanzania*, Dar es Salaam: Government Printer, LIV (26th October, 1973) No. 43 p. 4
14 'TANU, The Musoma Resolutions on Education' *Daily News* (6.1, 7.1, 8.1, 13.1 1975)
15 The United Republic of Tanzania 'The Institute of Education Act, 1975' *Acts Supplement to the Gazette of the United Republic of Tanzania* (August 12, 1975) pp. 115–126 Bibl. 94 For some reflections on the changing role of the Institute of Education see Mmari, G R V 'The Changing Role of the Institute of Education' in *Studies in Curriculum Development* 1975, Vol. 5 pp. 1–6
16 The United Republic of Tanzania 'The Institute of Adult Education Act, 1975' *Acts Supplement to the Gazette of the United Republic of Tanzania* (August 12, 1975) pp. 103–114 Bibl. 148 For its role in the past see Snyder, M C *The Role of the Institute of Adult Education in the Process of Development in Tanzania: A Study of its Direct Teaching Function in the City of Dar es Salaam* Ph.D. Dissertation Dar es Salaam: UDSM, 1971. For some future trends see Mbunda, D *The Institute of Adult Education and its Obligation to Tanzania* Bibl. 142
17 Nyerere, J K 'Our Education Must Be for Liberation'. p. 4 (See Notes 1 and 5)
18 Mwobahe, B L and Mbilinyi, M J (eds.) *Challenge of Education for Self-Reliance in Tanzania* p. 3 Bibl. 88
19 Mbilinyi, M J 'Education, Stratification and Sexism in Tanzania: Policy Implications' p. 332 Bibl. 83
20 Mbakile, E P R *The National Literacy Campaign: A Summary of Results of the Nation-Wide Literacy Tests* p. 38 Bibl. 158
21 Nyerere, J K *Freedom and Development* p. 60 (See Note 3) Bibl. 12
22 The article 'Manpower policy needs retouching' appeared in *Daily News* (25.3.1976)

Chapter 2 The Overall Educational Conception

2.1 Education for Self-Reliance
J K Nyerere

The first of the President's 'post-Arusha' policy directives on education issued in March 1967 in *Freedom and Socialism* by J K Nyerere pp. 267–290 Bibl. 11

... The educational systems in different kinds of societies in the world have been, and are, very different in organization and in content. They are different because the societies providing the education are different, and because education, whether it be formal or informal, has a purpose. That purpose is to transmit from one generation to the next the accumulated wisdom and knowledge of the society, and to prepare the young people for their future membership of the society and their active participation in its maintenance or development.

This is true, explicitly or implicitly, for all societies—the capitalist societies of the West, the communist societies of the East, and the pre-colonial African societies too.

The fact that pre-colonial Africa did not have 'schools'—execpt for short periods of initiation in some tribes—did not mean that the children were not educated. They learned by living and doing. In the homes and on the farms they were taught the skills of the society, and the behaviour expected of its members. They learned the kind of grasses which were suitable for which purposes, the work which had to be done on the crops, or the care which had to be given to animals, by joining with their elders in this work. They learned the tribal history,

17

and the tribe's relationship with other tribes and with the spirits, by listening to the stories of the elders. Through these means, and by the custom of sharing to which young people were taught to conform, the values of the society were transmitted. Education was thus 'informal'; every adult was a teacher to a greater or lesser degree. But this lack of formality did not mean that there was no education, nor did it affect its importance to the society. Indeed, it may have made the education more directly relevant to the society in which the child was growing up.

In Europe education has been formalized for a very long time. An examination of its development will show, however, that it has always had similar objectives to those implicit in the traditional African system of education. That is to say, formal education in Europe was intended to reinforce the social ethics existing in the particular country, and to prepare the children and young people for the place they will have in that society. The same thing is true of communist countries now. The content of education is somewhat different from that of Western countries, but the purpose is the same—to prepare young people to live in and to serve the society, and to transmit the knowledge, skills, and values and attitudes of the society. Wherever education fails in any of these fields, then the society falters in its progress, or there is social unrest as people find that their education has prepared them for a future which is not open to them.

Colonial Education in Tanzania and the Inheritance of the New State
The education provided by the colonial government in the two countries which now form Tanzania had a different purpose. It was not designed to prepare young people for the service of their own country; instead, it was motivated by a desire to inculcate the values of the colonial society and to train individuals for the service of the colonial state. In these countries the state interest in education therefore stemmed from the need for local clerks and junior officials; on top of that, various religious groups were interested in spreading literacy and other education as part of their evangelical work.

This statement of fact is not given as a criticism of the many individuals who worked hard, often under difficult conditions, in teaching and in organizing educational work. Nor does it imply that all the values these people transmitted in the schools were wrong or inappropriate. What it does mean, however, is that the educational system introduced into Tanzania by the colonialists was modelled on the British system, but with even heavier emphasis on subservient attitudes and on white-collar skills. Inevitably, too, it was based on the assumptions of a colonialist and capitalist society. It emphasized and encouraged the individualistic instincts of mankind, instead of his co-operative instincts. It led to the possession of individual material wealth being the major criterion of social merit and worth.

This meant that colonial education induced attitudes of human inequality, and in practice underpinned the domination of the weak by the strong, especially in the economic field. Colonial education in this country was therefore not transmitting the values and knowledge of Tanzanian society from one generation to the next; it was a deliberate attempt to change those values and to replace traditional knowledge by the knowledge from a different society. It was thus a part of a deliberate attempt to effect a revolution in the society; to make it into a colonial society which accepted its status and which was an efficient adjunct to the governing power. Its failure to achieve these ends does not mean that it was without an influence on the attitudes, ideas, and knowledge of the people who experienced it. Nor does that failure imply that the education provided in colonial days is automatically relevant for the purposes of a free people committed to the principle of equality.

The independent state of Tanzania in fact inherited a system of education which was in many respects both inadequate and inappropriate for the new state. It was, however, its inadequacy which was most immediately obvious. So little education had been provided that in December 1961, we had too few people with the necessary educational qualifications even to man the administration of government as it was then, much less undertake the big economic and social development work which was essential. Neither was the school population in 1961 large enough to allow for any expectation that this situation would be speedily corrected. On top of that, education was based upon race, whereas the whole moral case of the independence movement had been based upon a rejection of racial distinctions.

Action Since Independence

The three most glaring faults of the educational inheritance have already been tackled. First, the racial distinctions within education were abolished. Complete integration of the separate racial systems was introduced very soon after independence, and discrimination on grounds of religion was also brought to an end. A child in Tanzania can now secure admittance to any government or government-aided school in this country without regard to his race or religion and without fear that he will be subjected to religious indoctrination as the price of learning.

Secondly, there has been a very big expansion of educational facilities available, especially at the secondary school and post-secondary school levels.

The third action we have taken is to make the education provided in all schools much more Tanzanian in content. No longer do our children simply learn British and European history. Faster than would have been thought possible, our University College and other institutions are providing materials on the history of Africa and making these available to our teachers. Our national songs and dances are once again being learned by our children; our national language has been given the importance in our curriculum which it needs and deserves. Also, civics classes taken by Tanzanians are beginning to give the secondary school pupils an understanding of the organization and aims of our young state. In these and other ways changes have been introduced to make our educational system more relevant to our needs.

What Kind of Society Are We Trying to Build?

Only when we are clear about the kind of society we are trying to build can we design our educational service to serve our goals. But this is not now a problem in Tanzania. Although we do not claim to have drawn up a blueprint of the future, the values and objectives of our society have been stated many times. We have said that we want to create a socialist society which is based on three principles: equality and respect for human dignity; sharing of the resources which are produced by our efforts; work by everyone and exploitation by none. We have set out these ideas clearly in the National Ethic; and in the 'Arusha Declaration' and earlier documents we have outlined the principles and policies we intend to follow. We have also said on many occasions that our objective is greater African unity, and that we shall work for this objective while in the meantime defending the absolute integrity and sovereignty of the United Republic. Most often of all, our government and people have stressed the equality of all citizens, and our determination that economic, political, and social policies shall be deliberately designed to make a reality of that equality in all spheres of life. We are, in other words, committed to a socialist future and one in which the people will themselves determine the policies pursued by a government which is responsible to them.

It is obvious, however, that if we are to make progress towards these goals, we in Tanzania must accept the realities of our present position, internally and externally, and then work to change these realities into something more in accord with our desires. And the truth is that our United Republic has at present a poor, undeveloped, and agricultural economy. We have very little capital to invest in big factories or modern machines; we are short of people with skill and experience. What we do have is land in abundance and people who are willing to work hard for their own improvement. It is the use of these latter resources which will decide whether we reach our total goals or not. If we use these resources in a spirit of self-reliance as the basis for development, then we shall make progress slowly but surely. And it will then be real progress, affecting the lives of the masses, not just having spectacular show-pieces in the towns while the rest of the people of Tanzania live in their present poverty.

Pursuing this path means that Tanzania will continue to have a pre-dominantly rural economy for a long time to come. And as it is in the rural areas that people live and work, so it is in the rural areas that life must be improved. This is not to say that we shall have no industries and factories in the near future. We have some now and they will continue to expand. But it would be grossly unrealistic to imagine that in the near future more than a small proportion of our people will live in towns and work in modern industrial enterprises. It is therefore the villages which must be made into places where people live a good life; it is in the rural areas that people must be able to find their material well-being and their satisfactions.

This improvement in village life will not, however, come automatically. It will come only if we pursue a deliberate policy of using the resources we have—our manpower and our land—to the best advantage. This means people working hard, intelligently, and together; in other words, working in co-operation. Our people in the rural areas, as well as their government, must organize themselves co-operatively and work for themselves through working for the community of which they are members. Our village life, as well as our state organization, must be based on the principle of socialism and that equality in work and return which is part of it.

This is what our educational system has to encourage. It has to foster the social goals of living together, and working together, for the common good. It has to prepare our young people to play a dynamic and constructive part in the development of a society in which all members share fairly in the good or bad fortune of the group, and in which progress is measured in terms of human wellbeing, not prestige buildings, cars, or other such things, whether privately or publicly owned. Our education must therefore inculcate a sense of commitment to the total community, and help the pupils to accept the values appropriate to our kind of future, not those appropriate to our colonial past.

This means that the educational system of Tanzania must emphasize co-operative endeavour, not individual advancement; it must stress concepts of equality and the responsibility to give service which goes with any special ability, whether it be in carpentry, in animal husbandry, or in academic pursuits. And, in particular, our education must counteract the temptation to intellectual arrogance; for this leads to the well-educated despising those whose abilities are non-academic or who have no special abilities but are just human beings. Such arrogance has no place in a society of equal citizens.

It is, however, not only in relation to social values that our educational system has a task to do. It must also prepare young people for the work they will be called upon to do in the society which exists in Tanzania—a rural society where improvement will depend largely upon the efforts of the people in agriculture and in village development. This does not mean that education in Tanzania should be designed just to produce passive agricultural workers of different levels of skill who simply carry out plans or directions received from above. It must produce good farmers; it has also to prepare people for their responsibilities as free workers and citizens in a free and democratic society, albeit a largely rural society. They have to be able to think for themselves, to make judgements on all the issues affecting them; they have to be able to interpret the decisions made through the democratic institutions of our society, and to implement them in the light of the local circumstances peculiar to where they happen to live.

It would thus be a gross misinterpretation of our needs to suggest that the educational system should be designed to produce robots, who work hard but never question what the leaders in government or TANU are doing and saying. For the people are, and must be, government and TANU. Our government and our Party must always be responsible to the people, and must always consist of representatives—spokesmen and servants of the people. The education provided must therefore encourage the development in each citizen of three things: an enquiring mind; an ability to learn from what others do, and reject or adapt it to his own needs; and a basic confidence in his own position as a free and equal member of the society, who values others and is valued by them for what he does and not for what he obtains.

These things are important for both the vocational and the social aspects of education. However much agriculture a young person learns, he will not find a book which will give him all the answers to all the detailed problems he will come across on his own farm. He will have to learn the basic principles of modern knowledge in agriculture and then adapt them to solve his own problems. Similarly the free citizens of Tanzania will have to judge social issues for themselves; there neither is, nor will be, a political 'holy book' which purports to give all the answers to all the social, political and economic problems which will face our country in the future. There will be philosophies and policies approved by our society which citizens should consider and apply in the light of their own thinking and experience. But the educational system of Tanzania would not be serving the interests of a democratic socialist society if it tried to stop people from thinking about the teachings, policies or the beliefs of leaders, either past or present. Only free people conscious of their worth and their equality can build a free society.

Some Salient Features of the Existing Educational System

These are very different purposes from those which are promoted by our existing educational arrangements. For there are four basic elements in the present system which prevent, or at least discourage, the integration of the pupils into the society they will enter, and which do encourage attitudes of inequality, intellectual arrogance and intense individualism among the young people who go through our schools.

First, the most central thing about the education we are at present providing is that it is basically an elitist education designed to meet the interests and needs of a very small proportion of those who enter the school system.

Although only about 13 per cent of our primary school children will get a place in a secondary school, the basis of our primary school education is the preparation of pupils for secondary schools. Thus 87 per cent of the children who finished primary school last year—and a similar proportion of those who will finish this year—do so with a sense of failure, of a legitimate aspiration having been denied them. Indeed we all speak in these terms, by referring to them as those who failed to enter secondary schools, instead of simply as those who have finished their primary education. On the other hand, the other 13 per cent have a feeling of having deserved a prize—and the prize they and their parents now expect is high wages, comfortable employment in towns, and personal status in the society. The same process operates again at the next highest level, when entrance to university is the question at issue.

In other words, the education now provided is designed for the few who are intellectually stronger than their fellows; it induces among those who succeed a feeling of superiority, and leaves the majority of the others hankering after something they will never obtain. It induces a feeling of inferiority among the majority, and can thus not produce either the egalitarian society we should build, nor the attitudes of mind which are conducive to an egalitarian society. On the contrary, it induces the growth of a class structure in our country.

Equally important is the second point; the fact that Tanzania's education is such as to divorce its participants from the society it is supposed to be preparing them for. This is particularly true of secondary schools, which are inevitably almost entirely boarding schools; but to some extent, and despite recent modifications in the curriculum, it is true of primary schools too. We take children from their parents at the age of seven years, and for up to $7\frac{1}{2}$ hours a day we teach them certain basic academic skills. In recent years we have tried to relate these skills, at least in theory, to the life which the children see around them. But the school is always separate; it is not part of the society. It is a place children go to and which they and their parents hope will make it unnecessary for them to become farmers and continue living in the villages.

The few who go to secondary schools are taken many miles away from their homes; they live in an enclave, having permission to go into the town for recreation, but not relating the work of either town or country to their real life—

which is lived in the school compound. Later a few people go to university. If they are lucky enough to enter Dar es Salaam University College they live in comfortable quarters, feed well, and study hard for their degree. When they have been successful in obtaining it, they know immediately that they will receive a salary of something like £660 per annum. That is what they have been aiming for; it is what they have been encouraged to aim for. They may also have the desire to serve the community, but their idea of service is related to status and the salary which a university education is expected to confer upon its recipient. The salary and the status have become a right automatically conferred by the degree.

It is wrong of us to criticize the young people for these attitudes. The new university graduate has spent the larger part of his life separated and apart from the masses of Tanzania; his parents may be poor, but he has never fully shared that poverty. He does not really know what it is like to live as a poor peasant. He is more at home in the world of the educated than he is among his own parents. Only during vacations has he spent time at home, and even then he will often find that his parents and relatives support his own conception of his difference, and regard it as wrong that he should live and work as the ordinary person he really is. For the truth is that many of the people in Tanzania have come to regard education as meaning that a man is too precious for the rough and hard life which the masses of our people still live.

The third point is that our present system encourages school pupils in the idea that all knowledge which is worthwhile is acquired from books or from 'educated people'—meaning those who have been through a formal education. The knowledge and wisdom of other old people is despised, and they themselves regarded as being ignorant and of no account. Indeed it is not only the education system which at present has this effect. Government and Party themselves tend to judge people according to whether they have 'passed school certificate', 'have a degree', etc. If a man has these qualifications we assume he can fill a post; we do not wait to find out about his attitudes, his character, or any other ability except the ability to pass examinations. If a man does not have these qualifications we assume he cannot do a job; we ignore his knowledge and experience. For example, I recently visited a very good tobacco-producing peasant. But if I tried to take him into government as a Tobacco Extension Officer, I would run up against the system because he has no formal education. Everything we do stresses book learning, and underestimates the value to our society of traditional knowledge and the wisdom which is often acquired by intelligent men and women as they experience life, even without their being able to read at all.

This does not mean that any person can do any job simply because he is old and wise, nor that educational qualifications are not necessary. This is a mistake our people sometimes fall into as a reaction against the arrogance of the book-learned. A man is not necessarily wise because he is old; a man cannot necessarily run a factory because he has been working in it as a labourer or storekeeper for 20 years. But equally he may not be able to do so if he has a Doctorate in Commerce. The former may have honesty and ability to weigh up men; the latter may have the ability to initiate a transaction and work out the economics of it. But both qualifications are necessary in one man if the factory is to be a successful and modern enterprise serving our nation. It is as much a mistake to over-value book learning as it is to under-value it.

The same thing applies in relation to agricultural knowledge. Our farmers have been on the land for a long time. The methods they use are the result of long experience in the struggle with nature; even the rules and taboos they honour have a basis in reason. It is not enough to abuse a traditional farmer as old-fashioned; we must try to understand why he is doing certain things, and not just assume he is stupid. But this does not mean that his methods are sufficient for the future. The traditional systems may have been appropriate for the economy which existed when they were worked out and for the technical knowledge then available. But different tools and different land tenure systems are being used now; land should no longer be used for a year or two and then abandoned for up to 20 years to give time for natural regeneration to take place. The introduction of an ox-plough instead of a hoe—and, even more, the introduction of a tractor—means more than just a different way of turning over the land. It requires a change in the organization of work, both to see that the maximum advantage is taken of the new tool, and also to see that the new method does not simply lead to the rapid destruction of our land and the egalitarian basis of our society. Again, therefore, our young people have to learn both a practical respect for the knowledge of the old 'uneducated' farmer and an understanding of new methods and the reason for them.

Yet at present our pupils learn to despise even their own parents because they are old-fashioned and ignorant; there is nothing in our existing educational system which suggests to the pupil that he can learn important things about farming from his elders. The result is that he absorbs beliefs about witchcraft before he goes to school, but does not learn the properties of local grasses; he absorbs the taboos from his family but does not learn the methods of making nutritious traditional foods. And from school he acquires knowledge unrelated to agricultural life. He gets the worst of both systems!

Finally, and in some ways most importantly, our young and poor nation is taking out of productive work some of its healthiest and strongest young men and women. Not only do they fail to contribute to that increase in output which is so urgent for our nation; they themselves consume the output of the older and often weaker people. There are almost 25000 students in secondary schools now; they do not learn as they work, they simply learn. What is more, they take it for granted that this should be so. Whereas in a wealthy country like the United States of America it is common for young people to work their way through high school and college, in Tanzania the structure of our education makes it impossible for them to do so. Even during the holidays we assume that these young men and women should be protected from rough work; neither they nor the community expect them to spend their time on hard physical labour or on jobs which are uncomfortable and unpleasant. This is not simply a reflection of the fact that there are many people looking for unskilled paid employment—pay is not the question at issue. It is a reflection of the attitude we have all adopted.

How many of our students spend their vacations doing a job which could improve people's lives but for which there is no money—jobs like digging an irrigation channel or a drainage ditch for a village, or demonstrating the construction and explaining the benefits of deep-pit latrines, and so on? A small number have done such work in the National Youth Camps or through school-organized, nation-building schemes, but they are the exception rather than the rule. The vast majority do not think of their knowledge or their strength as being related to the needs of the village community.

Can These Faults Be Corrected?

There are three major aspects which require attention if this situation is to change: the content of the curriculum itself, the organization of the schools, and the entry age into primary schools. But although these aspects are in some ways separate, they are also inter-locked. We cannot integrate the pupils and students into the future society simply by theoretical teaching, however well designed it is. Neither can the society fully benefit from an education system which is thoroughly integrated into local life but does not teach people the basic skills—for example, of literacy and arithmetic, or which fails to excite in them a curiosity about ideas. Nor can we expect those finishing primary schools to be useful young citizens if they are still only twelve or thirteen years of age.

In considering changes in the present structure it is also essential that we face the facts of our present economic situation. Every penny spent on education is money taken away from some other needed activity—whether it is an investment in the future, better medical services, or just more food, clothing and comfort for our citizens at present. And the truth is that there is no possibility of Tanzania being able to increase the proportion of the national income which is spent on education; it ought to be decreased. Therefore we cannot solve our present problems by any solution which costs more than is at present spent; in particular we cannot solve the 'problem of primary school leavers' by increasing the number of secondary school places.

This 'problem of primary school leavers' is in fact a product of the present system. Increasingly children are starting school at six or even five years of age, so that they finish primary school when they are still too young to become responsible young workers and citizens. On top of that is the fact that the society and the type of education they have received both led them to expect wage employment—probably in an office. In other words, their education was not sufficiently related to the tasks which have to be done in our society. This problem therefore calls for a major change in the content of our primary education and for the raising of the primary school entry age so that the child is older when he leaves, and also able to learn more quickly while he is at school. . . . It is only a few who will have the chance of going on to secondary schools, and quite soon only a proportion of these who will have an opportunity of going on to university, even if they can benefit from doing so. These are the economic facts of life for our country. They are the practical meaning of our poverty. The only choice before us is how we allocate the educational opportunities, and whether we emphasize the individual interests of the few or whether we design our educational system to serve the community as a whole. And for a socialist state only the latter is really possible.

The implication of this is that the education given in our primary schools must be a complete education in itself. It must not continue to be simply a preparation for secondary school. Instead of the primary school activities being geared to the competitive examination which will select the few who go on to secondary school, they must be a preparation for the life which the majority of the children will lead. Similarly, secondary schools must not be simply a selection process for the university, Teachers' Colleges, and so on. They must prepare people for life and service in the villages and rural areas of this country. For in Tanzania the only true justification for secondary education is that it is needed by the few for service to the many. The teacher in a seven-year primary school system needs an education which goes beyond seven years; the extension officer who will help a population with a seven-years' education needs a lot more himself. Other essential services need higher education—for example, doctors and engineers need long and careful training. But publicly provided 'education for education's sake' must be general education for the masses. Further education for a selected few must be education for service to the many. There can be no other justification for taxing the many to give education to only a few.

Yet it is easy to say that our primary and secondary schools must prepare young people for the realities and needs of Tanzania; to do it requires a radical change, not only in the education system but also in many existing community attitudes. In particular, it requires that examinations should be down-graded in Government and public esteem. We have to recognize that although they have certain advantages—for example, in reducing the dangers of nepotism and tribalism in a selection process—they also have severe disadvantages too. As a general rule they assess a person's ability to learn facts and present them on demand within a time period. They do not always succeed in assessing a power to reason, and they certainly do not assess character or willingness to serve.

Further, at the present time our curriculum and syllabus are geared to the examinations set—only to a very limited extent does the reverse situation apply. A teacher who is trying to help his pupils often studies the examination papers for past years and judges what questions are most likely to be asked next time; he then concentrates his teaching on those matters, knowing that by doing so he is giving his children the best chance of getting through to secondary school or university. And the examinations our children at present sit are themselves geared to an international standard and practice which has developed regardless of our particular problems and needs. What we need to do now is think first about the education we want to provide, and when that thinking is completed, think about whether some form of examination is an appropriate way of closing an education phase. Then such an examination should be designed to fit the education which has been provided.

Most important of all is that we should change the things we demand of our schools. We should not determine the type of things children are taught in primary schools by the things a doctor, engineer, teacher, economist, or administrator needs to know. Most of our pupils will never be any of these things. We should determine the types of things taught in the primary schools by the things which the boy or girl ought to know—that is, the skills he ought to acquire and the values he ought to cherish if he, or she, is to live happily and well in a socialist and predominantly rural society, and contribute to the improvement of life there. Our sights must be on the majority; it is they we must be aiming at in determining the curriculum and syllabus. Those most suitable for further education will still become obvious and they will not suffer. For the purpose is not to provide an inferior education to that given at present. The purpose is to provide a different education—one realistically designed to fulfil the common purpose of education in the particular society of Tanzania. The same thing must be true at post-primary schools. The object of the teaching must be the provision of knowledge, skills and attitudes which will serve the student when he or she lives and works in a developing and changing socialist state; it must not be aimed at university entrance.

Alongside this change in the approach to the curriculum there must be a parallel and integrated change in the way our schools are run, so as to make them and their inhabitants a real part of our society and our economy. Schools must, in fact, become communities—and communities which practise the precept of self-reliance. The teachers, workers, and pupils together must be the members of a social unit in the same way as parents, relatives, and children are the family social unit. There must be the same kind of relationship between pupils and teachers within the school community as there is between children and parents in the village. And the former community must realize, just as the latter do, that their life and well-being depend upon the production of wealth—by farming or other activities. This means that all schools, but especially secondary schools and other forms of higher education, must contribute to their own upkeep; they must be economic communities as well as social and educational communities. Each school should have, as an integral part of it, a farm or workshop which provides the food eaten by the community, and makes some contribution to the total national income.

This is not a suggestion that a school farm or workshop should be attached to every school for training purposes. It is a suggestion that every school should also be a farm; that the school community should consist of people who are both teachers and farmers, and pupils and farmers. Obviously if there is a school farm, the pupils working on it should be learning the techniques and tasks of farming. But the farm would be an integral part of the school—and the welfare of the pupils would depend on its output, just as the welfare of a farmer depends on the output of his land. Thus, when this scheme is in operation, the revenue side of school accounts would not just read as at present—'Grant from government . . .; Grant from voluntary agency or other charity . . .'. They would read—'Income from sale of cotton (or whatever other cash crop was appropriate for the area) . . .; Value of the food grown and consumed . . .; Value of labour done by pupils on new building, repairs, equipment, etc . . .; government subvention . . .; Grant from . . .'.

This is a break with our educational tradition, and unless its purpose and its possibilities are fully understood by teachers and parents, it may be resented at the beginning. But the truth is that it is not a regressive measure, nor a punishment either for teachers or pupils. It is a recognition that we in Tanzania have to work our way out of poverty, and that we are all members of the one society, depending upon each other. There will be difficulties of implementation, especially at first. For example, we do not now have a host of experienced farm managers who could be used as planners and teachers on the new school farms. But this is not an insuperable difficulty; and certainly life will not halt in Tanzania until we get experienced farm managers. Life and farming will go on as we train. Indeed, by using good local farmers as supervisors and teachers in particular aspects of the work, and using the services of the Agricultural Officers and assistants, we shall help break down the notion that only book learning is worthy of respect. This is an important element in our socialist development.

Neither does this concept of schools contributing to their own upkeep simply mean using our children as labourers who follow traditional methods. On the contrary, on a school farm pupils can learn by doing. The important place of the hoe and of other simple tools can be demonstrated; the advantages of improved seeds, of simple ox-ploughs, and of proper methods of animal husbandry can become obvious; and the pupils can learn by practice how to use these things to the best advantage. The farm work and products should be integrated into the school life; thus the properties of fertilizers can be explained in the science classes, and their use and limitations experienced by the pupils as they see them in use. The possibilities of proper grazing practices, and of terracing and soil conservation methods can all be taught theoretically, at the same time as they are put into practice; the students will then understand what they are doing and why, and will be able to analyse any failures and consider possibilities for greater improvement.

But the school farms must not be, and indeed could not be, highly mechanized demonstration farms. We do not have the capital which would be necessary for this to happen, and neither would it teach the pupils anything about the life they will be leading. The school farms must be created by the school community clearing their own bush, and so on—but doing it together. They must be used with no more capital assistance than is available to an ordinary, established, co-operative farm where the work can be supervised. By such means the students can learn the advantages of co-operative endeavour, even when outside capital is not available in any significant quantities. Again, the advantages of co-operation could be studied in the classroom, as well as being demonstrated on the farm.

The most important thing is that the school members should learn that it is their farm, and that their living standards depend on it. Pupils should be given an opportunity to make many of the decisions necessary—for example, whether to spend money they have earned on hiring a tractor to get land ready for planting, or whether to use that money for other purposes on the farm or in the school, and doing the hard work themselves by sheer physical labour. By this sort of practice and by this combination of classroom work and farm work, our educated young people will learn to realize that if they farm well they can eat well and have better facilities in the dormitories, recreation rooms, and so on. If they work badly, then they themselves will suffer. In this process government should avoid laying down detailed and rigid rules; each school must have considerable flexibility. Only then can the potential of that particular area be utilized, and only then can the participants practise—and learn to value—direct democracy.

By such means our students will relate work to comfort. They will learn the meaning of living together and working together for the good of all, and also the value of working together with the local non-school community. For they will learn that many things require more than school effort—that irrigation may be possible if they work with neighbouring farmers, that development requires a choice between present and future satisfaction, both for themselves and their village.

At the beginning it is probable that a good number of mistakes will be made, and it would certainly be wrong to give complete untrammelled choice to young pupils right from the start. But although guidance must be given by the school authorities and a certain amount of discipline exerted, the pupils must be able to participate in decisions and learn by mistakes. For example, they can learn to keep a school farm log in which proper records are kept of the work done, the fertilizers applied, or food given to the animals, etc., and the results from different parts of the farm. Then they can be helped to see where changes are required, and why. For it is also important that the idea of planning be taught in the classroom and related to the farm; the whole school should join in the programming of a year's work, and the break-down of responsibility and timing within that overall programme. Extra benefits to particular groups within the school might then well be related to the proper fulfilment of the tasks set, once all the members of the school have received the necessary minimum for healthy development. Again, this sort of planning can be part of the teaching of socialism.

Where schools are situated in the rural areas, and in relation to new schools built in the future, it should be possible for the school farm to be part of the school site. But in towns, and in some of the old-established schools in heavily populated areas, this will not be possible. In such cases a school might put more emphasis on other productive activities, or it may be that in boarding schools the pupils can spend part of the school year in the classroom and another part in camp on the school farm some distance away. The plan for each school will have to be worked out; it would certainly be wrong to exclude urban schools, even when they are day schools, from this new approach.

Many other activities now undertaken for pupils, especially in secondary schools, should be undertaken by the pupils themselves. After all, a child who starts school at seven years of age is already fourteen before he enters secondary school, and may be twenty or twenty-one when he leaves. Yet in many of our schools now we employ cleaners and gardeners, not just to supervise and teach but to do all that work. The pupils get used to the idea of having their food prepared by servants, their plates washed up for them, their rooms cleaned, and the school garden kept attractive. If they are asked to participate in these tasks, they even feel aggrieved and do as little as possible, depending on the strictness of the teacher's supervision. This is because they have not learned to take a pride in having clean rooms and nice gardens, in the way that they have learned to take a pride in a good essay or a good mathematics paper. But is it impossible for these tasks to be incorporated into the total teaching task of the school? Is it necessary for head teachers and their secretaries to spend hours working out travel warrants for school holidays, and so on? Can none of these things be incorporated into classroom teaching so that pupils learn how to do these things for themselves by doing them? Is it impossible, in other words, for secondary schools at least to become reasonably self-sufficient communities, where the teaching and supervisory skills are imported from outside, but where other tasks are either done by the community or paid for by its productive efforts? It is true that, to the pupils, the school is only a temporary community, but for up to seven years this is the group to which they really belong.

Obviously such a position could not be reached overnight. It requires a basic change in both organization and teaching, and will therefore have to be introduced gradually, with the schools taking an increasing responsibility for their own well-being as the months pass. Neither would primary schools be able to do so much for themselves —although it should be remembered that the older pupils will be thirteen and fourteen years of age, at which time children in many European countries are already at work.

But, although primary schools cannot accept the same responsibility for their own well-being as secondary schools, it is absolutely vital that they, and their pupils, should be thoroughly integrated into the village life. The pupils must remain an integral part of the family (or community) economic unit. The children must be made part of the community by having responsibilities to the community, and having the community involved in school activities. The school work—terms, times, and so on—must be so arranged that the children can participate, as members of the family, in the family farms, or as junior members of the community on community farms. At present children who do not go to school work on the family or community farm, or look after cattle, as a matter of course. It must be equally a matter of course that the children who do attend school should participate in the family work—not as a favour when they feel like it, but as a normal part of their upbringing. The present attitudes whereby the school is regarded as something separate, and the pupils as people who do not have to contribute to the work, must be abandoned. In this, of course, parents have a special duty; but the schools can contribute a great deal to the development of this attitude.

There are many different ways in which this integration can be achieved. But it will have to be done deliberately, and with the conscious intention of making the children realize that they are being educated by the community in order that they shall become intelligent and active members of the community. One possible way of achieving this would give to primary school pupils the same advantages of learning by doing as the secondary school pupils will have. If the primary school children work on a village communal farm—perhaps having special responsibility for a given number of acres—they can learn new techniques and take a pride in a school community achievement. If there is no communal farm, then the school can start a small one of their own by appealing to the older members to help in the bush-clearing in return for a school contribution in labour to some existing community project.

Again, if development work—new buildings or other things—are needed in the school, then the children and the local villagers should work on it together, allocating responsibility according to comparative health and strength. The children should certainly do their own cleaning (boys as well as girls should be involved in this), and should learn the value of working together and of planning for the future. Thus for example, if they have their own shamba the children should be involved not only in the work, but also in the allocation of any food or cash crop produced. They should participate in the choice between benefit to the school directly, or to the village as a whole, and between present or future benefit. By these and other appropriate means the children must learn from the beginning to the end of their school life that education does not set them apart, but is designed to help them be effective members of the community for their own benefit as well as that of their country and their neighbours.

One difficulty in the way of this kind of reorganization is the present examination system; if pupils spend more of their time on learning to do practical work, and on contributing to their own upkeep and the development of the community, they will not be able to take the present kind of examinations—at least within the same time-period. It is, however, difficult to see why the present examination system should be regarded as sacrosanct. Other countries are moving away from this method of selection, and either abandoning examinations altogether at the lowest levels, or combining them with other assessments. There is no reason why Tanzania should not combine an examination, which is based on the things we teach, with a teacher and pupil assessment of work done for the school and community. This would be a more appropriate method of selecting entrants for secondary schools and for university, teacher training colleges and so on, than the present purely academic prodecure. Once a more detailed outline of this new approach to education is worked out, the question of selection procedure should be looked at again.

This new form of working in our schools will require some considerable organizational change. It may be also that the present division of the school year into rigid terms with long holidays would have to be re-examined; animals cannot be left alone for part of the year, nor can a school farm support the students if everyone is on holiday when the crops need planting, weeding or harvesting. But it should not be impossible for school holidays to be staggered so that different forms go at different periods or, in double-stream secondary schools, for part of a form to go at one time and the rest at another. It would take a considerable amount of organization and administration, but there is no reason why it could not be done if we once make up our minds to it.

It will probably be suggested that if the children are working as well as learning they will therefore be able to learn less academically, and that this will affect standards of administration, in the professions and so on, throughout our nation in time to come. In fact it is doubtful whether this is necessarily so; the recent tendency to admit children to primary schools at ages of five and six years has almost certainly meant that less can be taught at the early stages. The reversion to seven or eight years' entrance will allow the pace to be increased somewhat; the older children inevitably learn a little faster. A child is unlikely to learn less academically if the studies are related to the life he sees around him.

But even if this suggestion were based on provable fact, it could not be allowed to over-ride the need for change in the direction of educational integration with our national life. For the majority of our people the thing which matters is that they should be able to read and write fluently in Swahili, that they should have an ability to do arithmetic, and that they should know something of the history, values, and workings of their country and their government, and that they should acquire the skills necessary to earn their living. (It is important to stress that in Tanzania most people will earn their living by working on their own or on a communal shamba, and only a few will do so by working for wages which they have to spend on buying things the farmer produces for himself.) Things like health science, geography, and the beginning of English, are also important, especially so that the people who wish may be able to learn more by themselves in later life. But most important of all is that our primary school graduates should be able to fit into, and to serve, the communities from which they come.

The same principles of integration into the community, and applicability to its needs, must also be followed at post-secondary level, but young people who have been through such an integrated system of education as that outlined are unlikely to forget their debt to the community by an intense period of study at the end of their formal educational life. Yet even at university, medical school, or other post-secondary levels, there is no reason why students should continue to have all their washing up and cleaning done for them. Nor is there any reason why students at such institutions should not be required as part of their degree or professional training, to spend at least part of their vacations contributing to the society in a manner related to their studies. At present some undergraduates spend their vacations working in government offices—getting paid at normal employee rates for doing so. It would be more appropriate (once the organization had been set up efficiently) for them to undertake projects needed by the community, even if there is insufficient money for them to constitute paid employment. For example, the collection of local history, work on the census, participation in adult education activities, work in dispensaries, etc., would give the students practical experience in their own fields. For this they could receive the equivalent of the minimum wage, and any balance of money due for work which would otherwise have been done for higher wages could be paid to the college or institution and go towards welfare or sports equipment. Such work should earn credits for the student which count towards his examination result; a student who shirks such work—or fails to do it properly—would then find that two things follow. First, his fellow students might be blaming him for shortfalls in proposed welfare or other improvements; and second, his degree would be down-graded accordingly.

Conclusion

The education provided by Tanzania for the students of Tanzania must serve the purposes of Tanzania. It must encourage the growth of the socialist values we aspire to. It must encourage the development of a proud, independent, and free citizenry which relies upon itself for its own development, and which knows the advantages and the problems of co-operation. It must ensure that the educated know themselves to be an integral part of the nation and recognize the responsibility to give greater service the greater the opportunities they have had.

This is not only a matter of school organization and curriculum. Social values are formed by family, school, and society—by the total environment in which a child develops. But it is no use our educational system stressing values and knowledge appropriate to the past or to the citizens in other countries; it is wrong if it even contributes to the continuation of those inequalities and privileges which still exist in our society because of our inheritance. Let our students be educated to be members and servants of the kind of just and egalitarian future to which this country aspires.

2.2 Education Never Ends
J K Nyerere

This article combines the 1969 and 1970 New Year's Eve addresses to the nation. In *Adult Education and Development in Tanzania*, edited by National Adult Education Association of Tanzania pp. 1–15 Bibl. 145

The importance of adult education, both for our country and for every individual, cannot be over-emphasized. We are poor and backward, and too many of us just accept our present conditions as 'the will of God', and feel that we can do nothing about them. In many cases, therefore, the first objective of adult education must be to shake ourselves out of a resignation to the kind of life Tanzanian people have lived for centuries past. We must become aware of the things that we, as members of the human race, can do for ourselves and our country. We must learn to realize that we do not have to live miserably in hovels, cultivate with inadequate *jembes* (hoes), or suffer from many diseases; we must learn that we, ourselves, can change these things. The first job of adult education is to give us the ability to reject bad houses, bad *jembes*, and preventable diseases: it must make us recognize that we have the ability to attain better houses, better tools, and better health.

Of course, many people already know this. What they need to learn is how to bring about improvements in their lives. They need to know such things as the fact that dirty water makes their children ill, and that they can avoid such sickness by working together to bring clean water to their village, or even just by boiling water before drinking it. In other words, the second objective of adult education is to teach us how to improve our lives. We have to learn how to produce more on our farms and in our factories and offices. We have to learn about better food, what a balanced diet is and how it can be obtained by our own efforts. Every house-wife must learn that good food does not mean European cooking. We need to learn about modern methods of hygiene, about making furniture for ourselves out of local materials, about working together to improve the conditions in our villages and streets and so on.

But learning these skills is not enough. For we can only accomplish these things if all members of the nation work together for our common good. The third objective of adult education therefore must be to have everyone understand our national policies of socialism and self-reliance. We must learn to understand the plans for national economic advancement, so that we can ensure that we all play our part in making them a success, and that we all benefit from them. But what is adult education? Quite simply, it is learning about anything at all that helps us to understand the environment we live in and the manner in which we can use and change this environment in order to improve ourselves. Education is not just something that happens in classrooms. It is learning from others, and from our own experience of past successes or failures.

Education is learning from books, from the radio, from films, from discussions about matters that affect our lives, and especially from doing things. The question of learning by doing is very important. The best way to learn sewing is to sew; the best way to learn farming is to farm; the best way to learn cooking is to cook; the best way to learn how to teach is to teach; and so on. A child learns to walk by walking, not by reading a book on how to walk. We learn from the experience of doing.

Learning from experience should not be difficult for us to understand. In our traditional society, we did not have schools as we have now. But we learned from our parents and other elders about the society we lived in, about the methods of farming, and so on.

We learned about plants and animals; which were useful and which were dangerous. We learned which trees were useful for making bows or axe-handles or canoes; we learned which trees were useless for these purposes, but were very good for making charcoal. We learned how our tribe governed itself—and, indeed, we took our places in that government. This was education about the tribal society we lived in, even though there were no formal school and no teacher.

But our education was very limited, and it often discouraged us from asking ourselves questions and thinking out new ways of doing things. What was important, and what is still valuable, is that education in our traditional societies was part of life, not something separate, which a person took part in for just a short period in his lifetime. A man's education continued throughout his whole life; and this is how it should be, even these days. But we now live in very different kinds of society; we live in a village or town, as part of Tanzania, as part of Africa, and as part of the world. So we have very much more to learn now—and a much wider area from which we can learn. We must begin to ask questions about our lives, and to search for our own answers. Yet it is still true that the first education anyone ever gets is from his parents and his brothers and sisters, as he grows from infancy into childhood. . . . Second, there is formal education at school. . . .

Adult education is the third stage, and it can cover many of the subjects learned at school for those who never had the opportunity. It applies to every one of us, without exception. We can all learn more. Those who have never been to school, those who have just attended primary school, and those who have attended secondary school or university; there is much more that everyone can learn about our work and about areas of knowledge that they were not taught when they were at school.

I know that there are some of my literate fellow citizens who never read at all. Their purpose in going to school was to get a certificate, which they could use to get work. After getting the certificate and using it to obtain employment, they just put the certificate on the wall so that everyone could see it. But they never use the knowledge of reading and writing; they never read at all. This is a big mistake, arising from colonial attitudes of mind.

A very pleasant thing about adult education is that we can learn what we want to learn, what we feel would be useful to us in our lives. At school, children are taught the things that we adults decide they should be taught. But adults are not like children, who sit in classrooms and are then taught history or grammar or a foreign language. As adults, we can try to learn these things if we wish, but we do not have to do so. Instead, we can learn more about growing a particular crop, about the government, about house-building, about whatever interests us. We can build on the education we already have using the tools of literacy, a foreign language, or an understanding of scientific principles. Or, if we never went to school, we can start by learning about the things of most immediate importance to us—better farming methods, better child care, better feeding. We do not even have to start by learning to read and write!

For literacy is just a tool; it is a means by which we can learn more, more easily. This is its importance. It enables us to read the instructions that come with a bag of fertilizer, it enables us to read about new methods so that we do not have to rely on a teacher being near; it enables us to study our Party policy until we really understand it. And if we have not yet had the opportunity of learning to read and write, we can still learn and we should still learn, if we do not want to be left behind as we make progress.

For I repeat, education is something that all of us should continue to acquire from the time we are born until the time we die. This is important both for individuals and for our country as a whole. A country whose people do not learn, and make use of their knowledge, will stay very poor and very backward. The nation will always be in danger of losing its independence to stronger and more educated nations, and the people will always be in danger of being exploited and controlled by others.

This means that education is very important to a country like Tanzania. We want to improve our lives and maintain our freedom; we shall only be able to do this if we apply ourselves to learning as much as possible and as quickly as possible. Many of our farmers realize that a neighbour who does not keep his shamba (field) clean is both a disgrace and a danger to the whole village. He and his children live in poverty and sickness, and sooner or later the other villagers get angry with him because the weeds and insects from his plot spread disease to their shambas. Let our country not be like that farmer who, by his laziness, antagonizes neighbours who are bigger and stronger than he is. For the rest of the world is advancing all the time. Other countries are using new methods of production and are organizing themselves for their own benefit. They will not wait for us! Unless we determine to educate ourselves we shall get left behind again; we shall be at the mercy of other nations and peoples. Independence that is subject to the decisions of other peoples is not independence, it is an illusion.

We must change our conditions of life ourselves; and we can learn how to do this by educating ourselves. We must recognize that there is no use in demanding that someone else do something about it. Nor is there any use in the citizens simply sitting back and waiting. The government and the Party are simply organizations of citizens, a coming together of people for certain purposes. Neither the government not TANU can do anything apart from the citizens; nor can these organizations do everything that has to be done in our country. Every one of us, by improving his own education, can begin to make improvements in his own life and, therefore, in the lives of us all. By educating ourselves more each one of us can help to make our country stronger and our children's lives better.

But as well as being students, we all have to be willing to be teachers. We have to be willing to teach whatever skills we have by whatever methods we can—by demonstration and example, by discussion, by answering questions, or by formal classroom work. If we all play our part, both as students and teachers, we shall really make some progress. I would like to remind you of the promise of TANU members: 'I shall educate myself to the best of my ability and use my education for the benefit of all.' . . . Adult education is something which never stops. Whatever level of education we have reached, we can go on; there is always something new to learn. And if we have not begun to learn about the modern world, we can begin now. For education is like a big hill which climbs to the skies and gives a view over the surrounding countryside. And all of us can climb at least some of the way up, so that all of us can gradually extend our vision and learn more of the things which affect our lives, or which can be made to help our lives. In fact, we are like the people of olden times who used to climb the nearby hill—or a tree if there was no hill—to see what was passing, or what was approaching them, so as to be ready to welcome the guests, or to protect themselves against invaders. We who live in the twentieth century world, in which the activities of all the countries affect all the others, need to go on climbing this hill so as to get away from the danger of floods, to get away from the disease and misery we used to live in, and to take advantage of all mankind's knowledge for our own welfare. . . .

As I have already said, adult education means adults learning about anything which interests them. It is possible to learn from talking with others, from the example of others, from the radio. But a tool which is essential if anyone is to make very much progress, is the ability to read and to write. Literacy is almost the first step up this hill of modern knowledge, and it is the key to further progress.

We have had many literacy campaigns in the past, and many adults are now able to read and write for themselves, although as children they never had a chance to go to school. We must increase this number, for a socialist Tanzania cannot be created if some people are very highly educated and others are completely illiterate. The illiterate ones will never be able to play their full part in the development of our country or of themselves; and they will always be in danger of being exploited by the great knowledge of others. Therefore it is necessary that we should plan to overcome the existing high level of illiteracy. We must help as many of our people as possible on to this first step up the hill; afterwards they will be able to climb further by using this basic knowledge to read and study more.

There is no useless knowledge, no useless learning. There are only priorities of learning. As a nation we have said that our priorities must be learning about agriculture, about better food, better health, greater skills for production, and greater understanding of our national policies of socialism and self-reliance. In these areas whatever help is possible will be given. But this is a very wide field and each man and woman, once literate, can determine his own priorities—he can choose for himself what he wants to learn next. He can also use his literacy to learn other things, from a foreign language to the movement of the stars in the universe—there are books, at least in English, about everything. Or he can read just for enjoyment—to read stories about our past and about the lives of other peoples, just as we once used to listen to story tellers or travellers as they visited our villages and sat around the fire of an evening.

Let me sum up. We must increase the production of goods of all kinds in Tanzania, and we must develop our nation along socialist lines so as to enable every man and woman to develop in freedom and without being exploited. In the rural areas this means we must increase the number of ujamaa villages, and we must expand the co-operative production in all of them. But we must also begin now to organize our own social and cultural activities in these villages and in our towns and hamlets. Even though we must still give first priority to production, we can begin slowly to benefit from the greater social life and greater cultural life, which living in villages and working together makes possible.

2.3 Relevance and Dar es Salaam University
J K Nyerere

Speech held at inauguration of the University of Dar es Salaam on 29 August,
1970. In *Freedom and Development* pp. 192–203 Bibl. 12

It is with great pleasure that I have come to this campus today to preside over the
formal inauguration of the University of Dar es Salaam. On the good foundation
built by the University College of Dar es Salaam, which was a constituent part of
the University of East Africa, we are now embarking upon our independent
existence as a university. This is therefore an occasion for rejoicing. It is also an
occasion which calls for re-dedication and renewed endeavour by all those
involved. For it is now our responsibility to shape this institution so that it gives
the maximum service to the people of Tanzania and their socialist objectives.

To do this effectively, however, it is first necessary that we should be clear in
our own minds about the function of a university in the modern world, and about
the particular tasks of the first University in Tanzania. Only when we have done
this can we avoid the twin dangers, on the one hand, of considering our
university in the light of some mythical 'international standard', or, on the other
hand, of forcing our university to look inwards and isolate itself from the world in
which we live.

. . . A university is an institution of higher learning; a place where people's
minds are trained for clear thinking, for independent thinking, for analysis, and
for problem solving at the highest level. This is the meaning of 'a university'
anywhere in the world. Whatever it may be called, an institution is a university
only if that definition can be truly applied to it.

Given this definition, a university has, in my opinion, three major and
important social functions. From one generation to the next it transmits
advanced knowledge, so that this can serve either as a basis of action, or as a
spring-board for further research. Second, a university provides a centre for the
attempt to advance the frontiers of knowledge: it does this by concentrating in
one place some of the most intellectually able people who are not preoccupied by
day-to-day administrative or professional responsibilities, and through its
possession of good library and laboratory facilities. And third, a university
provides, through its teaching, for the high-level manpower needs of the society.

It is in the context of this definition, and these functions, that young and
backward nations seek to establish their own universities—Tanzania being no
exception. For although a university is, by its nature, inevitably expensive to
establish and to maintain, the full value of university activity can only be
obtained when the university and the society it serves are organically linked
together. A nation without a university can be served by graduates from foreign
universities; specific research needs can often be met by scholars based at a good
foreign institution. Tanzania knows this by experience. But these are short-term
expedients; they help a society while it is establishing or strengthening its own
institutions, but they cannot replace them.

For learning of all kinds has a purpose: that purpose is to increase man's power
over himself and his environment. In other words, the function of learning is the
development of men, and of mankind. And development must start from where

you are. You cannot teach calculus to an illiterate peasant—he first has to learn to read and write and to understand numbers. Similarly, a university is wasting time and effort if it ignores the society in which its student grew and learned his preliminary lessons. . .

Quite apart from the learning process itself, however, there is another way in which university education is linked to the community. It is provided at the expense of the community as a whole. I know that we who have received education do not like being reminded of this fact; but it is better to remind ourselves than to be reminded by others. The peasants and workers of a nation feed, clothe, and house both the students and their teachers, they also provide all the educational facilities used—the books, test-tubes, machines, and so on. The community provides these things because it expects to benefit—it is making an investment in people. It believes that after their educational opportunity the students will be able to make a much greater contribution to the society, they will be able to help in the implementation of the plans and policies of the people.

The community's investment will, however, have been a bad one if the student is ill-equipped to do any of the jobs required when he is called upon to make this contribution. In such a case the university will have failed in its task. The same is true if the graduate is unwilling to fulfil his responsibilities without demanding further privileges from the community. For, I repeat, the purpose of learning is the advancement of man. Knowledge which remains isolated from the people, or which is used by a few to exploit others, is therefore a betrayal. It is a particularly vicious kind of theft by false pretences. Students eat the bread and butter of the peasants because they have promised a service in the future. If they are unable or unwilling to provide that service when the time comes, then the students have stolen from the peasants as surely as if they had carried off their sacks of wheat in the night.

Thus, new nations establish their own universities because they need a type of higher education appropriate to their problems and their aspirations. This is not to deny that much knowledge is international. The laws of chemistry apply everywhere: an economic analysis is valid or invalid wherever it is made. But the kind of problems which are examined at a university—the means through which advanced and theoretical knowledge is taught—do and should vary according to the background, and the anticipated requirements, of the students. Is more time spent studying the chemistry of ice formation, or of volcanic eruptions? Are the tools of economic analysis acquired by considering mostly developed or developing, capitalist or co-operative societies? In a tropical new nation which aims to build socialism, the emphasis at the university will be very different from that applied in highly industrialized and capitalist nations with temperate climates.

The kind of intellectual skills taught and practised is, however, only one of the reasons for having a national university. Another is that an educational process inevitably encourages the development of certain social attitudes and beliefs. It is certainly true that university education must encourage the students to think for themselves. But the ethos of the university and the surrounding society does have an automatic and unavoidable influence on the students. . .

Our nation has decided to divert development resources from other potential uses because we expect to benefit by doing so. We believe that through having our own higher educational institution in this country, we shall obtain the kind of high-level manpower we need to build a socialist society, and we shall get the emphasis we need on investigating the particular problems which face us. In other words, we expect that our university will be of such a nature that all who pass through it will be prepared both in knowledge and in attitude for giving maximum service to the community.

In its teaching activities, and in its search for new knowledge, therefore, the aim of the University of Dar es Salaam must be service to the needs of a *developing socialist Tanzania*. This purpose must determine the subjects taught, the content of the courses, the method of teaching, and the manner in which the university is organized as well as its relations with the community at large.

Thus our university, like all others worthy of the name, must provide the facilities and the opportunities for the highest intellectual enquiry. It must encourage and challenge its students to develop their powers of constructive thinking. It must encourage its academic staff to do original research and to play a full part in promoting intelligent discussion of issues of human concern. It must do all these things because they are part of being a university; they are part of its reason for existence.

And because this is a Tanzanian university, it must do these things in such a manner that the thinking is done in the framework of, and for the purpose of serving, the needs of Tanzania's development towards socialism. The University of Dar es Salaam must be a university; and it must be *our* university—relevant to the present and future society of Tanzania.

In this connection I must add that we have a past error to correct, and a present danger to avoid. For we have always recognized that Harvard University must try to understand American society, and be understood by it, in order to serve America. And we have always known that London University and Moscow University must each try to understand, and be understood by, their respective societies in order to serve their nation's people. Yet it is only recently that we have realized a similar necessity in Africa. Our universities have aimed at understanding Western society, and being understood by Western society, apparently assuming that by this means they were preparing their students to be—and themselves being—of service to African society.

This fault has been recognized, and the attitude it involved has been in the course of correction in East Africa—and particularly in Dar es Salaam—for some time. But there is now the danger of an understandable—but nevertheless a foolish—reaction to it. This is that the universities of Africa which aim at being 'progressive' will react by trying to understand, and be understood by, Russian, East European, or Chinese society. Once again they will be fooling themselves into believing that they are thus preparing themselves to serve African society. Yet surely it is clear that to do this is simply to replay the old farce with different characters. The truth is that it is Tanzanian society, and African society, which this university must understand. It is Tanzania, and the Tanzanian people, who must be able to comprehend this university. Only when these facts are firmly grasped will the University of Dar es Salaam be able to give full and proper service to this society. The University of Dar es Salaam has not been founded to turn out intellectual apes whether of the Right or of the Left. We are training for a socialist, self-respecting and self-reliant Tanzania.

What is Relevance in the University?

. . . To plan is to choose. On what basis, then, shall we determine the kind of disciplines, the kind of knowledge taught at our university? On what basis should the university syllabuses be determined?

The answers to these question can be deduced from an understanding of our present national circumstances and national goals. Tanzania is a backward and poor country, most of whose people live in the rural areas. Our economy depends upon agriculture, but we need to diversify it. We aim to revolutionize the conditions in which our people live, so that everyone is assured of the basic necessities of life and is able to live in decency and dignity. But we are not only trying to develop; we are determined to do this on the socialist basis of human equality. We want to establish a free society where all citizens are equally assured of justice. And while doing all this, we need to safeguard our national independence against all external or subversive attacks.

It follows that at our university the implications of these conditions and these ambitions must be studied and taught. Students must learn to anticipate the kind of problems which might arise from any combinations of these circumstances and desires. And they must have their minds orientated towards solving such problems; analysis has to be followed by action, and a university education must lead to a positive and constructive approach to the difficulties which might face our nation in future. Further, while the students acquire this understanding and this problem-solving approach, they must also be learning the skills necessary for the implementation of policies. For it is not enough to work out that the solution to a problem of underdevelopment in one area is to build a particular bridge. We must also have the ability—the skill—necessary to construct that bridge.

Thus, university 'relevance' is not a question of drawing up syllabuses which talk about 'Tanzania' all the time. It is a question of intelligent and knowledgeable tutors relating their discipline to the student's, and the society's, past, present, and anticipated future experience. It is a question of the teaching being oriented towards solving the problems of Tanzania—as they are, and as they can reasonably be expected to be in the future.

When determining whether a particular subject should be offered, the university should therefore be asking itself: 'What contribution can a study of this subject make to Tanzania's future?' Similarly, when a tutor is preparing his syllabus, his lecture or seminar, he should first ask himself: 'What needed understanding, or what new information, am I trying to convey to the students?'; he should then go on to ask: 'What knowledge of, or from, our own society is relevant to this matter?' And finally: 'What has mankind's heritage of knowledge to teach us in this connection?' If the university authorities, and the professors and lecturers, always bear in mind the reason for the existence of the university, the principles on which our society is based, and the purposes of our policies, then their courses will be relevant, and the institution itself will be relevant.

. . . And ultimately, the community has to judge the university by results. When a fruit tree is growing, the farmer can tell whether it is being attacked by pests, whether it is in danger of dying from lack of water or nutrients, or whether its shoots look healthy. He can tell from the leaves whether it is the kind of fruit he wanted, or whether he planted the wrong seed by mistake. But he can only tell whether it is a good tree when, year after year, it has produced a great deal of large and sweet fruit. If he tries to examine its roots while it is still growing, or to transplant it every year, he is more likely to destroy than to improve it.

The same thing is true of our university. Having made clear why we are establishing it, and what we expect from it, and having done our best to select administrators and teachers capable of fulfilling our intentions, we have then to trust those we employ and those we select to attend it. We can watch and warn. We can demand that they should explain what they are doing and why—and we can tell them to change if that is necessary! We can instruct the staff to examine themselves and their work every year—to conduct 'post-mortems' with the students at the end of every course and to use the experience as they gain it. But we should be stupid to try to bind the university staff hand and foot, and move them like puppets.

The university must be allowed to experiment, to try new courses and new methods. The staff must be encouraged to challenge the students and the society with arguments, and to put forward new suggestions about how to deal with the problems of building a socialist Tanzania based on human equality and dignity. Further, they must be allowed, and indeed expected, to challenge orthodox thinking on scientific and other aspects of knowledge—it is worth remembering that Galileo was very unpopular when he first argued that the world went round the sun! The staff we employ must lead in free debate based on a concept of service, on facts, and on ideas. Only by allowing this kind of freedom to our university staff will we have a university worth its name in Tanzania. For the University of Dar es Salaam will be able to serve our socialist purposes only if we accept that those whom we are paying to teach students to think, must themselves be allowed to think and speak their thoughts freely.

Conclusion

In conclusion, therefore, I simply want to say that every single individual working or living on this campus, as well as very many people outside it, has a part to play in the work ahead. For this will be a socialist university in a socialist country only if all members of the community recognize their common involvement and their mutual responsibility to each other and to the society at large. And it must be remembered that the community extends from the men who look after the grounds, or wash the dishes, or type the letters, to the Vice-Chancellor and his staff, as well as the students.

Of course, we shall not have a socialist university after today's ceremony, any more than we have a socialist society because of the 'Arusha Declaration': indeed it is impossible for the university to be fully socialist unless the society in which it operates is fully socialist. But I believe that the University of Dar es Salaam can help our people to attain their goals, both by its work and by its example. Let us commit ourselves to the attitudes, the organization, and the work, which this requires.

2.4 Our Education Must be for Liberation
J K Nyerere

Opening speech for a two-week seminar on 'Education and Training and Alternatives in Education in African Countries' on 20 May, 1974, organized by the Dag Hammarskjold Organization and the Institute of Development Studies in Dar es Salaam. *The Tanzania Education Journal* 3 (1974), No. 8 pp. 3–8.

. . . In 1967 I defined the purpose of education as 'to transmit from one generation to the next the accumulated wisdom and knowledge of the society, and to prepare the young people for their future membership of the society and their active participation in its maintenance or development'.

Today, seven years later, I still think that this is a good definition. But it was a definition intended to cover all kinds of societies—it was designed to be universal, objective, and descriptive. As a guide for action it therefore needs some expansion and emphasis, especially for Africa. And I believe that the necessary emphasis can be stated very simply: the primary purpose of education is the liberation of man.

To 'liberate' means to 'set free', and to 'set free from something'. It implies impediments to freedom having been thrown off; it can therefore be a matter of degree, and of a process. Thus, when a man succeeds in untying his wrists and liberating his arms, he can use his hands to liberate his feet from the shackles which bind them. But a man can be physically free from restraint and still be unfree if his mind is restricted by habits and attitudes which limit his humanity.

Education has to liberate both the mind and the body of man. It has to make him more of a human being because he is aware of his potential as a human being, and is in a positive, life-enhancing relationship with himself, his neighbour, and his environment. Education has therefore to enable a man to throw off the impediments to freedom which restrict his full physical and mental development. It is thus a matter of attitudes and skills—both of them. Education is incomplete if it only enables man to work out elaborate schemes for universal peace but does not teach him how to provide good food for himself and his family. It is equally incomplete and counter-productive if it merely teaches man how to be an efficient tool-user and tool-maker, but neglects his personality and his relationship with his fellow human beings.

What I am suggesting is that a liberated nation, in Africa or elsewhere, is not just a nation which has overcome alien occupation. That is an essential first part of liberation, but it is only the first. Liberation means more than that. A truly liberated nation is a self-reliant nation, one which has freed itself from economic and cultural dependence on other nations, and is therefore able to develop itself in free and equal co-operation with other members of the world community.

Similarly for man. The first essential of a liberated man is an awareness of two things: his own manhood, and the power of man to use circumstances rather than to be used by them. He must have overcome any ingrained feelings of inferiority, or superiority, and therefore be able to co-operate with other men, on the basis of equality, for their common purposes.

In this sense a man can be liberated while his country is still colonized, and—theoretically at least—while he himself is still physically unfree. Indeed it is only

43

after men have been to some degree liberated mentally that the struggle for physical liberation can be waged with a hope of success. The man who believes himself to be inferior to others because of his birth will remain inferior to them in the organization of society. A man who has been so far liberated that he rejects the concept of slavery and colonialism, as well as his own status as a slave, has taken the first steps towards overthrowing his slavery and his colonialism. For no man's freedom is secure while slavery exists: it is not possible to be a free man in a slave society without working against slavery. A liberated man in an unfree society will inevitably be working for freedom: and he will be turning even the most unfavourable circumstances to his ends. Even if, for example, he is conscripted into the colonial army, he will learn how to use weapons, and how his enemy fights, and in due course he will make an opportunity to use this knowledge for the cause of national liberation.

And when his country has thrown out an alien occupation, a liberated man will recognise that his task is not yet ended. For he will reject poverty and disease and ignorance in the same way as he rejects slavery, knowing that these are as effective in destroying the humanity of man as an overseer with a whip. A liberated man will work with others to defeat these evils, and will again use whatever resources are to hand. These resources may be his own knowledge, the knowledge of others, the land, the water, or simply his own sweat. By this kind of self-reliant struggle, a man will be further liberating himself, because by fighting the things which degrade humanity he will be expanding humanity.

It is the task of education in Africa to effect this mental liberation, or at least to begin it. Education has to liberate the African from the mentality of slavery and colonialism by making him aware of himself as an equal member of the human race, with the rights and duties of his humanity. It has to liberate him from the habit of submitting to circumstances which reduce his dignity as if they were immutable. And it has to liberate him from the shackles of technical ignorance so that he can make and use the tools of organization and creation for the development of himself and his fellow men.

The purpose of education is therefore liberation through the development of man as a member of society. The purpose is not the development of objects— whether they be pyramids, or irrigation ditches, railways, or palaces. The development of things—what is usually called economic development—can be involved in the development of man. It is so involved in Africa. But the purpose of education is not to turn out technicians who can be used as instruments in the expansion of the economy. It is to turn out men who have the technical knowledge and ability to expand the economy for the benefit of man in society.

That is not merely a play upon words. Nor is it a distinction of no importance. It is certainly true that Africa has great need of men with technical knowledge, and that our freedom is restricted by the absence of such men. I am not arguing against technical training in favour of what are sometimes called the liberal arts. On the contrary, in Tanzania just now we are engaged in a major exercise aimed at giving our education a practical and technical bias. What I am trying to do is to make a serious distinction between a system of education which makes liberated men and women into skilful users of tools, and a system of education which turns men and women into tools. I want to be quite sure that our technical and practical education is an education for creators, not for creatures. I would like to be quite sure that our educational institutions are not going to end up as factories turning out marketable commodities. I want them to enlarge men and women, not convert men and women into efficient instruments for the production of modern gadgets.

I do not think that in saying these things I am giving an unnatural extension to the word liberated. For I am talking about the liberation of man's humanity. Nor do I accept that education has liberated a man who regards his knowledge as a tool for the exploitation of others. For such an attitude means that he is seeking to suck sustenance from society without a greater, or even a comparable, contribution to the society. He is thinking of his knowledge as having taken him out of society, as having put him on a pinnacle. They are not free, those who do not value the freedom and humanity of others as they value their own freedom and their own humanity.

For man is a social animal. A man in isolation can be neither liberated nor educated; the words are meaningless in relation to an abandoned child brought up by wolves. And education is a social activity, with a social purpose. It is individuals who are educated. But they are educated by their fellows, for the common purpose of all members of the society. The intention is to develop them as human beings who are part of mankind.

These things are difficult to express in positive terms simply because each individual is unique as well as being part of mankind. Therefore each man's liberation will lead to a unique kind of contribution to the totality of humanity. But the antithesis of education in the sense that I am trying to describe can be easily understood. As I have already indicated it is the kind of education which teaches an individual to regard himself as a commodity, whose value is determined by certificates, degrees, or other professional qualifications.

Yet this antithesis of education is still too often the effect of what we call education in Africa—and in Tanzania. There are professional men who say: 'My market value is higher than the salary I am receiving in Tanzania.' But no human being has a market value—except a slave. There are educated people in positions of leadership in government, in parastatals, and still seeking jobs, who say: 'I am an educated person but I am not being treated according to my qualifications—I must have a better house, or a better salary, or a better status, than some other man.' But the value of a human being cannot depend on his salary, his house, or his car; nor on the uniform of his chauffeur.

When such things are said, the individuals saying them believe that they are arguing for their 'rights', as educated people. They believe that they are asserting the value of their education—and of themselves.

In reality they are doing the opposite. For in effect they are saying: 'This education I have been given has turned me into a marketable commodity, like cotton or sisal or coffee.' And they are showing that instead of liberating their humanity by giving it a greater chance to express itself, the education they have received has degraded their humanity. For they are arguing that as superior commodities they must be exchanged with commodities of equal value in an open market. They are not claiming—or not usually claiming—that they are superior human beings, only that they are superior commodities. Thus their education has converted them into objects—into repositories of knowledge like rather special computers. It is as objects, or commodities, that they have been taught to regard themselves and others.

With such an attitude a person will inevitably spend his life sucking from the community to the maximum of which is capable, and contributing the minimum he is able to contribute and live as he desires to live. He sucks from the local community as he is fed, clothed, housed, and trained. He sucks from the world community when he moves like a parcel of cotton to where the price is highest for his acquired skill.

Such a person is not a liberated human being. He is a marketable commodity.

We condemn such a person, or feel sorry for him as one of society's failures. But it would be much more appropriate to condemn the system which produces such people, and then to change that system.

For it is the education we are now giving in Africa, and the social values on which it is based, which is creating the people we condemn. It is our educational system which is instilling into young boys and girls the idea that their education confers a price tag on them, and which makes them concentrate on this price tag. It is our educational system which ignores the infinite and priceless value of a liberated human being, who is co-operating with others in building a civilization worthy of creators made in the image of God.

In thus describing what our education is doing, and what it should be doing, two things become very clear.

The first is that we in Africa have a definite responsibility to challenge the social values, and the educational system which produces people who look upon themselves as commodities, and who we must regard as social failures. This should not be a matter of political attacks on Africa's current leaders; for our present system is a product of history. But we leaders will be—and should be—criticized in the future if we now refuse to acknowledge the need for change. We will be, and we should be, condemned by later generations if we do not act now to try to find and institute an educational system which will liberate Africa's young people.

The second point is that education cannot be considered apart from society. The formal school system cannot educate a child in isolation from the social and economic system in which it operates. Of course it is a commonplace to say that education must be part of society. But the truth is that education is unavoidably part of society. Children, like adults, learn more from their experience of life than from their books and teachers.

Only a moment's reflection is needed to confirm this. Suppose a child is taught in school that the supreme virtue is co-operation with others, and help to those with greater difficulties than himself. What happens if selection for a privileged place in the society—whether it be higher education or some other economic or social benefit—is then based solely upon academic knowledge? The child who has learned his lessons well will fail to qualify. For the good pupil will have spent time working with others so as to raise the general standard of knowledge, while the bad pupil will have concentrated on his own learning of the things which are to be the basis for selection. The facts of life will thus teach all the pupils that while co-operation may be a religious virtue, the pursuit of self-interest is what determines a man's status, his income, and his power. Two things will have taught this lesson. First, the very existence of privilege in the society; and second, the basis on which selection is made for that privilege.

Formal education in a school or adult classes system is no substitute for the informal education provided by life experience. Nor can a formal system operate effectively in opposition to the social practices. Yet Africa needs change; and change has to start somewhere.

Without venturing into the wider debate, it is quite clear that in Africa at any rate the problem of integrating education with the society cannot be solved by abandoning a formal education structure. We cannot go back to an exclusive dependence on the traditional system of what I previously called 'learning by living and doing'. We cannot go back because modern knowledge is not dispersed in our societies. Even the social values of co-operation have in many places been undermined by the effects of imported capitalism. And the techniques of modern production, exchange, and organisation, were unknown in traditional Africa; they are still unknown by the majority of our adults.

Thus we have the position where a formal school system, devised and operated without reference to the society in which its graduates will live, is of little use as an instrument of liberation for the people of Africa. And at the same time, learning just by living and doing in the existing society would leave us so backward socially, and technologically that human liberation in the foreseeable future is out of the question.

Somehow we have to combine the two systems. We have to integrate formal education with the society. And we have to use education as a catalyst for change in that society. That, I believe, is our task. It is one which various African nations, or groups within nations, have been trying to fulfil over the last decade. Interesting work has been done, and valuable experience gained. We need to examine this carefully, and to implement the things which it teaches us. . . .

I think we admit that we have not done all that is necessary. We have been too timid—too unliberated—to effect the required radical transformation of the system we inherited. We have made important changes, especially in the curriculum and syllabi. But we are still mentally committed to 'international standards' in education. We still apparently believe that a Tanzanian is not educated unless his education takes a form recognizable by, and acceptable to, other countries—and in particular the English-speaking countries. It is from others that we see our certificates of respectability.

So the first problem we have not solved is that of building sufficient self-confidence to refuse what we regard as the world's best (whatever that may mean), and to choose instead the most appropriate for our conditions. In education, industry, agriculture, and commerce, we all too often prefer blind imitation to relevant initiative or rational adaptation.

The second problem is our apparent inability or unwillingness to really integrate education and life, and education and production. I am not suggesting that we have made no advances in this direction. Nor am I suggesting that our failure to advance further can be attributed simply to the prejudices of our educationalists. Parents, politicians, and workers, as well as educators, are suspicious of, or hostile to, the educational innovations required. But the total result is that few of our schools are really an integral part of the village life, except in the sense that they occupy village children for so many hours a day. And what is true in the villages is even more true of the towns. Further, few schools—if any—can really claim that their production makes any large contribution even to their own upkeep, much less to the society in general.

Our third failure is in not overcoming the belief that academic ability marks out a child or an adult as especially praise-worthy, or as deserving a privileged place in the society. We still have the idea that a child who is not selected for secondary school has 'failed'. And that idea will persist until we have eradicated the idea that a person who does receive post-primary education must receive a greater monetary income just because of that extra education, and regardless of how he uses it. For it is this practice of fixing wage rates according to the final year of education which epitomizes the concept of education as the processing of human raw material into refined commodities.

Once again, this is not just a failure within the formal education system. It is a failure of the society as a whole. Indeed, the educationalists have advanced in these matters more than other sections of the community. We have therefore down-graded examination results in selecting pupils for secondary school; we have included course work assessment in determining degree awards. But our society has not accepted that character, co-operativeness, and a desire to serve, are relevant to a person's ability to benefit from further training. We have not really begun to consider the value of experience with small jobs as a necessary preliminary to more advanced training. You cannot enter a Tanzanian secondary school except straight from primary school. Even mature entry to university is often regarded as a concession to political doctrine rather than a valuable system in its own right! . . .

All that I have been saying is that the function of education is the liberation of man. I have not been arguing that academic training is bad, unnecessary, or unimportant. I have not been saying either that technical and professional training are unimportant. What I have been trying to suggest is that education must not be thought of only, or even primarily, as a matter for schools, or as an instrument for academic and technical advance.

The dissemination of academic, professional, and technical knowledge is important, and indeed vital to Africa. But it is vital only because it is a necessary part of the education which liberates man, and enables him to work as an equal with his fellow men for the development of mankind.

2.5 Adult Education and Development
J K Nyerere

Address to the participants of the international conference on 'Adult Education and Development' organized by the International Council for Adult Education and held at the University of Dar es Salaam, 21–25 June, 1976.

... Development is for Man, by Man, and of Man. The same is true of education. Its purpose is the liberation of Man from the restraints and limitations of ignorance and dependency. Education has to increase men's physical and mental freedom—to increase their control over themselves, their own lives, and the environment in which they live. The ideas imparted by education, or released in the mind through education, should therefore be liberating ideas; the skills acquired by education should be liberating skills. Nothing else can properly be called education. Teaching which induces a slave mentality or a sense of impotence is not education at all—it is attack on the minds of men.

This means that adult education has to be directed at helping men to develop themselves. It has to contribute to an enlargement of Man's ability in every way. In particular it has to help men to decide for themselves—in co-operation—what development is. It must help men to think clearly; it must enable them to examine the possible alternative courses of action; to make a choice between those alternatives in keeping with their own purposes; and it must equip them with the ability to translate their decisions into reality.

The personal and physical aspects of development cannot be separated. It is in the process of deciding for himself what is development, and deciding in what direction it should take his society, and in implementing those decisions, that Man develops himself. For Man does not develop himself in a vacuum, in isolation from his society and his environment; and he certainly cannot be developed by others. Man's consciousness is developed in the process of thinking, and deciding and of acting. His capacity is developed in the process of doing things.

But doing things means co-operating with others, for in isolation Man is virtually helpless physically, and stultified mentally. Education for liberation is therefore also education for co-operation among men, because it is in co-operation with others that Man liberates himself from the constraints of nature, and also those imposed upon him by his fellow men. Education is thus intensely personal in the sense that it has to be a personal experience—no-one can have his consciousness developed by proxy. But it is also an activity of great social significance, because the man whom education liberates is a man in society, and his society will be affected by the change which education creates in him.

There is another aspect to this. A man learns because he wants to do something. And once he has started along this road of developing his capacity he also learns because he wants to *be*; to be a more conscious and understanding person. Learning has not liberated a man if all he learns to want is a certificate on his wall, and the reputation of being a 'learned person'—a possessor of knowledge. For such a desire is merely another aspect of the disease of the acquisitive society—the accumulation of goods for the sake of accumulating them. The accumulation of knowledge, or worse still the accumulation of pieces of paper which represent a kind of legal tender for such knowledge, has nothing to do with development.

So if adult education is to contribute to development, it must be a part of life—integrated with life and inseparable from it. It is not something which can be put into a box and taken out for certain periods of the day or week—or certain periods of a life. And it cannot be imposed: every learner is ultimately a volunteer, because however much teaching he is given, only he can learn.

Further, adult education is not something which can deal with just 'agriculture', or 'health', or 'literacy', or 'mechanical skill', etc. All these separate branches of education are related to the total life a man is living, and to the man he is and will become. Learning how best to grow soy-beans is of little use to a man if it is not combined with learning about nutrition and/or the existence of a market for the beans.

This means, therefore, that adult education will promote changes in men, and in society. And it means that adult education *should* promote change, at the same time as it assists men to control both the change which they induce, and that which is forced upon them by the decisions of other men or the cataclysms of nature. Further, it means that adult education encompasses the whole of life, and must build upon what already exists.

Changes and Adult Education

In that case, the first function of adult education is to inspire both a desire for change, and an understanding that change is possible. For a belief that poverty or suffering is 'the will of God' and that Man's only task is to endure, is the most fundamental of all the enemies of freedom. Yet dissatisfaction with what *is* must be combined with a conviction that it can be changed: otherwise it is simply destructive. Men living in poverty or sickness or under tyranny or exploitation must be enabled to recognize both that the life they lead is miserable, and that they can change it by their own action, either individually or in co-operation with others.

Work of this kind is not often called 'adult education' and it is not usually regarded as a function of Adult Education Associations or Departments. But neither is teaching a child to walk, or to speak, usually regarded as 'education'! It is only when a child does not learn these primary functions as it grows out of infancy that organized education takes over the task of teaching them in 'special Schools' for the deaf or the otherwise handicapped. Similarly, whether or not institutions of adult education ought to be doing this fundamental work of arousing consciousness about the need for, and the possibility of change, will depend upon the circumstances in which they are operating. In Third World countries such work often has to be done by someone, or some organization. It will simply be a matter of organization and efficiency whether it is done by people called 'Community Development Workers', or 'Political Education Officers', or 'Adult Teachers'. What is important is that it is done, and that all should recognize it as a necessary basis for all other developmental and educational activities.

The same thing is true of what I would call the second stage of adult education, that is, helping people to work out what kind of change they want, and how to create it. For example: it is not enough that the people in a village should come to recognize that something can be done about their endemic malaria—that it is not an evil which has to be endured. They also have to learn that malaria can be treated with drugs, or prevented by controlling mosquitoes, or that malaria can be dealt with by a combination of curative and preventive action. And all this must be followed up with action.

Thus we have a whole series of educational activities all of which involve a learning process—an expansion of consciousness. The combination of them all is required if the development—of men and the environment—is to be life-enhancing. And all of them can be assisted by the activities of an educator.

The Scope of Adult Education

Adult education thus incorporates anything which enlarges men's understanding, activates them, helps them to make their own decisions, and to implement those decisions for themselves. It includes training, but is much more than training. It includes what is generally called 'agitation' but it is much more than that. It includes organization and mobilization, but it goes beyond them to make them purposeful.

Thinking of adult education from the point of view of the educators, therefore, one can say that they are of two types—each of whom needs the other. The first are what one might call the 'generalists'. They are the political activists and educators—whether or not they are members of, and organized by, a political party or whether they are Community Development workers or religious teachers. Such people are not politically neutral; by the nature of what they are doing they cannot be. For what they are doing will affect how men look at the society in which they live, and how they seek to use it or change it. Making the people of a village aware that their malaria can be avoided, for example, will cause them to make demands upon the larger community in which they live. At least they will demand drugs, or insect spray, or teachers; they will no longer be passive beings who simply accept the life they know. And if people who have been aroused cannot get the change they want, or a substitute for it which is acceptable to them, they will become discontented—if not hostile—towards whatever authority they regard as responsible for the failure. Adult education is thus a highly political activity. Politicians are sometimes more aware of this fact than educators, and therefore they do not always welcome real adult education.

The work of these 'generalists' is fundamental to adult education. It is after their work has been done—that is after a demand has been generated and a problem identified—that what might be called the 'specialists' can become effective. If you go into a village and explain how to spray stagnant water, you may be listened to with politeness; but your effort has been wasted, and nothing will happen after you have left unless the villagers first understand what the spraying will do, and why it is important. Of course, it is possible for the 'health educator' to give this explanation himself—he should certainly be capable of doing so, and prepared to do so. But his specialized knowledge can be more effective—and can be spread among a larger number of villages—if the people have already discussed and absorbed the reasons for anti-mosquito spraying, and developed a desire to learn how to do it for themselves.

It is at the level of this 'specialist' adult education that the division into health, agriculture, child care, management, literacy, and other kinds of education, can make sense. But none of these branches can be self-contained; their work must be co-ordinated and linked. The work of the agricultural specialist must be linked with that of the nutritionist and that of the people who train villagers to be more effective in selling or buying; and he may himself find the need to call upon—or lead the villagers towards—the person who can teach literacy. Adult education in fact must be like a spider's web, the different strands of which knot together, each strengthening the other, and each connected to the others to make a coherent whole.

But in saying that I do not wish to imply that adult education has a beginning and an end, or that it is necessary for a particular community or individual to travel along all the various branches of learning at a fairly simple level. The point I am trying to make is that mass adult education—which is what most of us are concerned with in our working lives—must not be thought of as being in self-contained compartments, nor must it be organized into them. If the people's felt need is improved health, the health specialist must lead them into an awareness of the need for improved agricultural techniques as he teaches the elements of preventive medicine, or helps them to lay the foundations of a curative health service. And the health specialist must have organizational links with the agriculture teacher, so that this new interest can be met as it is aroused—and so on.

But certain individuals or communities will wish to pursue particular interests further. The mass education must be of a kind as to show that this can be done, and to provide the tools with which it can be done. For example, it must lead to literacy (if it does not start with that); and it must incorporate access to books of different levels, even if it cannot include provision for more formal teaching. The mass education should also show people how to learn from the use of resources which are locally available—like a nearby dispensary, a good farmer, local school teachers, and so on.

For mass adult education must be seen as a beginning—a foundation course on which people can build their own structures according to their own interests and own desires. And the adult educator must demonstrate this function in his own activities—that is, by continuing to expand his personal knowledge through reading, listening to the radio, informal discussions, participation in physical development activities, and attendance at such other organized education courses as may be available.

The Methods of Adult Education
For all these are methods of adult education, and must be understood as such. Which one, or which combination, is appropriate at a particular time will depend upon many things. But one fundamental fact must underlie the choice made. A mother does not 'give' walking or talking to her child; walking and talking are not things which she 'has' and of which she gives a portion to the child. Rather, the mother helps the child to develop its own potential ability to walk and talk. And the adult educator is in the same position. He is not giving to another something which he possesses. He is helping the learner to develop his own potential and his own capacity.

What all this means in practice is that the adult educator must involve the learners in their own education, and in practice, from the very beginning. Only activities which involve them in doing something for themselves will provide an on-going sense of achievement and mean that some new piece of knowledge is actually grasped—that it has become something of 'theirs'. It does not matter what form this involvement takes; it may be a contribution to a discussion, reading out loud, or writing, or making a furrow of the required depth and width. What is important is that the adult learner should be learning by doing, just as—to go back to my earlier example—a child learns to walk by walking.

There is a second very fundamental determinant of adult education method. It is that every adult knows something about the subject he is interested in, even if he is not aware that he knows it. He may indeed know something which his teacher does not know. For example, the villagers will know what time of the year malaria is worse and what group of people—by age or residence or work place—are most badly affected.

It is on the basis of this knowledge that greater understanding must be built, and be seen to be built. For by drawing out the things the learner already knows, and showing their relevance to the new thing which has to be learnt, the teacher has done three things. He has built up the self-confidence of the man who wants to learn, by showing him that he is capable of contributing. He has demonstrated the relevance of experience and observation as a method of learning when combined with thought and analysis. And he has shown what I might call the 'mutuality' of learning—that is, that by sharing our knowledge we extend the totality of our understanding and our control over our lives.

For this is very important. The teacher of adults is a leader, a guide along a path on which all will travel together. The organizers and teachers in an adult education programme can be no more than that; to be effective therefore they have consciously to identify themselves with those who are participating in it primarily as learners. Only on this basis of equality, and of sharing a task which is of mutual benefit, is it possible to make full use of the existing human resources in the development of a community, a village, or a nation. And it is within this context of sharing knowledge that all the different techniques of teaching can be used.

The most appropriate techniques in a particular case will depend upon the circumstances, and the resources, of the learning community and of the nation in which it lives. For it is no good spending time and money on elaborate visual aids which need skilled operators and electricity, if either the skilled operator or the electricity is lacking in the village which wants to learn! It is no use relying upon techniques which need imported materials if you are working in a country which has a permanent balance of payments problem. And in a poor country the techniques used must be of very low cost, and preferably capable of being constructed out of local materials, at the place where the teaching will be done, and by the people who will teach and learn. Self-reliance is a very good educational technique as well as being an indispensable basis for further development!

The Organization of Adult Education

This need to become increasingly self-reliant in adult education, as in other aspects of development, will have to be reflected in the organization of adult education activities. Obviously there is no 'ideal' adult education organization pattern to which all nations could, or should, aspire. The type of organization has to reflect the needs, and the resources, of each country, as well as its culture and its political commitment.

The one unavoidable thing is that resources have to be allocated to adult education. It will not happen without them! There is a regrettable tendency in times of economic stringency—which for poor countries is all the time—for governments to economize on money for adult education. And there is a tendency also, when trained people are in short supply, to decide that adult education must wait—or to pull out its best practitioners and give them more prestigious jobs and administration.

It would certainly be a mistake to try to duplicate for adults the kind of educational establishment we have for children—either in staff or buildings. The most appropriate adult teachers are often those who are also engaged in another job—who are practitioners of what they will be teaching. But it is necessary to have some people whose full-time work is teaching adults, or organizing the different kinds of adult education. And these people have to be paid wages and given the equipment, and facilities, which are needed to be effective. How many of them there should be, and whether they should be in one educational hierarchy or under different specialized Ministries or Departments, will depend upon local factors, and will probably vary from time to time. Certainly we in Tanzania have not solved this kind of organizational problem to our satisfaction.

All this means that adult education has to be given a priority within the overall development and recurrent revenue allocations of governments or other institutions. And what priority it obtains is perhaps one of the most political decisions a government will take. For if adult education is properly carried out, and therefore effective, it is the most potent force there can be for developing a free people who will insist upon determining their own future.

Education arouses curiosity and provokes questioning—the challenging of old assumptions and established practices. An educated ujamaa village, for example, will neither allow nor tolerate dishonesty among its accountants, or authoritarianism among its leaders. An educated population will challenge the actions of its elected representatives—including its President. Maybe this is why adult education is generally the cinderella of government departments, or why its function is captured by newspaper, cinema, and television owners and editors with a personal axe to grind! And do not let me pretend that Tanzania is an exception to any of this. Our policy of commitment to adult education is clear. But our practice, and our practitioners, are—to put it mildly—not above criticism!

But of course, even if a top priority is given to adult education, there are priorities within that priority still to be determined. Resources are always limited. In poor and backward countries they are laughably small in relation to the need. So choices have to be made between such things as generalized education, different kinds of specialized mass education, the radio, mass circulation of subsidized literature, residential education, the training of the educators and an increase in teachers untrained in techniques—and so on.

Once again, there is no 'best' choice or balance among all these necessary activities. What is appropriate will depend upon the existing level of knowledge and understanding in different fields, and upon the existing resources in men, materials, and equipment. In Tanzania, for example, we have now broken through the stage where miserable conditions were regarded as 'The Will of God'. Our present task is therefore primarily that of helping people to acquire the tools of development—the literacy, the knowledge of health needs, the need for improved production, the need to improve dwelling places, and the basic skills necessary to meet all these needs.

We are finding that the organization of this second stage is much more difficult, with our limited resources, to ensure that when people have learned a skill, the ploughs, and the carpentry equipment, and the survey levels etc., are also where they are wanted and at an accessible price level!

But there is a saying that nothing which is easy is worth doing, and it could never be said that adult education is not worth doing! For it is the key to the development of free men and free societies. Its function is to help men to think for themselves, to make their own decisions, and to execute these decisions for themselves.

Chapter 3 The Integration Approach in Tanzania

3.1 Towards the Integration of Formal and Non-formal Education
Y O Kassam

Ever since Independence in 1961, Tanzania has been trying to overhaul its total educational system, which was inherited from the colonial system, in order to match it with its *own* new goals, aspirations, concepts and challenges of development. By far the most revolutionary re-appraisal of the purpose and the whole system of education began with the proclamation of the 'Arusha Declaration'[1] in 1967 which is a blueprint for the Tanzanian policy of socialism and self-reliance, and with the publication of President Nyerere's policy document on 'Education for Self-Reliance'[2] also in 1967. Since then one can perceive three main trends in the educational policy of Tanzania. First, increasing importance and priority is attached to the development of non-formal education which can reach the masses and provide a more functional type of education. Second, formal education is undergoing a gradual transformation both in content and structure. And third, attempts have been made to integrate formal and non-formal education. This paper focusses on the different ways and means which have been used in integrating formal and non-formal education[3] in Tanzania, the rationale for this kind of integration, and the problems involved in the process of effecting it.

1. The rationale for integration

The objective of the high priority that adult education enjoys in Tanzania is to develop human resources on a mass scale and as rapidly as possible. At the same time the provision of mass adult education is designed to reduce the social inequalities and the wide gap between the overwhelming majority of the people who are either illiterate or have had little education, and the small educated elite which is mainly the product of formal education. In particular, emphasis is placed on improving the living conditions of the rural population, which constitutes more than 90 per cent of the total population and forms the backbone of the economy which is based on agriculture. The formal system of education caters for only about 50 per cent of the children of school-going age, of whom only about 6 per cent get places in secondary schools. Given the scarce education resources of a poor developing country like Tanzania, adult education on a mass scale can only be provided by maximizing the utilization of existing resources of the formal system of education. Such a utilization of resources can be effectively made by institutional, structural and oragnizational integration of the formal system of education with non-formal or adult education.

But the rationale for integrating formal and non-formal education goes beyond the logistic and economic considerations. In the minds of many people, 'education' has traditionally been regarded as being synonymous with formal schooling. Consequently, any kind of education that is provided outside the formal system of education is not considered worthwhile or valuable. Such a misconceived notion can be eliminated if the institutions of formal education are made to function simultaneously as centres of adult education or non-formal education. In any case, since education is recognized as a continuing and lifelong process, it is unrealistic to have artificial barriers between formal and non-formal education.

Lastly, while provision of non-formal education on an extensive scale is greatly facilitated by being integrated with the system of formal education, formal education in its turn undergoes positive changes by the impact of non-formal education. This point can be illustrated by citing some of the criticisms that have been levelled at formal schooling. For example, 'Education for Self-Reliance' pointed out that formal education in Tanzania was highly elitist and academic-oriented and was not geared towards helping the vast majority of students to live usefully and happily in a predominantly rural society. Formal education is also marked by the rigidity of its curriculum and is not integrated with work. By contrast, non-formal education is largely characterized by its functional and utilitarian orientation, by flexibility in programming and participatory pedagogical methods. Its integration with formal education therefore assists the latter in transforming itself in the light of the kind of criticisms that have been made against it.

2. The nature of integration between formal and non-formal education

Non-formal education in Tanzania, as Elsewhere, is charactcrized by a wide spectrum of different programmes under a wide assortment of agencies and institutions, both government and non-government, as well as voluntary agencies. A large number of non-formal education programmes, such as those in agricultural extension and community development, had been in existence long before the proclamation of the 'Arusha Declaration'. However, since the 'Arusha Declaration' the further development of non-formal education has become a top priority. New organizational and administrative structures have been set up, and new and closer relationships between formal and non-formal education have been fostered.

3. The incorporation of adult education within the Ministry of National Education

A significant step towards the integration of formal and non-formal education was taken in 1969 when the responsibility of directing, administering and co-ordinating adult education was transferred from the Ministry of Rural Development and Regional Administration to the Ministry of Education, and consequently, the latter was renamed Ministry of *National* Education. Up to that time, the Ministry of Education had been only concerned with formal education, and this had led to a sharp distinction between formal and non-formal education.

As a result of this transfer of powers, a new Directorate of Adult Education was established in this Ministry on the same footing as other Directorates dealing with the various levels of formal education. In the following year the Ministry for the first time appointed a new cadre of adult educators known as Education Officers in charge of Adult Education for every district in the country. These officers, whose main responsibility is to organize and co-ordinate adult education programmes and activities in their districts, work together with and on the same level as education officers in charge of formal education. Between 1970 and 1972, more adult education officers were appointed at different administrative levels such as the Regional Co-ordinators, Divisional Co-ordinators and Ward Co-ordinators.

4. The committee structure

In addition to the appointment of these officers, an elaborate committee structure for non-formal education has been set up since 1970 (See Chart 3.1). It is designed to provide a horizontal co-ordination between various agencies of non-formal education programmes on the one hand, and a co-ordination of non-formal education programmes with institutions of formal education on the other. The Regional Adult Education Committee is chaired by the Regional Secretary of TANU, with the Regional Co-ordinator of Adult Education acting as Secretary. The members of the Committee include the Heads of Departments of Ministries involved in adult education, such as Agriculture, Health, co-operatives, etc., representatives of UWT, NUTA and TAPA as well as representatives of missionary and other voluntary agencies. A similar composition of membership characterizes the District Adult Education Committee. The Ward Adult Education Committee chaired by the TANU Branch Chairman comprises Heads of formal education institutions such as the primary school, secondary school, College of National Education, etc., as well as Heads of other institutions that may exist in the ward such as a national service camp, prison, factory, etc. Finally, every school and college and all other institutions are supposed to have their own adult education committees.

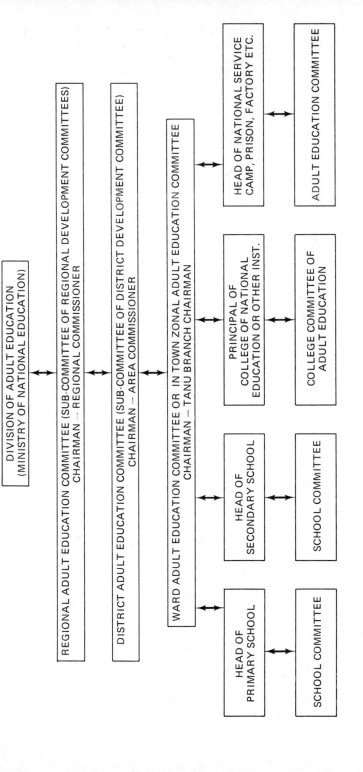

Chart 3.1

The Committee Structure of Adult Education Under the Ministry of National Education

Although the importance of having such a committee structure is undeniable, its effectiveness is sometimes hampered by a number of problems. For example, some of the ward, district and regional committees do not meet very regularly, some members do not maintain a regular attendance, and at times the decisions and plans made by the committees are not implemented.

One of the main tasks of the Ministry of National Education has been to mobilize and co-ordinate all possible resources, human and material, for carrying out non-formal education on a nation-wide scale. In this connection, the Ministry has been trying to stress the guiding principle that the task of providing non-formal education rests on the co-operation and participation of as many Ministries and organizations as possible. Table 3.1 illustrates the number of teachers from different organizations who are involved in teaching various non-formal education programmes as at December, 1973. Table 3.2 shows the number of participants in the various programmes.

Table 3.1

Number of People from Various Organizations Teaching in Non-formal Education Programmes Organized by the Ministry of National Education, December 1973.

Organization	No. of teachers
Primary school teachers	20672
Secondary school students	2893
TANU	3310
Ministry of Agriculture	1129
Ministry of Health	1575
Prime Minister's Office	4449
Religious bodies	644
Others (mainly Volunteers)	59590
	94262 Total

Source: Ministry of National Education: Adult Education Statistics.

5. Primary schools as centres of adult education

Another significant development in the relationship between formal and non-formal education occurred with the launching of the Second Five-Year Development Plan (1969–74) which required every primary school in the country, without exception, to operate as a centre of adult education in addition to providing primary education for the children. Such a step can be looked upon as the first practical attempt to harmonize and integrate in some form and degree formal and non-formal education. To quote the relevant section of the Plan:

'The general principle is to place the main organizing responsibility (for adult education) on the primary school. The school will then become a community

Table 3.2

The Number of Participants by Subject in Non-formal Education Organized by the Ministry of National Education, December 1973.

Subjects	No. of participants
Political Education	1 272 080
Agriculture	1 370 000
Health	1 171 606
Literacy	2 586 702
Home Economics	750 335
Kiswahili ⎫	
Arithmetic ⎬	2 203 933
History ⎭	
Typing	43 375
English	224 701
Technical subjects	81 046
Economics	81 999

Source: Ministry of National Education: *Adult Education Statistics*. (An individual may be enrolled for more than one subject.)

educational centre, at which the provision of primary education is only one function. A school so conceived will increasingly become a focal point for the total educational needs of the community, rather than serving as a somewhat detached institution for the education of children.'[4]

The person charged with the general responsibility for the adult education activities of the centre is the Headmaster who is required to identify community needs, find suitable instructors from various adult education agencies at the local level as well as other competent and knowledgeable individuals from the neighbourhood, and arrange the necessary classes. All primary school teachers also have to teach adults and other non-school-goers as an integral part of their duties, for which they receive no additional remuneration.

The subjects taught in the non-formal education programme of the centre cover a wide range. The main emphasis according to the Plan should be on rural development:

'It will include simple training in agriculture techniques and craftsmanship, health education, housecraft, simple economics and accounting, and education in politics and the responsibilities of the citizen.'[5]

In order to enable primary schools to run non-formal education programmes, they are given a small additional grant for equipment and materials. But the main reliance is on maximum utilization of their existing resources.

In addition to the primary schools, a wide range of other places also function as centres of adult education. These include dispensaries, community centres, TANU offices, the backyard of an individual's house or the space under a large tree, and so on. The classes organized at such centres are normally run by voluntary teachers, a large majority of whom are primary school leavers. A large number of these volunteers, particularly those teaching functional literacy in the four northern regions of Tanzania where the UNDP/Unesco work-oriented adult literacy pilot project had been operating, have been trained in functional literacy methods. Secondary schools and teacher training colleges also operate as centres of adult education.

Although a positive kind of relationship has been forged between non-formal education and primary schools, there are several problems involved in this relationship. First, although primary school teachers have generally acquired a high degree of political consciousness and have readily responded to the national call for adult education, they sometimes complain of being overloaded with work since they have to teach children during the day and teach adults in the afternoons and evenings. The situation is aggravated by the general shortage of primary school teachers which results in incomplete staffing of the schools. Furthermore, it has not always been easy to get instructors from other organizations and institutions to come and teach at the centres. Second, while primary education has, on the whole, an adequate and suitable supply of teaching materials, non-formal education is generally critically short of suitable materials except for literacy primers. Third, in many schools the small-size desks, chairs and benches originally designed for school children are obviously unsuitable for adults, both physically and psychologically. Fourth, the voluntary teachers for adult education who are supposed to receive an honorarium of Tshs 30 per month sometimes do not get it all, and very often its payment is delayed for several months due to financial and administrative problems. Furthermore, payment of an 'honorarium' and not of a salary is interpreted by some people to mean that non-formal education is an inferior kind of education.

6. Community education centres

The new plan of the government to set up what will be known as 'community education centres' is an extension of the idea of the existing system of primary schools functioning as adult education centres. It is also an attempt to integrate formal with non-formal education on the one hand, and primary school with the community on the other. The source of inspiration for this new proposal has been the Kwamsisi ujamaa village in Tanga Region, where a pilot project of integrating the work and curriculum of the primary school with the activities of the village, especially through the village's self-help activities, has shown encouraging results. At Kwamsisi, the traditional and generally unsuitable type of academic study is giving way to a meaningful, relevant and practical preparation for village life. The pupils themselves are involved in the planning and implementation of their self-help activities in the village, and the villagers, besides attending various non-formal education classes at the primary school, also have a say in what they think should be taught to their children.[6]

7. The training of cadres for non-formal education
Another relationship between formal and non-formal education in Tanzania lies in the training of cadres for non-formal education. All colleges of National Education (i.e., teacher training colleges) have incorporated compulsory training in adult education methodology in their curriculum. In other words, all teacher trainees are trained to teach primary school children as well as adults and youths in non-formal education. Besides the theoretical training, the practical training involves the teacher trainees in carrying out teaching practice in both primary education and adult education.

The University of Dar es Salaam also offers a number of courses to meet the increasing demand for professional adult educators, who are needed for an increasing number and variety of non-formal education programmes and institutions. The Institute of Adult Education of the University of Dar es Salaam has been offering a professional Diploma Course in Adult Education since 1969.[7] The Diploma Course is a residential course lasting for one academic year and is designed to provide professional training in adult education to people already working in the field of adult education in Tanzania, including extension services in rural development, agriculture, co-operation, health, etc. . . ., and also to people working in other organizations and agencies dealing with non-formal education in general.

Two courses in adult education at the degree level are also offered at the University of Dar es Salaam. The first is an optional course for third year education students who, in addition to their teaching duties in formal education, will be involved with teaching and organizing adult education programmes in and around secondary schools and teacher training colleges. The second course, which was initiated in 1974, is designed to train a small group of second year education students in planning and organizing adult education programmes. The graduates of this course are absorbed by the Ministry of National Education in various programmes and institutions of adult education.

By training various cadres for both formal and non-formal education at the same level the University of Dar es Salaam has recognized the importance of non-formal education. However, since the training for non-formal education is a fairly recent introduction at the university, it is sometimes subjected to pressures from stereotyped and rigid requirements that go with the training of teaching cadres for formal education and also, to a certain extent, to the scepticism of the traditional and conservative formal educationalists.

Training of adult educators in seminars is also carried out by the adult education officers of the Ministry of National Education at the regional, district and divisional levels. In addition, every region has what is known as a permanent regional training team which conducts training mainly in functional literacy methods. The training team consists of a total of six representatives from the Ministry of National Education, Ministry of Agriculture, Ministry of Health, College of National Education, Prime Minister's Office and National Service. However, these training teams have not been functioning effectively, mainly due to frequent transfers of their members to different regions or different jobs.

8. Abolition of 'direct entry' into the university
The most recent and revolutionary step towards changing the whole system of

education in Tanzania and bringing about a more harmonious relationship between formal and non-formal education is the abolition of direct admission of Form VI leavers to the University with effect from 1975. This step has been taken in one of the resolutions, popularly known as the 'Musoma Resolutions', passed by the National Executive Committee meeting of TANU in Musoma in November, 1974. This resolution requires all Form VI leavers to work first in offices, factories and villages. Only when they have proved their work competence and other abilities and attitudes, and obtained recommendations from their work places and TANU Branches, will they be considered for university education. Such a step, which is, in effect, an implementation of some of the ideas put forward in the policy of 'Education for Self-Reliance', is intended to integrate education with work and to de-emphasize the paper qualifications of formal education. In other words, the ability to pass examinations in formal education will no longer be considered to be the only criterion in selecting people for further education. Such a process as de-emphasizing purely academic abilities and formal examinations and enhancing and upgrading the value and importance of non-formal education will, it may be hoped, contribute to the development of a more positive and harmonious relationship between formal and non-formal education.

However, a distinction and conflict between formal and non-formal education that is still to be reckoned with as far as salaried employment is concerned lies in the very issue of credentials of formal education. Job opportunities almost invariably require qualifications of formal education at some level. As a result, non-formal education frequently comes under pressure for certification and grading that could 'correspond' with the various levels of formal education. Although of late vacancies for employment advertized in the local newspapers tag on the words 'or equivalent' to a list of formal educational qualifications, the essential conflict remains largely unresolved. On the other hand, exposure to non-formal education has been one of the entrance requirements for those wishing to pursue undergraduate studies at the university under what is known as the 'mature age entry scheme'. Similarly, previous participation in teaching adult education classes is one of the entrance qualifications for primary Grade VII leavers who wish to join the Grade C teacher training course.

Conclusions

This paper has presented and analyzed a number of innovative steps that have been taken to integrate formal and non-formal education in Tanzania. This integration which has developed in the process of the very rapid growth and expansion of non-formal education derives its great strength from the very nature of Tanzania's political ideology of socialism and self-reliance.[8] While non-formal education has gained considerable advantages for its own development, formal education has begun to turn to non-formal education for answers to some of its problems. Of course, a number of problems still exist in the relationships between formal and non-formal education, and they are by no means easy to surmount. But since Tanzania has taken bold steps in the right direction, it may be hoped that the problems will in time be solved.

Notes

1 Nyerere, J K *Freedom and Socialism* pp. 231–256 Bibl. 11
2 *Freedom and Socialism* pp. 267–290
3 The definition adopted for non-formal education in this paper is that given by Philip H Coombs in *New Paths to Learning For Rural Children and Youth*. New York: International Council for Educational Development, 1973: 'Non-formal education is any organized educational activity outside the established formal system—whether operating separately or as an important feature of some broader activity—that is intended to serve identifiable learning clienteles and learning objectives.' Formal education as defined by Coombs is: 'the hierarchically structured, chronologically graded "educational system" running from primary school through the university and including, in addition to general academic studies, a variety of specialized programmes and institutions for full-time technical and professional training.' p. 11
4 The United Republic of Tanzania. *Tanzania Second Five-Year Plan for Economic and Social Development* . . . Vol. I, pp. 231–256
5 See Note 4, Vol. I, p. 157
6 For further details see the article by Ishumi in this chapter, p. 86
7 For a study of the graduates of the Diploma Course in Adult Education see Kassam, Y O *The Training and Functions of Full-Time and Professional Adult Educators in Tanzania*. Dar es Salaam: UDSM, 1973 (M.A. thesis)
8 See Kassam, Y O 'Political Education vis-à-vis Adult Education in Tanzania: The Dynamics of their Interaction'. *Convergence*. VII (1974), No. 4 pp. 40–50

3.2 Community Centres in Tanzania: Their Development and Scope
A G M Ishumi
Introduction

The place and role of Community Centres in a changing society has been, and still is, a subject of discussion both in the developed and in the developing regions of the world today. This is reflected not only in the changing conception of the nature and function of such centres over the years, but also in the shifting emphasis in the very definition of a community centre and the process of community development in general.

Two principal views have dominated the trend of thinking about community centres and their role in social development. The first, older view originated from the technologically developed countries, where such centres have been designed as meeting places for various groups, mostly for cultural and recreational activities such as games, dancing, choirs, orchestra, opera, theatre, or debate. In these countries there are many centres of this type located in cities and in the countryside to meet the various needs and interests of the urban and/or 'urbanizing' population.[1]

The majority of these centres were established through the initiative of individuals or groups and gradually gained the support of either statutory bodies such as the central government, local authorities, etc., or voluntary agencies such as churches and foundations. They are what has often been referred to as 'community welfare centres'. Because of their admirable physical and structural set-up and individualized interests, they were 'copied' in many of the underdeveloped colonial territories. For instance, most of the community centres found in Tanzania and many other developing countries today were conceived along this line, with distinguished physical structures and characterized mainly by sectional leisure functions such as indoor games and jazz.

A second, and belated conception of community centres stems from more recent and more radical thinking in several countries and groups in the Third World. This conception, which is in fact a revolt against the traditional view, attaches more significance to the institutionalized educative-productive aspect of a community centre than to its physical structure. That is to say, greater emphasis is placed on stimulating a group of individuals within a given locale to engage in a problem-solving activity in order to improve their condition or welfare. Such problem-solving action would presumably be based on a common group awareness of environmental hazards which the members of the community could tackle—regardless of whether there are 'buildings' for the purpose or not.

While the debate has been revolving mainly around these two views—not only in Tanzania but also in several other countries in Africa—it may be important to strike a balance between them and emphasize the relevance of a merger of their characteristics. While it is essential that discussion of environmental problems, programming of social or community action, and planning of community development projects be stimulated and supported, a building or a set of buildings becomes equally essential, *not* for ornamental purposes but for the specific purposes of institutionalizing such community activities and of providing safe custody to the materials and tools that are to facilitate such processes. In such a situation, community centres become functional community industries rather than simply leisure or ornamental facilities.

Against this integrated conception of their role in social development, community centres should be defined as institutionalized 'congregational' centres set up for socially approved activities (cultural, developmental, educational, etc.), communally performed by residents of a particular locality in response to their felt need for their own self-improvement and progress. The functions and continuity of such centres should therefore determine both their physical location and their symbolic 'rituals', which should correspond to the kind of activities consonant with the community's aspirations. They should further be characterized by a comprehensive programme or programmes relating to the community's ameliorative and self-improvement needs; by participation of all or the majority of the members in a communally perceived undertaking; and by a democratic decision-making process which draws on the input by each one of the participants. As such the processes within community centres must be *educative* as well as *creative* towards community progress. A community development centre must therefore be a community education centre.

1. Historical development of community centres in Tanzania

Community centres in Tanzania date back to the beginning of the idea of 'community development' in the middle years of the British colonial period.

Soon after the Second World War, the necessity arose to re-absorb into their territorial community those African servicemen who had been on military assignment in India, Burma, Egypt and other battlefields abroad alongside the British, and who had therefore been accustomed to social amenities which were not readily available back at home. Thus, social centres were set up by the British administration in urban locations throughout the territory, principally to provide some of the amenities these ex-servicemen had become used to during their war careers. This programme was conceived of by government as part of the general rehabilitation process after the tense war years.[2] The centres, consisting of one or two buildings with a hall, were used almost exclusively for leisure activities, especially indoor games and western jazz. Then the idea was extended to meet the need for stimulating local initiative and providing mass education as part of the community development process. This was expressed in 1947 by the 'Advisory Committee on Education in the Colonies', which recommended that:

'Means must be found and found quickly whereby the people as a community can understand and appreciate the forces which have changed and are changing their lives so radically. Mass education should, as it spreads and develops, be able to give this knowledge and at the same time call out the ability and the will to share in the direction and control of the social, economic, and political forces.'[3]

In spite of this new thinking in colonial official circles, however, little headway was made. For the next four years of the projected ten-year development plan (1947–56), only one mass education officer was appointed; and a total of only 220 social welfare staff were charged with the enormous responsibility of community development in general. Clearly, this figure was too small to make an impact on the large territory comprising thousands of mostly rural communities. Moreover, nearly all of the staff were stationed in towns, leaving the rural areas uncatered for. The situation was further worsened by the lack of adequate educational and professional preparation for the staff. Most of them were women who had completed primary education or dropped out of school and had had no chance of continuing with post-primary education or training.[4] As for community centres, they did not increase in number, and continued to pursue the old 'rehabilitational' and leisure activities for the few to whom they were accessible.

It was in 1961, at the peak of political consciousness attendant on national independence, that a more rigorous, more long-sighted and more action-oriented programme was conceived. This is reflected in the parliamentary speech of the then Minister for Local Government in which he emphasized as principal objectives in community development: attacking illiteracy; women's education in home economics, child care and general hygiene; stimulating the formation of village development committees and higher agricultural production; and 'combined' multi-disciplinary operations for quicker rural development.

Accordingly, social welfare staff workers were given a more definitive position as 'community development workers who should be engaged in bringing to small communities an understanding of the part they can play in the building of a new nation and in reaching a higher living standard for themselves'.[5] Their role was defined operationally as:

'. . . firstly, explaining to the people what needs to be done to improve their agriculture, health or education; secondly, suggesting ways in which the people can tackle these problems themselves, with sponsoring the setting up of the necessary local organizations.'[6]

Further, all local authorities were called upon to set up community welfare centres to facilitate the dissemination of the new ideas to the surrounding rural communities. However, although this resulted in a fairer distribution of community centres from the few principal urban locations (such as Dar es Salaam, Tanga, and Arusha) to a larger number of locations in the periphery, they were, up to the middle and even late sixties, limited to towns and never reached the rural populations. The same applies to material incentives and facilities such as Unicef assistance, vehicles, film shows, and handicraft and cooking materials which were intended to strengthen the work of the centres in disseminating developmental innovations.

There were further problems and weaknesses in connection with community centres and with the whole approach to community development in a newly independent nation. Firstly, neither the instructors nor the participants at the centres knew precisely what the objectives or goals of the activities were. Nor, indeed, was there a precise or well-defined programme of activities (partly, at least, because of the professional inadequacy of the staff, as will be observed later). The staff seemed to conceive of their role as just another cosy job, and the general population had little information as to what the centres existed for.

Secondly, the monotonous activities (almost invariably cooking, knitting and child care) could not for long sustain a spirit of seriousness and creativity in terms of new and challenging learning or practical development projects. This in turn meant a drop in the rate of attendance and a further reduction of the number and variety of 'programmes' that could be offered. Moreover, the reputation of the centres was undermined because they came to be associated with 'disguised unemployment' and/or idleness. The general public tended to regard them as centres for townswomen's gossip, and even suspected them of being hide-outs for women of easy virtue. In fact, the few women who had secure employment in government or elsewhere shunned the centres altogether.

Thirdly, the 'community development' activities at the centres provided no opportunities for men to contribute towards the development of their respective localities. To most of them these centres appeared to be inferior institutions fit only 'for semi-responsible or otherwise undignified' females. Consequently they stayed away and kept their wives away from them.

Lastly, the whole community development process, as it was then, was designed for the small urban sector of the population and in response to problems of urban life.[7] The predominant rural population (about 98 to 99 per cent of the total national population in the early sixties) were out of the picture and almost out of consideration. It was only after 1967 that a more rural orientation of national objectives and programmes was systematized. The change in the name and structure of government ministries and in the official designation from 'Social Welfare' staff to 'Rural Development' staff and, after the 1970s, 'Ujamaa' and 'Co-operative' staff workers reflects a heightening concern for rural community development.

2. The current situation

While it has to be acknowledged that since the mid-1960s, and more particularly the 1970s, the Tanzanian Government has emphasized the need to develop the rural sector economically and educationally, practical and concrete achievements have yet to be evidenced. This is not surprising since most of the investments in human and material development have tended to be long-term or medium-term rather than short-term. As such, they cannot be expected to show immediate returns upon which a sound judgment could be made. Nonetheless, an analysis of the current situation may be attempted, particularly with regard to community centres which, as an institution, have been in existence in the country for almost three decades. In the following these institutions will, therefore, be examined from both a quantitative and a qualitative point of view.

Presently, there are about 958 community centres in Tanzania[8] with an average distribution of one to two centres per district, both or at least one of them located in the urban sector. Besides this uneven distribution across the country, the total number is very small and inadequate when considered against the country's total population of 15 million, scattered over an area of 362 819 square miles and divided into 20 administrative regions with a total of 88 administrative districts, not to mention the hundreds of smaller divisional, and thousands of village communities, each of which would ideally require at least one centre. Thus, from a purely statistical point of view, the community centres presently operating in the country are too few to have an adequate impact upon the mass of the population.

Table 3.3

Arusha, Bagamoyo and Masai Districts: Distribution of Community Centres and Community Development Staff as in 1974

District (With area and population)	Divisions	Community Centres	Staff Attached to Community Centres	Other Community Development Staff
Arusha (1 150 sq. miles) (Pop. 175 671)	Enaboishu	1	8	9
	Moshono (Adjacent to Enaboishu)	0	0	6
	Poli	1	2	0
	Mkulat	0	0	0
	King'ori	1	1	0
	Mbuguni	0	0	0
		(3)	(11)	(15)
Bagamoyo (3 800 sq. miles) (Pop. 116 300)	Mwambao	1	4	7
	Yombo	3	4	0
	Msata-Kiwangwa	0	0	1
	Msoga	1	3	0
	Miono	1	2	0
	Kwaruhombo	0	0	2
		(6)	(13)	(10)
Masai (24 350 sq. miles) (Pop. 104 313)	Kissongo	1	3	0
	Loliondo	0	0	1
	Ngorongoro	0	0	2
	Manyara	2	3	0
	Longide	0	0	1
	Naberera	0	0	2
	Kibaya	0	0	4
		(3)	(6)	(10)

Source: A recent study by the author.

The first division on the list of divisions for each district houses the district's administrative headquarters. It is therefore in large part an urban location or is in the process of urbanization. In Arusha District, Enaboishu and Moshono form one predominantly urban area and for practical purposes Moshono is well-served in terms of community facilities, by Enaboishu.

Table 3.3 presents three sample districts, one of which (Arusha)[9] represents the relatively developed or advanced districts in the country, while the other two (Bagamoyo and Masai) represent the relatively backward areas. As can be seen from the table, in none of the districts is the number of community centres adequate for the total population or the total area. Nor is it equitably distributed across the smaller divisions within the district. The table further shows that while urban divisions are relatively over-represented in terms of number of centres and community development workers attached, the rural areas are clearly under-represented.

In terms of quality and effectiveness, community centres as one of the developmental bases in Tanzania have been below the standard expected of them. As has already been pointed out in connection with their distribution, they have almost always catered for the needs and tastes of urban residents or else for people within the circumference of semi-urban 'central' locations. The majority of people in the rural periphery have hardly known of their existence, or have shunned them. Even in the urban regions, community centres have tended to represent the needs and tastes of only a small selection of the population—the working and earning 'middle class'. (Hence the regular western-type balls, indoor games, especially darts, and 'closed-door bar' drinking—the few main activities for which urban community centres have often been known.)[10]

A recent study by the author[11] shows clearly that town-based and 'central' community centres are richer in facilities, such as physical structures and furniture, recreational equipment and reading materials, than peripheral centres in rural locations. It further indicates that only one quarter of the community centres in the sample districts covered by the research seem to sponsor diversified activities or programmes—political, economic, educational. The other 75 per cent engage in only one or two activities with any degree of consistency. In all centres, jazz and ballroom dancing seems to be the dominant activity. In fact it boosts attendance at the centres in the 75 per cent category, which is otherwise rare, irregular and unpredictable. Recently the community centres have begun to feel the responsibility for adult literacy training and

Table 3.4

Community Development Staff in Arusha, Bagamoyo and Masai: Formal Education Background.

District	Total staff in district	Level of formal education				
		Primary Standard	Secondary (Form II)	Secondary (Form IV)	Secondary (Form VI)	University
Arusha	26* (100%)	11 (42.3%)	9 (34.6%)	5 (19.2%)	1 (3.8%)	0
Bagam-oyo	23* (100%)	10 (43.9%)	10 43.9%	3 (13.0%)	0	0
Masai	16* (100%)	7 (43.8%)	6 (37.5%)	3 (18.7%)	0	0

Source: The data are derived from researches by the author (1947).

*Detailed percentages for each of the sample districts may not add up to 100 because of rounding off.

DISTRICT	TOTAL STAFF IN THE DISTRICT	HAD NO PREPARATORY (PRE-SERVICE) TRAINING	HAD PREPARATORY (PRE-SERVICE) TRAINING PRIOR TO RECRUITMENT FOR				HAVE HAD IN-SERVICE TRAINING COURSE OR HAVE ATTENDED PROFESSIONAL RELEVANT SEMINARS DURING PERIOD OF EMPLOYMENT FOR				HAVE HAD NEITHER PRE-SERVICE NOR IN-SERVICE TRAINING NOR REFRESHER COURSES
			Not more than 4 months	Up to 6 months	Between 6 & 12 months	More than one year	Not more than 4 weeks	Between 1 and 2 months	Between 3 and 6 months	More than 6 months	
ARUSHA	26 (100%)	5 (19.2%)	11	4	1	–	3	–	–	–	2 (7.7%)
			16 (61.5%)				3 (11.5%)				
BAGAMOYO	23 (100%)	8 (34.8%)	1	3	–	–	6	1	–	–	4 (17.4%)
			4 (17.3%)				7 (30.4%)				
MASAI	16 (100%)	6 (37.5%)	–	3	–	–	5	1	–	–	1 (6.3%)
			3 (18.1%)				6 (37.5%)				

Table 3.5

Community Development Staff in Arusha, Bagamoyo and Masai: Professional Training Levels

Source: The data are derived from researches by the author (1974)

general adult education, but even then attendance is generally poor or at best modest, just as it is in a number of 'open-air' adult education centres. However, home economics and general political discussion are becoming popular with a small section of women, most of whom tend to be middle-aged wives of higher-status public officials.

Leadership at the community centres and generally in the districts covered by this study leaves much to be desired. As Tables 3.4 and 3.5 indicate, the formal educational attainment of most of the development workers, whether assigned to community centres or working elsewhere in the districts, was low, and their professional preparation in terms of training was also inadequate. If it is reasonable to believe that a person's level of education (knowledge) and the extent of his/her professional preparation (skill) have a direct bearing on their occupational performance, then it can be argued that the performance of community development workers in Tanzania, and through them of the community centres, has not been a distinguished one. There is a clear need for both well-educated and well-trained community development/community education workers to stimulate the development potential within the many communities in the country.

3. Prospects

Despite the somewhat disappointing picture that is presented by the research data above, the hope for improvement in this vital area of Tanzania's development struggle is far from unrealistic. For the problem of rural under-development has spurred the government and TANU to take immediate action to introduce ameliorative and innovative programmes that would combine knowledge acquisition (through mass education) with skill acquisition and productivity (through practical problem-solving challenges). Two particular programmes should be mentioned:

With the financial and technical assistance of the World Bank, the Ministry of National Education is establishing *community education centres* with the express purpose of effecting 'integrated rural development centred on the school' and of meeting the educational needs of the whole population including pupils, youths, adults and other non-school-goers.[12] The plan is to transform the primary schools into all-embracing educational institutions that will provide basic functional knowledge and skills for every member of the community—young and old alike.

It is therefore envisaged that all existing primary schools will be extended to include facilities for the other sectors of the community around them. New buildings are being constructed with integrated facilities: formal classrooms, library, handicraft workshops, school offices, a community hall, convertible rooms. Five such community education centres are being built in Dodoma region (with a concentration around the site of the new capital). It is hoped that in due course more such centres will be set up in all regions and that an equitable distribution will have been achieved when all primary schools have been transformed into community education centres. The whole idea is to combine theoretical learning with skill training and production, which, in turn, would draw on the different talents available in the community, namely *bona fide* school teachers, community 'teachers' (i.e. villagers with specialized practical skills that are economically and/or culturally beneficial to the community) and every other able-bodied member of the larger community. Faster progress towards this goal may be expected now that the Universal Primary Education (UPE) programme demands such centres for its eventual effectiveness. Not only these community education centres and primary schools but also the existing formal community centres will certainly be called upon to take up the challenge of educating the community for its self-improvement and progress.

The second innovation is the establishment of *folk development colleges*. They are to serve three main purposes, namely to 'stimulate and motivate learning of adults, men and women'; to 'facilitate and ease the follow-up activities related to literacy campaigns and the need for improving the standard of general education—including Standard VII (primary school) leavers'; and to provide 'knowledge and various skills . . . useful in the development of rural life.'[13] These centres are being set up with financial and technical aid from the Swedish Government. They will run both short-term and long-term courses pertaining to one of three areas—general education (including political, economic and social sciences, mathematics, the pure sciences, agriculture, nutrition and hygiene); skill training (in various crafts, agriculture, domestic science, carpentry, masonry, etc.); and cultural training (in music, folk song, traditional dancing and drama).

The programme officially began in December 1975 when, for the first phase, 25 colleges were constructed. In the financial year 1976–77 their number will rise to at least two in each region, except in Dar es Salaam where there will be only one. Some of the 36 centres are already offering courses and training to a considerable number of adults and youths. The target is to establish a total of 85 folk development colleges for the whole country. There is also a scheme of stocking these centres with extensive libraries and follow-up materials so as to make them institutions not only for theoretical knowledge production but also for practical skill application.

These two practical projects are convincing evidence of Tanzania's renewed concern and effort in the direction of community development at all levels.

Notes

1 The general tendency in the industrialized societies of the West has been 'urbanizing the countryside' rather than the opposite process of 'ruralizing'. See, for instance, Hendriks, G 'Community Development in Western Europe' *Community Development Journal*, 7 (April 1972) No. 2 pp. 76–77

2 Although it is worth noting that the programme was also a way by which the colonial government hoped to control and pacify ex-soldiers who had been in contact with all sorts of people and revolutionaries and who might have developed 'subversive' tendencies—as did their counterparts in India, for instance.

3 *A Ten-Year Plan for the Development of African Education*. Dar es Salaam: Government Printer, (1947) p. 17

4 Apart from the problem of a poor educational level and lack of thorough professional training, quite a number of young unmarried women on the staff found themselves in the contradictory position of instructing mothers on child care, hygiene and housekeeping, while they themselves had difficulties in caring for their own illegitimate children.

5 Quoted in Ministry of Information and Tourism (Tanzania Government), *Tanzania Today*, Nairobi: University Press of Africa, (1968) p. 95

6 See Note 5.

7 From the mid-fifties and well into the sixties, the drift into towns was increasing as urban job seeking, among other factors, was heightening. For instance, Dar es Salaam's urban population has been rising rapidly from 51 000 in 1948 to 92 330 in 1957, to 150000 in 1962, to 272 821 in 1967; see Ishumi, A G M *East African Cities: Some Persistent Problems of Modernization*, Dar es Salaam: University of Dar es Salaam, (1975) (mimeo). The resulting problems included unemployment or underemployment, more particularly among women, and lack of sufficient facilities to promote activities that could keep the growing urban population busy and psychologically relaxed. See also Leslie, J A K *A Survey of Dar es Salaam*, Nairobi: Oxford University Press, (1963) pp. 121–130, 203–208, Little, K *African Women in Towns*. London: Cambridge University Press, (1973) pp. 6–48.

8 The figure is taken from official sources in the Department of Rural Development. In actual fact, the total is smaller, since a number of new districts which were created following the government decentralization scheme adopted in 1972, took over urban community centre buildings for their headquarter offices. Also, some of the community centres on the official list are in fact no longer operating or even existing.

9 Since 1975, Arusha district has been further divided into two districts—the rural Aru-Meru district and Arusha urban district. For the purpose of analyzing the data, which were collected before the division, Arusha is here treated as one district as distinct from Masai district which, together with the former, makes up the larger Arusha Region.

10 The inadequacy of these community 'welfare' centres in terms of number and quality partly explains the relative rise of specialist 'middle class' social centres and clubs in towns, with similar but higher-quality facilities.

11. Ishumi, A G M *Community Education and Development*. Dar es Salaam: University of Dar es Salaam, (1974). (Ph.D. dissertation.)

12 See Directorate of Planning and Development, Community Education Centres: Ministry of National Education, *Proposals for Improvement of Internal Efficiency in the Primary Education System*. Dar es Salaam: (1973).

13 See Sectoral Planning Unit: Ministry of National Education, *Establishment and Equipment of Folk Development Colleges in Tanzania—A Project Proposal for External Financing*. Dar es Salaam: (1975).

Chapter 4 Experience in Schooling and Teacher Training

4.1 History of Formal Schooling in Tanzania
M L Mbilinyi

1. Indigenous education

Pre-colonial African societies had their own education systems related to the various kinds of existing production system. Division of labour by sex corresponded to separate formal and informal education for the boys and girls, informal education beginning at a very early age. Young girls were instructed by their mothers, elder sisters and grandmothers on proper techniques of crop cultivation, on the processing and preparation of food, on child care, and some learned special skills and knowledge of medicine and ritual, basket weaving and pottery making. Young boys were taught animal husbandry, house construction, tool manufacture and some also learned special skills and knowledge of medicine, of government, of blacksmithing and other crafts. Certain aspects of these areas of knowledge and technology were taught informally while the child was actively engaged in doing what he/she was to learn about. The girl learned crop cultivation by helping her mother in the fields. The boy learned animal husbandry by tending calves at an early age.

Most societies also had formal education institutions, the most common being the 'schools' set up separately for boys and girls at the time of puberty to initiate them into the adult ranks of their society. Certain elders were assigned to teach the boys or the girls about tribal history, religion and all the skills and knowledge which an adult man or woman was expected to possess to function intelligently in his/her life. The period of instruction lasted for as long as three years in some places, and was never less than several weeks. The young people and their teachers resided together in separate 'camps' or temporary isolated villages. The whole time could therefore be concentrated on intense instruction, though much of it involved physical endeavour at sports and the practical elements of the knowledge being learned. Circumcision was the final stage in most of these schools, after which the boy or girl returned home with a new status, a young adult.

2. Mission education and Islamic schools during German colonial rule

The ideological institutions which the German colonial administrators first depended upon were, however, not indigenous ones, but rather the mission and Islamic educational and religious institutions.[1] Missionaries had penetrated the interior of the Tanganyikan territory prior to formal colonial rule, setting up churches, schools, workshops and trading centres. The missionaries as well as their metropolitan sponsors (finance capital) did not separate their religious role of converting the native to Christianity from their economic role of establishing commercial agricultural production and externally oriented trade. All this was perceived to be a part of their 'civilizing' mission in Africa. For example, the University Missions to Central Africa were set up to be: 'centres of Christianity and civilization for the promotion of true religion, agriculture and commerce'.[2]

Once the colonial state was established, the role of the missions in reproducing the colonial economy and the colonial superstructure was strengthened. The following resolution of a German mission congress in 1886 is illustrative: 'German missions, Evangelical and Catholic alike, should be encouraged to take an active part in the realization of a national colonial programme; in other words they should not restrict their activities to mission work but should help to establish German culture and German thought in the colonies'[3]

The German colonial administration also made use of Islamic educational and political institutions in order to create the *akida* and *liwali* system of Direct Rule. Initially, literate products of Islam Quran schools of relatively high social standing became *akidas* and *liwalis*, and others became members of the colonial army and police. Later, government schools were relied upon to produce African administration officials, but the Islamic political institutions symbolized by the *akidas* and *liwalis* remained. The Swahili language was relied upon for official correspondence as well as for dealing with local matters, and it rapidly spread inland.

Most schools were under the control of the missions, although in 1913 the government began to subsidize missions and also increasingly relied on mission schools for the training of government personnel. Mission schools were mainly bush schools with classes of one to two years' duration, in which was taught literacy, numeracy, and catechism in the vernacular. These schools were staffed mainly by African catechists and received very little if any direct 'missionary' supervision. They were built by local people, on land the people provided, and the catechist teacher depended for a living on his own household's agricultural production plus contributions from the local people.

In addition, missions had central, usually boarding schools, of up to four standards, and later six, or more. Only a very small proportion of the youths entered central mission schools, which produced catechists, artisans, teachers and modern farmers. Most of the curriculum was vocational—masonry, carpentry, tailoring, road construction, agriculture—depending on the economic needs of the specific mission. Students worked for the mission throughout their schooling period, making roads, houses, clothes; farming etc. As one Trappist Missionary noted in 1901: 'The black people must be taught through work and prayers.'[4] Manual work in school was perceived as instrumental in fostering adaptation to work relations of exploitation and domination in later life. This is illustrated by a government statement which referred to government education but could also relate to the mission system: 'These works of the school are of great value in accustoming the natives to regular physical labour from youth onwards.'[5]

The few government schools which were built were related to specific manpower needs, for skilled labourers, teachers, clerks, etc. Courses were mounted for specific vocational needs. In line with this policy, government training was restricted to boys, corresponding to the sexist relationships which were further developed in the colonial economy. Like the educational systems of the missions, the government schools had a pyramidal structure but with a very narrow base compared to the missionary bush school foundation. The government central schools like some mission central schools were mainly for sons of chiefs and/or wealthy Africans, which contributed to the stratification processs among the African labour force. And as in the case of missions, students were responsible for building government schools and in other ways providing *necessary* manual labour.

The objective function of the schools therefore included training in specific skills, reproduction of colonial relations of production (a small number of Africans delegated to semi-skilled and skilled manual work, clerical positions and low level teaching and pastoral work, and the majority peasant producers), and the internalization of colonial ideology. Caning was as important as the teaching of German history in producing submissiveness and acceptance of the colonial system.

'. . . colonial schools are the cradle of German culture in Africa. . . . The true process of civilization has to be internalized if it is to be effective. The purpose of the schools cannot be merely to teach a trade to a few people. Rather it must be to bring up a new generation that will have accepted the new civilization internally as well as externally.'[6]

The new civilization of course was underdeveloped capitalism, and the schools were to foster internalization of bourgeois work ethics and racist ideology. This ideological function of schools continued under the English colonial administration.

'Our objective is . . . an educational system which will provide for African needs and at the same time produce a virile and loyal citizen of the Empire . . . where character, health, industry and a proper appreciation of the dignity of manual labour rank as of first importance . . . the school . . . is the centre of all government propaganda work.'[7]

3. British colonial schooling
(i) Separate racial school systems
Three distinctly different school systems developed—African, Asian and European. They were separated from each other on a racist basis and divided internally into education for the 'leaders' and education for the 'masses'. The European and Asian communities had a much more highly developed education pyramid than the Africans. The European one was rooted in the metropolitan system and the children received their higher levels of schooling in Europe. Primary and secondary education developed at a faster pace for Asians than for Africans, with more primary school leavers entering secondary school. The Asian school systems developed primarily through the financial support of the Asian communities themselves and concentrated on bookish literary education. African education was limited to Standard VI until 1937, with limited expansion beyond Standard VIII thereafter. African schools were vocational. They used vernacular (or Swahili) as the medium of instruction at the elementary level and Swahili for most Central School advanced courses (Standards IV–VI) until 1945.

The form and content of these different education systems corresponded to the different positions the racial groups had in the colonial economy. The African was the producer (peasant and productive worker) but had no control over the system. A bare minimum of skills and knowledge were sufficient to reproduce a productive producer—given the perpetuation of the precapitalist form of production under colonialism and the low level of technology, the productive forces required only *basic* education.

The socialization which took place through school rituals, and authority relationships—flag-raising, caning, standing at attention when the teacher entered the classroom—was given as much attention by colonial educators as the subject matter, and was called 'character training'. The African education system functioned to produce submissiveness, a sense of inferiority, an orientation towards extrinsic rewards and punishments, and an ideological acceptance of capitalist work demands. Even for the majority who never had formal schooling, the education system functioned to reproduce ideological acceptance of the superiority of those who *were* educated and their 'right' to a superior position in the colonial economy.

There were explicit political reasons for maintaining a racially segregated school system. When asked by the Governor (Cameron) to state his opinion on integration of the Asian and African schools, the Director of Education, Rivers-Smith opposed integration for the following reasons:

'. . . there is the political aspect which in all schemes of education should be kept constantly in view. With the knowledge of political developments during the last few years in India, we cannot afford to ignore the possibility of an unfortunate African political repercussion in future years as a result of the development of a closer liaison between the two races which might be a result of co-education.

At present we have a healthy rivalry and a growing race-consciousness amongst the Africans and a certain feeling of resentment that the Asiatics get so many of the 'plums'. In my opinion co-education might conceivably weaken this healthy and natural rivalry and eventually lead to making common cause for political ends.

For facility of educational administration and from the financial point of view, co-education offers many advantages. There is, however, this political aspect, whether in years to come it may deprive the Administration of a very valuable asset.'[8]

The political technique of 'Indirect Rule' used by the British to administer the territory also influenced schooling. At the local level, 'Native Authorities' were relied upon. These positions were filled by either traditional chiefs or headmen or else by individuals selected by the colonial administration. Tribalism was deliberately promoted in order to facilitate domination and hamper the growth of militant 'detribalized' Africans who might start a nationalist movement. Governor Sir Donald Cameron gave the following explanation for the policy:

'If we aim at indirect administration through the appropriate Native Authority—Chief or Council—founded on the people's own traditions and preserving their own tribal organization, their own laws and customs purged of anything that is repugnant to justice and morality, we shall be building an edifice with some foundation to it, capable of standing the shock which will inevitably come when the educated native seeks to gain possession of the machinery of government and to run it on Western lines.'[9]

Both the policies of racial segregation and polarization and of Indirect Rule reveal how class contradictions and class struggle were developed in the colonial society through the creation of contradictions between the colonial administrators representing the metropolitan capital and the African progressive petty bourgeois elements ('educated native') as well as of intra-class contradictions between the Native Authorities and the educated petty bourgeoisie, and between the Asian and the African petty bourgeoisie. Clearly the school was an instrument of class struggle.

In line with the policy of Indirect Rule, the medium of instruction at the elementary levels was the vernacular, and the special schools for sons of chiefs were continued. The 'experiments' made by Mumford, the first English Government Education Officer in Bukoba, in developing indigenous programmes within the government school system at Bukoba and later Malangali were oriented towards the preservation of certain tribal customs. Separate dormitories for pupils from different tribes, their separate instruction in 'tribal lore' by elders brought from their respective 'homelands'—all these and other aspects of Mumford's work served the function of tribalism, Indirect Rule and divide and rule.[10]

Government promotion of Native Authority school systems was in line with the same policy. Between 1919 and 1923, Native Authorities were financially responsible for more elementary schools than was the Department of Education.[11] In Shinyanga in the 1930s, 'Kaya' boarding schools were set up under Chief Wamba, who provided land, cattle, food and payments for teachers.[12] In 1941 a government inspector of schools in Mwanza pointed out that the aim of the Kaya schools was: 'rural education for boys and girls on *strictly tribal lines* . . . the principal object of the school is to give an education which will not take the youth of Usukuma away from the land'.[13] Mason, one of the more influential administrators, noted that these schools 'should be considered as purely agricultural schools, designed to meet the requirements of children of rich cattle owners, progressive peasants, headmen and the like'.[14]

The Kaya schools were thus serving the immediate interests of the rich peasant stratum and the traditional rulers of the area, and at the same time coincided with the interests of the colonial administration in maintaining pre-capitalist *forms* of production, even as capital penetrated them and oriented production towards the metropolitan capitalist system.

(ii) Changing directions for similar ends

Later emphasis on 'community education' or 'mass education' also served the function of maintaining the pre-capitalist forms of production. Constant struggle is recorded between different emerging classes among the African population and the colonialists over content, which remained at the level of basic skills in handicrafts and agriculture, and over control of the education system itself.

One example of such conflict is that between Mumford and the Bukoba Native Authorities. When Mumford arrived in Bukoba in 1923, he found a well-organized system of district schools known as the Sultan's schools. The children were housed and fed by the chiefs and supervized by local teachers. In 1924, Mumford 'relieved' the chiefs of all responsibility for school buildings and maintenance of the students,[15] and established a vocational curriculum including agriculture, industrial skills and handicrafts. As a result, the chiefs as well as many parents rejected the school programme and children were not enrolled in school as before. A Bukoba government official noted: 'in respect of his revival of basket and mat weaving, chiefs and parents were later preported as expressing the view that they did not sent their children to a "European school" for such instruction'.[16]

Colonial emphasis on elementary basic education for Africans is reflected in the structure of the education system. By 1924–25, there were 72 government primary schools in rural areas, two central schools in Tanga and Dar es Salaam, and schools for sons of chiefs in Tabora and Bukoba (up to Standard VI) and Mwanza (Standards I–IV). The central schools primarily consisted of 'industrial' courses (carpentry, tailoring, ploughing, masonry, boot-making and road construction) together with reading, writing and arithmetic.

There can be no doubt that the policies of the colonialists in charge of education both in London and in Dar es Salaam served the objective interests of finance capital, which was to maintain and at the same time *penetrate* the pre-capitalist production system. The difference in the treatment of chiefs and 'commoners' represents more than simply a political policy of Indirect Rule. In order to maintain and exploit peasant production, a class of comprador petty bourgeoisie was necessary, whose existence depended upon an underdeveloped economy and superstructure. As already noted, deliberate efforts were made to 'win over' the 'Native Authorities' to the side of the colonialists and to set them against the 'educated petty bourgeoisie', the future nationalistic elements. The promotion of a 'comprador' class of petty bourgeoisie is reflected in the sons of chiefs' schools as well as in streaming practices within schools. For example, at Bukoba Central School, two distinctly different curricula were developed for the students by 1923:

'Two broad divisions have been made in the school, forming a 'General side' and a 'Special side'. The first consists chiefly of sons of Sultans, Chiefs and wealthy landowners who receive a general all-round training consisting of academic subjects such as *English*, Mathematics, Geography, Hygiene and practical subjects such as Agriculture, Animal Husbandry, Elementary Carpentry and Tailoring, and Native Handicrafts (such as Drum-making, etc.) The second will consist of apprenticeship to various trades, carpentry, tailoring, etc.'[17]

The form and content of education at Tabora School, established in 1925 as a special central school, is also illustrative. Again recruiting first from 'sons of chiefs' or wealthy 'tribesmen', the school was organized on tribal lines. Students were housed in dormitories according to tribe, and were taught tribal customs. At the same time, students learned 'book-keeping, typing and office routine in *preparation for taking up jobs in government offices*'.[18] House competitions and the prefect system, the authoritarian nature of teacher-student, Headmaster-teacher-student relationships and teaching methodology promoted a hierarchical, competitive set of role relationships. The products of such a school would be able to adapt to a hierarchical, bureaucratic organization of work, and at the same time 'feel' they were a 'special' group of people, an African 'elite'.

After the Depression a period of retrenchment developed. The colonial administration was criticized by the Retrenchment Commission in 1931 for 'too rapid expansion of social services to the African population', namely education.[19] This is a remarkable judgment given the minuscule number of Africans who received even two years of primary schooling.

Expenditure on African education was reduced drastically and for a much longer period than other social services, and remained low long after the economy had picked up again in the later 1930s. Isherwood, the new Director of Education, spearheaded the drive to expand vernacular elementary education (Standards I–IV) and diminish what little of post-elementary levels of education still remained. The number of English courses was reduced and several former central schools were downgraded to become vernacular elementary schools, or else became specialized agricultural schools. For example, the Bukoba Central School was dropped and Nyakato Central School later became an agricultural school. The Native Authorities of Bukoba, as well as the local branch of the African Association, attacked this change in policy as a move to further the oppression of the African. Dissatisfaction with the course at Nyakato grew among parents and students, and culminated in student efforts to block the return of the first Head, A E Haarer. A report by the Acting Provincial Commissioner stated:

'Pupils had complained that instead of receiving scheduled lectures they had been given manual work of a non-instructional nature.'[20]

The elementary school syllabus for the territory was eventually extended to cover six years, with a strong handicraft bias. At some schools it was to be followed by a three-year rural industrial course. This constituted a definite policy switch from specialized industrial courses leading to wage employment, to village handicrafts thought more suitable for African producers in rural areas.

(iii) 'Education for adaptation'

Rural vocational education for Africans was called 'education for adaptation'. Although adaptation of students to their place as peasant producers had already characterized government and mission education in the German period, it received added impetus from the Phelps-Stokes Commission, led by a white 'leader' of Negro education in the United States, Dr Thomas Jesse Jones, which published two reports on Africa in 1922 and 1925. The principles of the Commission's approach were based on the form and content of 'Negro education' most often identified with Booker T Washington. In the United States agricultural education was justified by the argument that it was the most relevant type of education for African Americans since the vast majority of them were agricultural producers. The curricular content consisted of health, home life training, industry (meaning mainly agricultural) and recreation. As noted by King: 'Industrial education had originally been introduced as a guarantee that the Negro would continue to provide a low-level labour supply for the white South . . .'.[21]

Colonial administrators and missionaries were sent to the United States on 'study tours' to observe Negro education institutions, and praised the *relevance* and *practicality* of what they saw, its relevance being, of course, to the objective of producing docile and productive workers or peasants. Ideas about African intelligence were always related to the African's place in production. One Agriculture Officer in Shinyanga, for example, criticized schooling because it was too academic and 'divorced the pupils from *normal native agricultural pursuits*'.[22] In 1925 the Director of Agriculture stated that only 5 per cent of all African students were 'sufficiently intelligent to profit from academic instruction.'[23] The Superintendent of Education for Bukoba stated in the 1931–32 *Annual Report* that:'No Native I have met can teach English or Geography. The limits of their mental experiences prohibit them.'[24] And in 1931, the Director of Agriculture stated that 'the African is a peasant farmer at heart and should be trained rather then educated'.[25]

At the same time as the retrenchment policy which signified low level 'basic' education for the vast majority of schooled children was implemented, the colonial administration was faced with increasing demands for better qualified Africans to work in government departments and in private business. The central school curriculum was therefore 'improved' so that some Africans could enter Makerere secondary level courses. In 1934 Tabora Central School and St Mary's School at Tabora were upgraded to junior secondary schools. In 1936, six out of eight candidates passed the Makerere entrance examination. Secondary courses also began at Kibosho, Tosamaganga and Minaki, soon to be followed by other schools. The curriculum of secondary schools was literary and used English as the medium. Vernacular and vocational 'basic' education was restricted to lower levels of education. The Cambridge Syndicate was relied upon by Tanganyika, as well as Uganda and Kenya, for setting and marking of examinations at Form IV and finally Form VI level, which reinforced bourgeois control over secondary school form and content.

By 1945, there were 1 000 primary schools, 18 secondary schools and 24 teacher training centres in Tanganyika. The total secondary school enrolment was 1 000, teacher training 1 100, and there were 27 students at Makerere following a pre-senior secondary course.[26] In the same year the Ten-Year Plan 1946–1955, the first planning operation for the territory, was introduced. With respect to education, the focus of the plan was on primary education, with a stated aim of getting 36 per cent of the primary school age group enrolled in Standards I–IV. District day boarding middle schools were planned to include Standards V and VI, one-fifth of the Standard IV output being expected to enter Standard V. In 1946, the number of students in 'real' secondary school (Standards IX–XII) was 917, all of them boys. There was a very high degree of wastage throughout the educational pyramid; two-thirds of the Standard I intake in 1949 had dropped out by Standard IV.[27]

(iv) The last phase of colonial education
The principle of 'education for adaptation' continued, in the form of an agriculture syllabus for *rural primary and middle schools* introduced in 1952. However, since the policy met with strong resistance from parents and students alike, it was never implemented in several schools and was withdrawn by 1959. As noted by Nkonoki[28] some reasons for the failure of the agriculture syllabus were: it only applied to Africans and therefore seemed to be designed to perpetuate the colonial class structure; it was imposed with no consultation of African leaders, or else agreed to by 'Native Authorities' who increasingly lacked political legitimacy during this period of growing political consciousness because their role as compradors was too obvious; parents expected their children to get wage-earning jobs and not to become peasants like themselves; youths could not readily apply new ideas on agriculture given the traditional land tenure system; agriculture was not an examinable subject, which belittled its material importance; agricultural work was used as a punishment in schools; agriculture instructors had lower educational qualifications and therefore less prestige and authority among both teachers and students, which affected the subject as well; the syllabus, designed in the central headquarters, was too rigid and did not allow for specific situations to be considered; agriculture instruction consisted in practice mainly of manual work in the fields with little scientific or other subject content. Moreover, urban schools did not have a similar bias, but were academically oriented. This meant urban students were inevitably better prepared for the academic examinations which all students (urban or rural) had to take. Owing partly to differences among the colonial administrators themselves, training facilities for the special needs of agriculture instruction were inadequate. By 1956, only 85 out of 232 middle schools had even one trained agriculture instructor.[29]

The Ten-Year Plan's emphasis on primary education reflected heightened class contradictions in the African Colonies at this time. It followed the lead of the Advisory Committee on Education in the Colonies which pointed out in a 1944 policy paper, *Mass Education in African Society*, that growing political conciousness among the natives was of primary concern. Character training (socialization of obedience, submissiveness, passiveness, punctuality and hard work) in the mission schools was praised. In correspondence among Tanganyikan government officials, many of whom had previously served in India, frequent reference was made to that colony. The creation in India of: 'a fully developed primary and secondary educational system' was partly blamed for

Table 4.1

Enrolment in the Educational System in 1956 (Voluntary Agencies, Government and Native Authorities Combined).

	Total	Girls
Primary School (Standard I–IV)	336 000	105 000
Middle School (Standard V–VIII)	28 000	4 900
Secondary School (Standard IX–XII)	2 409	204

Source: Morrison, D R 'Education and Political Development. The Tanzanian Case'. University of Sussex, Ph.D. diss. (1970) for total enrolment figures, and Cameron, J and Dodd, W A *Society, Schools and Progress in Tanzania* (Bibliography No. 64), for girls' enrolment.

Table 4.2

1956 Percentage Targets for Enrolment of Children Aged Seven to Eleven and Percentage Enrolment in 1953, by Provinces.

Province	Percentage target for 1956	Percentage enrolment in 1953
Tanga	50	53
Northern	50	46
Southern	40	39
Eastern	40	29
Southern Highlands	30	23
Lake	30	20
Western	30	20
Central	30	18

Source: Department of Education, Annual Report 1953, in: Morrison, D R *Education and Political Development. . .*, p. 107

problems of rural stagnancy (!) as well as for the emergence of the nationalist movement.[30] The pyramid structure of the Tanganyikan education system resulting from the Ten-Year Plan is evident from the 1956 enrolment figures given in Table 4.1, which also illustrates the perpetuation of unequal educational opportunities for girls. Table 4.2 shows the uneven regional development of schools.

In the Five-Year Development Plan, 1956–1961 which led up to the period of Independence, there was a shift in emphasis from lower primary education to middle and post-primary education for Africans. Primary expansion was restricted, so that by 1961 only 45 per cent of the primary school age population would be enrolled compared to 40 per cent in 1957. Middle school places were to be increased by 50 per cent, secondary enrolment was to be expanded and a Higher School Certificate course introduced. The Plan was, however, never implemented, ostensibly due to lack of funds. Nevertheless, by 1959 secondary enrolment was 4200 and middle school enrolment 44700. Two hundred Tanganyikan students were at Makerere or Royal College (Nairobi). By 1960 three secondary schools offered higher school certificates and there were 1000 students overseas, mainly in university programmes. Whereas the middle school curriculum still retained a somewhat vocational agricultural bias in rural areas, the secondary and higher school curriculum was bookish and academic. The majority of post-primary teachers and principals, as well as the top officials in the Department of Education, were English. Cambridge 'O' and 'A' levels ensured that the system retained its peculiar class and cultural bias.

Conclusion

The history of formal schooling in colonial Tanganyika shows that schools functioned as ideological agents for the ruling class of the colony, the metropolitan bourgeoisie. The schooled and the non-schooled alike accepted the 'superiority' of those with formal European schooling and therefore their legitimate 'right' to positions carrying relatively higher income, power and prestige. Assumptions about innate intellectual differences reinforced the supposed legitimacy of a system based on examinations as selective mechanisms. The pyramid structure of the education system, with its broad base and very restricted top, reflected on the one hand the perpetuation of peasant commodity production and on the other the emerging petty bourgeoisie, who would eventually fill the positions of the colonial administrators, teachers, managers, etc. and the small number of *workers* on plantations, mines and factories. If a nationalist and progressive petty bourgeois 'group' emerged, it was *in spite of* the colonial education system and not because of it. The persistence of a bourgeois ideology among the highly educated up to the present time is an indication of the 'success' achieved by the colonial ideological state apparatus formal schooling.

Notes

1 Hirji, K 'Colonial Ideological Apparatuses in Tanganyika Under the Germans' in *The Colonization of Tanganyika* by M Kaniki.
2 Oliver, R *The Missionary Factor in East Africa* London: Longmans (1952) p. 13, cited in Hirji (see Note 1), p. 1, n. 3
3 Hellberg, K J *Missions on a Colonial Frontier West of Lake Victoria* Uppsala: Gleerup (1956) p. 92
4 *Annual Report on Development in German East Africa* (1901/02), Supp. A.IV, p. 39–40, cited in Hirji (see Note 1), p. 18
5 *Annual Report on Development in German East Africa* 1908/09, p. 189, cited in Hirji (see Note 1), p. 20, n. 49
6 Schilunk, M 'German Education Policy: The School System in the German Colonies' in *Traditions of African Education* edited by P Scalon New York: Columbia Teachers College Press (1964) p. 32
7 Education Department, Tanganyikan Territory *Annual Report (1924)*
8 Confidential letter from Rivers-Smith to Chief Secretary (24 July 1925) cited in Morris-Hale, W *British Administration in Tanganyika from 1920 to 1954* Geneva: University of Geneva (1969) (Ph.D. dissertation)
9 Circular from the Chief Secretary to Administrative Office (18 May 1925) cited in Morris-Hale (see Note 8), p. 265
10 For detailed discussion of education for adaptation and Mumford's work in particular, see Thompson, A *The Adaptation of Education to African Society in Tanganyika under British Rule* London: University (1968) (Ph.D dissertation)
11 See Note 10, Chapter 9
12 Tanganyika National Archives (TNA), SMP 215/1552, Vol. I, p. 217

13 'Letter from Blumer to Senior Agriculture Officer' (the italics are his emphasis) in TNA, SMP 215/1655, Vol. I

14 See Note 12, p. 220

15 See Note 7, Appendix III, p. 26

16 See Note 10, p. 107

17 See Note 7, p. 28 (The italics are my emphasis.)

18 Nkonoki, S *A Study of the Philosophy of Education for Self-Reliance and Its Implementation in Tanzania Secondary Schools with Special Reference to Students Attitudes Towards the Organization of Self-Reliance Activities* Dar es Salaam: University of Dar es Salaam (1972) (Draft of dissertation)

19 See Note 10, p. 191

20 See Note 10, p. 231

21 King, K *Pan-Africanism and Education: A Study of Race Philanthropy and Education in the Southern States of America and East Africa* Oxford: Clarendon Press (1971)

22 See Note 12 (the italics are my emphasis)

23 Saul, P 'Agricultural Education in Tanganyika: the Policy, Programmes and Practices, 1925–1955' in *Agricultural Research for Rural Development* edited by S Mbilinyi Nairobi: East African Literature Bureau (1973)

24 TNA, SNS 215/787, Vol. I, p. 787

25 See Note 23

26 Cameron, J and Dodd, W W *Society, Schools and Progress in Tanzania* p. 71 Bibl. 64

27 See Note 26

28 See Note 18

29 See Note 23

30 'Letter from Mason to King, 21 April 1939' in TNA, SMP 215/1552, Vol. I, p. 233

4.2 Primary Education Since 1961
F L Mbunda

1. Early post-independence education

Primary education has been continuously expanding since formal schooling was first introduced by the missionaries and the colonial governments, and this expansion explains the existence of what we have today in Tanzania. When the missionaries came to Africa, they met an educational system that was authentic and clear in its objectives. Unfortunately, these missionaries did not realize the authenticity of the system and replaced it with one that encouraged wrong attitudes on education and life in general.

At Independence the masses, through TANU, had already realized the unfair distribution of primary education among the ethnic groups, and in fact some steps had been developed, though slowly, to improve the situation. For example, the number of primary schools had increased from 2 192 in 1954 to 3 238 in 1961, that of pupils from 275 628 to 486 470 (public schools only,) and the number of teachers from 4 693 to 9 190.[1]

After achieving Independence (9th December, 1961) the major task of the new nation was to embark on an all-level development of education. The major need being self-sufficiency in manpower, greater stress was placed on the expansion of secondary education. It was therefore imperative to correct some of the major shortcomings of the primary education built up during the colonial period, so as to set up a strong foundation for those who would join secondary education. Since then, primary education has been developing rapidly to cater for the needs and interests of the people of Tanzania.

The Education Ordinance of 1961 which became operational in 1962 called for several changes in the system. The tripartite system of education was abolished so that all primary schools were integrated. It became unlawful to prevent a child from being admitted to any school (African, Asian or European) on racial grounds. The new policy catered for all learners irrespective of their racial, religious or economic origins. This meant a step forward toward equal opportunity for all children and for African children in particular. The Ordinance also provided for firmer government control of all schools. Employment of teachers, provision of equipment, admission of pupils, syllabi and other educational matters were put under the control of the Ministry of Education even though the Local Authorities and the Voluntary Agencies were allowed to continue running their schools. The establishment of Local Education Authorities, Boards of Governors and School Committees in the 1961 Ordinance gave the people powers to decide on the conduct of primary education appropriate to the local needs.

The curriculum was changed so as to include Tanzanian history, with emphasis on national heroes who fought for emancipation from colonial rule, and a Tanzanian interpretation of the country's contact with the foreign colonial powers. The Swahili language was given a more prominent status and became the medium of instruction throughout primary school, replacing English as the medium in middle schools. Local culture was revived and began to receive more attention. The main objective at the time was to provide an education that was more meaningful and relevant to national needs.

Another change towards expansion of primary education was elimination of the division between lower and upper primary schools by introducing a full eight-year course for all primary schools. As a first step the existing lower primary courses were extended to six years duration, and as more children were then admitted into the lower primary schools, the number of places in the upper primary had to be increased also. The Five-Year Plan for African Education (1957–61) stipulated that 200 new middle schools for boys and 38 for girls were to operate by 1962, so that the proportion for boys moving from standard IV to V would be increased from 20 per cent to 30 per cent and the proportion of girls from 12 per cent to 16 per cent.

Several other steps were taken to develop and expand primary education during the period from Independence to 1967, the year of the Arusha Declaration. The Local Authorities were encouraged to build more middle schools. They were also advised to reduce costs by making the schools day institutions. One important measure was the phasing out of Standard VIII. With continuous education in one school the programme could easily be adjusted in such a way that the standards reached at the end of primary VII would not be inferior to those previously reached at primary VIII. The reorganization envisaged free primary education, and an education complete in itself. It ensured that all who entered primary I would finish primary VII, and that education was no longer a selective process at the primary stage. The old system of a break at primary IV or VI and a transfer to different schools for primary V made education elitist, not because of normal wastage, but because of the promotion or entrance examinations at these levels. The following table shows the position in 1962.

Table 4.3

Enrolment in Primary Schools in 1962

Year	Enrolment in Year I	Enrolment in Year IV	Enrolment in Year V	Enrolment Year VIII
1962	125 251	98 139	26 803	13 730

Source: Burns, D G *African Education* London: Oxford University Press (1965) p. 39

The phasing out of Standard VIII started in 1965 and ended in 1967. Provision of complete primary education in one school was also effected. The so-called extended primary schools (Standards I–VI) and the former lower primary schools became full primary schools (I–VII). By 1968 the entrance examination to Standard V was abolished, so that a child who entered Standard I was assured of education for the full seven years.

The number of children attending public primary schools rose from 486 470 in 1961 to 753 114 in 1967. Schools were increased by 627, and the teaching force grew from 9 190 to 16 271 during the same period.

Some of the drawbacks experienced during that time were as follows:

As the number of children enrolled in these schools fluctuated, the schools were not always filled to capacity. There was a lot of wastage due not only to selection and examinations for promotion, but also to economic and social factors, such as inability to pay school fees, unfavourable geographical location of schools, villages or homesteads, apathy to schooling by parents and children alike, and early marriage in some societies. In such cases a monetary allowance had to be given to those repeating and to those promoted to higher classes.

The emergence of English-medium primary schools, which were intended to cater for children of European and Asian groups, was not quite in line with the Tanzanian policy of equality. Some of the top African leaders sent their children to these schools.

With the expansion of primary schools in terms of numbers of children, the country could not cope with the problem of school leavers. Although the number of secondary school places had increased, it was not possible to absorb the large primary school output. The majority of these flocked into towns from their villages in the hope of securing jobs, an indication that the type of education provided was still white-collar-job-oriented.

The traditional mode of teaching where knowledge and work were blended was neglected, and education continued to be elitist. It was competitive and examination-oriented. Only those who did very well in examinations got places in post-primary institutions, or managed to secure a job.

Through the localization of school management, competition grew up among the various Local Education Authorities. Whilst the richer authorities were easily able to expand, the less fortunate districts remained almost at a standstill. There was also conflict between Local Authorities and Voluntary Agencies, as well as among the different Voluntary Agencies.

The education offered was still divorced from society in the sense that the children were too much away from home, and that what they learned at school was not applicable or relevant at home. Hence the influx of school leavers into towns.

Apart from the above criticisms, the progress made since the time when the educational system had been inherited from the colonial administration was very considerable.

2. The 'Arusha Declaration' and after

The 'Arusha Declaration' in 1967, which defined the broad and clear national goals of Socialist Democratic Republican Government, was also an important milestone on the road from the colonial educational system to a system of national education. In his document 'Education for Self-Reliance' (see pp. 17–32 above), Mwalimu Nyerere outlines such broad educational aims as:

acquisition of basic concepts and content so that the child will be able to apply that knowledge to his ever-changing environment;

mastering of basic skills such as reading, writing, and numeracy;

development of self-confidence and provision of opportunities for self-directed instruction, study evaluation and formulation of goals and standards;

development of an enquiring mind so that the child can process information and become a self-educating adult;

development of the child's co-operative involvement with peers and the community as a whole;

provision of experience that will develop and demonstrate human values such as equality, honesty, trust, courage, responsibility and respect for others.

However, this policy statement was at first interpreted in different ways. Some implemented it by focusing on the idea of economic independence, others by endeavouring to increase the output of the schools' 'productive activities' (agricultural, handicrafts, etc.), commodities, and some, thinking that it was a policy for raising the schools' prestige as an end in itself, provided activities of no relation whatsoever with those of the community at large. All that confusion was engendered by the communication gap between the Ministry of Education and the schools concerned. The policy only came as a directive without regard to the feasibility of its implementation in individual primary schools; nor were the teachers told how to implement it.

'Education for Self-Reliance' also demanded changes in the existing curricula. This was done. New syllabi and new teaching materials were developed, but again these were sent to schools without proper instructions on their use. So many were the changes that in some instances the schools opted to carry out their own kind of implementation. A study made by Besha reveals some of the consequences:

'One does not wonder therefore to see that self-reliance activities in schools do not produce the required effect. The fact that so much is done in the schools already shows that our teachers have tried to do what they can under the circumstances. Because from the beginning nobody has sat down to think out or analyze how best, in details, these self-reliance activities can be carried out and integrated into the school curriculum, they have been taken in isolation and they have not been seen as part and parcel of the education system.'[2]

Nevertheless, the policy paper was introduced at the right time and set specific and clear objectives. Its emphasis was to prepare the children of Tanzania for a useful role in society.

'"Education for Self-Reliance" is now the major aim of the Arusha Declaration. The Primary School child is prepared for life in the village for which agriculture occupies special priority and more local content is included in all subject syllabi. Science studies and technical training are given far greater attention than formerly in order to solve the problem of manpower shortage.'[3]

With the above objectives in mind drastic measures were taken to change the inherited educational system. The reorganization of primary schooling from eight to seven years has already been mentioned. Other developments included full-day instead of half-day schooling in Standards III and IV. Two hundred and fifty schools with full-day schooling in Standards III and IV were opened by 1968. More Standard I and V classes were provided so that by the same year over 40 per cent of Standard IV pupils could get places in Standard V. In accordance with the country's policy of equal opportunity, these developments concentrated on districts with less than 50 per cent provision of Standards I–IV and Standard V. The position of enrolment is summarized in Table 4.4.

Table 4.4

Enrolment in Public and Private Primary Schools by 1968

All Regions	Std I	Std II	Std III	Std IV	Std V	Std VI	Std VII
Public	155 802	148 188	142 353	136 449	67 417	57 579	57 381
Private	29 575	24 910	5 704	4 504	1 205	1 340	1 491
Total	185 377	173 098	148 057	140 953	68 622	58 919	58 872

Source: Ministry of National Education. *Annual Report* Dar es Salaam, 1976, p. 28

The number of pupils in primary schools had risen considerably as compared with that of 1961, cited at the beginning of this chapter. Altogether there was a total of 833 898 pupils, of whom 512 554 were boys and 321 344 were girls. The teaching force too had increased to 17 584, of whom 1 970 were Grade A, 1 721 Grade B, 12 803 Grade C, 768 with permits to teach, and 322 others.

The Education Act of 1969 marked the end of about eighty years of mission participation in public education. As a result, education became the sole responsibility of the state. To make this possible, the Ministry had spent 49.98 per cent of its budget on primary education compared with 39 per cent in 1968.[4]

Teaching materials were improved in order to meet the interests of the nation. New syllabi, designed to implement the policies stated in 'Education for Self-Reliance', and new textbooks were introduced from 1968 onwards, Social studies, history, geography and civics were taught in such a way as to motivate pupils politically and to make them proud of their past, present and future.[5] Skills for rural living were incorporated and farming, poultry keeping and other agricultural projects were reintroduced. Swahili became the medium of instruction throughout primary school.

In line with these developments the teacher training programme had to be expanded and improved. Training of Grade A and C teachers increased considerably. For instance, by the end of 1969 there were 2 878 Grade A teachers in primary schools (as against 1 970 in 1968), and in-service courses were organized to familiarize teachers with the new materials. From the same year no further primary school teachers were recruited from outside the country. Table 4.5 shows the increase in schools, pupils and teachers from 1967–1975.

This increase was due to the fact that more rooms were available for Standards I and V, and to the nation's target of Universal Primary Education by 1989 (now 1977 after the Musoma Resolution of 1974). The abolition of school fees in 1972 also played a significant part; the number of newly enrolled pupils in 1973 was more than double that of 1972.

Table 4.5

Numbers of Schools, Pupils and Teachers, 1967 to 1975 (Public Schools only)

Year	Number of Schools	Number of Pupils	Number of Teachers
1967	3865	753114	16271
1968	3852	765169	15725
1969	3811	776109	16577
1970	4070	827984	17790
1971	4133	902619	19786
1972	4495	1003596	21926
1973	4838	1106387	23168
1974	5185	1228886	25000
1975	5804	1589008	28752

Source: Statistics Section, Planning Division. Dar es Salaam: Ministry of National Education

Other important features have helped the development of primary education towards 'Education for Self-Reliance'. The school entry age was raised to seven years so that pupils will be a year older on completing their education, and hence better able to assume an effective role in village life, the more so as primary education is designed to be complete in itself. The 'villagization' in progress and the decentralization of the primary education system will permit all children of school age to enjoy school facilities and a more relevant type of education. The schools have been brought closer to the community, and parents and the community at large have a bigger role to play. As experiments with community schools such as the Kwamsis project in Tanga region have proved very successful, they are now being extended to other regions in a joint effort by Unicef, Unesco and Tanzania.

3. The 'Musoma Resolution' and after

At the sixteenth meeting of the TANU National Conference (September 1973) it was regretfully noted that only 48.6 per cent of the school age children were in schools although there were places for 55 per cent. Considering that the people were responding to the government's appeal to live in villages, it seemed unfair to provide educational facilities for some and leave the others unprovided for. The TANU NEC held at Musoma in November 1974 therefore resolved that by 1977 arrangements should be made to enable every child of school age to go to school. Action to implement this resolution started almost immediately. The UPE programme would need an additional 13121 teachers to assist the existing 89745 teachers, and 26286 additional classrooms, as shown in Tables 4.6 and 4.7.

The Ministry of National Education has already prepared 2296 ward co-ordinators (primary school and adult education supervisors). These impart the basic teaching skills to the Standard VII leavers who are prospective teachers, by

Table 4.6

(a) Additional Teachers Needed for Universal Primary Education

Year	Grade C	Grade A	Total
1975–76	1947	1493	3440
1976–77	4546	1222	5768
1977–78	2914	999	3913
Total	9407	3714	13121

Table 4.7

(b) Additional Classrooms Needed for UPE at Standard I

Year	Classrooms
1975–76	6075
1976–77	9298
1977–78	10913
Total	26286

Source: Unesco/Unicef, *Report of a Conference-Workshop on Teacher Education for Basic Education*. Basic Education Resource Centre for Eastern Africa, 1976

training them on the job, coaching them in correspondence courses coupled with special radio broadcasts, and also assess their academic and practical skills. According to the Ministry of National Education projection and figures, up to 829 993 children were enrolled for UPE in 1975–1976, 848 293 are expected to enter Standard I in 1976–77[6] about 867 793 in November 1977, and 491 000 in 1978. This will bring the total up to 100 per cent of the school age children.[7]

The training of teachers is not limited to the preparation provided by the 31 colleges of National Education throughout the country and the arrangements mentioned above. Elements of pedagogy are also taught in Forms III and IV of the secondary school, and these students will help to teach in nearby primary schools to overcome the shortage of teachers. In this way the Ministry will also be able to identify prospective teachers.

The trend towards Universal Primary Education has been extended to disabled children. In his speech on the 1975–76 budget in Parliament, the Minister of National Education noted that there were three schools for the blind, six schools for the blind mixed with ordinary pupils, two schools for the deaf and one school for pupils with other physical handicaps. As this is insufficient to cope with the number of disabled pupils, every effort is being made to provide special schooling for all of them, and it is hoped to achieve this goal with the help of external aid in the form of materials and training facilities.

Since the aim of primary school education in Tanzania is to improve the economic and social conditions in the rural areas where about 90 per cent of our people live, a change in the curriculum was necessary. The new curriculum areas may be grouped under the following headings:

a) Literacy and Numeracy
b) Intermediate technology including mathematics and science
c) Agriculture including animal husbandry
d) Business education involving pupils in the activities of village co-operatives
e) Development studies including civics, history, health, sanitation
f) Cultural activities

This suggestion is not an easy one to carry out. Its implementation will require changing the existing materials and personnel and employing new teaching techniques such as the unit system.

The Musoma meeting also realized that the schools placed too much emphasis on academic subjects and examinations, neglecting work as part of the learning activity. It therefore resolved that work must be an integral part of education in all institutions in order to build up socialist attitudes and habits among the pupils. To implement the resolution, the Ministry of National Education through its curriculum development tools has suggested three types of timetable for the primary schools, namely heavy, medium and light work timetables; which of these is to be chosen will depend upon the geographical locations of the schools. As for examinations, the trend now is to de-emphasize them and to assess a pupil on his day-to-day progress in class and outside class. Furthermore, the primary school leaving examination has been decentralized, so that it can be made more relevant to the pupils' environment.

4. Observations and conclusion

Tanzania has achieved a great deal in terms of development of primary education. One of the problems still unsolved is that of selecting pupils for further education. With the growing number of pupils who complete Standard VII, and with the regional differences created in the colonial era, it will be very difficult to attain the equality of opportunity we are striving for. Although the problem of selection has been attenuated by the introduction of the District quota system, its full solution will require an expansion of secondary schools at district and regional levels.

The introduction of post-primary institutions with a technical bias in every district will alleviate the problem of school leavers, and at the same time help to develop the rural economy. Whilst private initiative to open such institutions is welcome, consideration will also have to be given to those unable to attend them. It is therefore suggested that other kinds of post-primary institution—teaching, agriculture, veterinary, community development and the like—be established so that the primary school leavers might render better services to their communities.

The growing number of pupils in schools calls for more teachers, buildings and teaching materials. The present emphasis on the use of local resources will only produce good results if teachers and tutors are continually trained and retrained. It is to be hoped that the TANU call for priority to be given to school projects will help all schools to obtain enough funds for their buildings and teaching materials. Equality of opportunity implies that there should be no difference in treatment in terms of teachers, buildings or materials.

The disparity between boys and girls in primary schools should also be reduced with the current move from isolated homesteads to villages, though parents and the society at large still have to be educated politically to attach the same importance to girls' education as they do to that of boys. UPE must mean compulsory education for both sexes from the start to the end.

Lastly, the masses in general and the privileged workers in particular must be politically oriented so that they change their attitudes on the expectations of their children after completing primary school education.

'. . . For we have recognized that, for the foreseeable future, the majority of our primary school pupils will not go to secondary school, and the majority of our secondary school pupils will not go to University. In Tanzania they will leave full time learning and become workers (not necessarily wage earners) in our villages and towns.'[8]

Notes

1 See Ministry of National Education Statistics Section, Planning Division. *Twenty Years Since the Birth of TANU* Dar es Salaam: Ministry of National Education, (1974).

2 Besha, M R *Education for Self-Reliance and Rural Development* Dar es Salaam: Institute of Education, (1973) p. 31

3 Ministry of National Education *Annual Report* (1968) Dar es Salaam: Printpak/MTUU, (1976) p. 4

4 Ministry of National Education *Annual Report (1969)*. Dar es Salaam: Printpak/MTUU, (1976) p. 6

5 See Note 3, p. 8

6 See *Daily News* (17.6.1976) p. 4

7 For some financial estimates of UPE and the whole of primary education see the article 'Teacher Training in Tanzania' by G R V Mmari, pp. 119–131 of this book.

8 Nyerere, J K 'Ten Years after Independence' in *Freedom and Development* by J K Nyerere, p. 298 Bibl. 12

4.3 Secondary Education
M J Mbilinyi

Introduction

Secondary education has developed and changed in response to the interests of different, often opposing, classes both internal and external to Tanzanian society. Initially colonial administrators representing the interests of metropolitan capitals (German, then English) blocked the expansion of secondary and higher education for Africans, despite the latters' growing demands for education 'equal' to that of Europeans and Asians. Later, the English colonialists provided for limited expansion of secondary education, especially after 1950, one aim being the promotion of (and ideological hegemony over) a comprador ruling class which would represent the interests of the metropolitan capital after independence.

Very little *qualitative* change in the overall education system took place immediately after independence, but there was rapid expansion of secondary and higher education in order to 'fill' high and middle level manpower positions. The definition and structure of these positions had already been established by the colonial administrators and experts, and followed the bureaucratic and hierarchical pattern typical of capitalist organization. As President Nyerere has noted:

'In a peaceful transfer of power, the colonial instruments of government exist. They are passed to the nationalist leaders. No other instruments of government have been created during the independence struggle. Colonial development objectives are also taken over. No alternative objectives have been thought out.'[1]

The 'Arusha Declaration' and various policy measures thereafter established TANU's policy of socialism and self-reliance, but Tanzania has found the path towards the goals of socialism and self-reliance a tortuous one. Although the 'Arusha Declaration' called for development based on local resources, dependence on foreign capital for the development budget has increased from 63 per cent in 1972–73, to over 70 per cent in 1974–75. In order to obtain the foreign exchange needed to repay loans and buy manufactured goods, Tanzanian agricultural products are used mainly for export rather than for internal processing or consumption. In 1974 they accounted for 80 per cent of the total export value. Agriculture remains the basis of the economy. Eighty-five per cent of the economically active population engage in agricultural production, the majority as smallholder peasant producers. They are increasingly dependent on the market for their basic needs and commodities required for production, and at the same time suffer from unequal terms of trade between the rural and urban sector. Poverty levels of existence in rural areas are the major explanation for the rural-urban migration which is so closely identified with the 'primary school leaver problem' and, since the expansion of secondary education, the 'secondary school leaver problem'. Secondary school leavers can no longer be assured of wage employment, let alone further training opportunities.

Basic education reform has developed partly to confront the effects of underdevelopment, e.g. unemployment and underemployment, the low levels of productivity in the agricultural production system, urban-rural disparities, etc. In order to comprehend the meaning and limitation of education reforms, it is essential to understand reform in the context of such economic and political factors.[2]

The first section of the paper will discuss the historical development of secondary education in the colonial and immediate post-independence periods. The second section outlines the policy of 'Education for Self-Reliance' and other policies since, with special attention to secondary education. Section 3 'Secondary Schools Today', concentrates on the structure of school and classroom, the curriculum, access to schooling and motivational outcomes for students and teachers. The final section is a conclusion based on the foregoing.

1. Historical development

As the chapter on the historical development of formal schooling has shown, there were separate education systems for Europeans, Asians and Africans, reflecting their different places in the production system. Very few Africans received any formal schooling, and of these few the majority received only one or two years of *basic* education (reading, writing, arithmetic, vocational training, catechism). Post-elementary education was geared to manual vocational training: carpentry, masonry, road construction, farming, etc. The explicit intention of post-elementary, agricultural training, as well as of elementary education, was to *adapt* the peasant to his place as peasant producer in an underdeveloped capitalist system of exploitation. Post-elementary training was mainly reserved for children of chiefs and wealthy peasants or traders, in line with the policy of developing a comprador class to administer the people at the local level.

African education at post-elementary levels was highly restricted. Expansion of junior secondary education in the 1930s was a result of growing manpower demands due to the depression in the worldwide capitalist system, which led to the need to use Africans in place of Englishmen at middle levels of administration. At the same time, expansion at this level met African demands for more education. Junior secondary schools fulfilled most government and private manpower demands for clerks, teachers, etc., and in 1945 only one full secondary school (Minaki) had a programme up to Standard XII, with six pupils. By 1946, Tabora Government Secondary School and Tabora White Fathers had also established full programmes.[3] There was relatively rapid expansion of secondary education thereafter, relative that is to the complete absence of any secondary programme before. Girls began to find their way into secondary schools, although the proportion of girls in total enrolment remained very small up to the time of independence.

The 1955 syllabus for four years' coursework included English, mathematics, biology, physics, chemistry (for girls, domestic science took the place of the three science subjects), history, civics, geography, Swahili, religion, art/handicrafts and current affairs. This basic curriculum content of secondary education continued up to the present time, as the later section on curriculum will show. The subjects were taught in a bookish way, the teacher's role being to cram the students' heads with isolated facts needed to pass competitive and bookish examinations. The Cambridge Overseas School Certificate was relied upon to evaluate secondary school performance at Form IV and later Form VI level.

By 1961 and Independence, a total of 16691 students were enrolled in secondary schools, compared with 9883 in 1957 and 1529 in 1947.[4] A limited number of high school courses had been established. Nevertheless, only 245 Africans had Secondary School Certificates in 1959 on the eve of Independence. Only 15 of the 116 graduate teachers in African secondary schools in 1959 were African, and there were few other local graduates to take over senior administrative posts. The pool of more highly educated teachers was utilized to take over government positions, increasing the lack of local teachers in secondary schools.[5] Table 4.8 on enrolment in 1961 is illustrative of the education pyramid at that time.

2. Post-Independence educational policies

One of the first reforms in education after Independence was the integration of the school system in order to eliminate racial and religious barriers to schooling. The Education Ordinance of 1961 established the policy of a racially integrated school system managed by government and voluntary agencies. Fees were controlled in order to foster the integration of high-cost schools, though inevitably access to them was restricted to high-income families. Another mechanism was reliance on the Primary School Leaving Examinations for selection to secondary school, thus eliminating race as a 'qualifier' but stressing the selective function of examinations. In addition, English and Swahili became the sole media of instruction in 1965. By 1968 Swahili became the medium for all primary schools although a few 'English' primary schools continue to exist and to serve high income Tanzanian households.

Table 4.8

School Enrolment Figures in 1961

		Public	**Private**
Primary School Standard	I	121 386	23 334
	IV	95 391	4 206
	V	19 721	3 120
	VIII	11 732	757
Secondary School Form	I	4 196	—
	IV	1 603	—
High School	V	326	—
	VI	176	—

Source: T L Maliyamkono, *Major Educational Reforms: A Tanzanian Case*. Dar es Salaam: University of Dar es Salaam (1976) (Mimeo.) Table A.1, p. 92 and Table B.1, p. 100

In both the Three-Year Development Plan, 1961–1964 and the Five-Year Plan, 1964–1969 expansion of secondary and higher education was given priority. The Five-Year Plan called for expansion of all four-year primary schools to reach Standard VII, and Standard VIII was phased out. The majority of secondary schools were academic, the major exceptions being Ifunda and Moshi Technical

Schools. A 'crash' programme was begun at the University College of Dar es Salaam, under the Department of Education, to produce Tanzanian graduate teachers for secondary schools and teacher training colleges. The Second Five-Year Plan also shifted emphasis toward science education, employing a science/arts ratio of 2:1 in high school and therefore also in lower secondary education. Emphasis on science was in line with the kinds of knowledge and skill necessary for economic development.

In the new curricula developed after Independence, national and African history and geography were given more attention, and the former study of 'English kings and queens' was eradicated. Efforts were made to provide local and relevant examples and exercises in different school subjects. Swahili became a compulsory subject at Form IV level. Eventually one could not get a Form IV Certificate without a pass in Swahili. There was no fundamental change, however, in the nature or method of the social sciences taught. Political education, history and economics were descriptive and historical, typical of the bourgeois ideology which permeated first the colonial and later the post-independence educational process.

In 1964, secondary school fees were abolished, a very important step towards providing more equal access to secondary schooling for all children. However, as primary school fees remained until 1973, access to schooling was limited to the children of richer peasants and traders in the rural areas. Poor peasant households required their children's labour at home, so that even abolition of fees could not 'free' all of them to go to school.[6] Unequal access to primary school inevitably led to unequal access to secondary school.

Expansion of secondary education must be seen in relation to the expansion of post-secondary education. In 1961, the University College of Dar es Salaam opened with a Faculty of Law. Full bursaries including free tuition, free room and board, and money for clothing, books and travel were provided to students. University selection was wholly based on Form VI examination performance, and Form V (high school) entry in turn depended on performance in Form IV examinations. Other post-secondary and post-high school training institutions also selected on the basis of examination performance. As a result, examinations had a significant back-wash effect on the curriculum and especially on the teaching methods and organization of work in schools and classrooms. The integral relation between education and work strengthened the potency of examinations. The national examinations (earlier Cambridge) were deliberately structured to select the 'best' from the majority, based on *assumptions* of the normal curve. The examination system was mystified at the fact that it *produced* failure, and was structured intentionally to fail the majority. As a result those who 'failed' were convinced that their failure was due to personal weakness or stupidity. The Standard VII Primary School Leaving Examination served the same function with respect to access to secondary schooling. This mystification process, which affects those in control of the system as well as those being controlled, was particularly crucial after primary schools began to expand and secondary school enrolment was restricted. The decreasing percentage of Standard VI leavers entering Form I became a political issue labelled 'primary school problem'. It was essential for the people to accept the legitimacy of the educational pyramid structure, especially to accept that the basis of selection to

Form I was 'objective' and fair. For a time, Standard VII Examination fulfilled this purpose.[7]

In 1967 TANU proclaimed the 'Arusha Declaration', a major ideological statement of the national policy of socialism and self-reliance. 'Education for Self-Reliance' was declared soon after in order to ensure that the educational institutions were in line with socialism and self-reliance and in order to confront other basic economic problems of underdevelopment, such as unemployment of primary school leavers.

In brief, 'Education for Self-Reliance' proposed the following changes in the education system: it should be oriented to rural life; teachers and students should engage together in 'productive activities', and students should make all the major decisions about what to produce and how to do it and what to do with the proceeds; productive work should not be alienated work as it had been in colonial days but should become a regular part of school curricula and provide meaningful learning experience; examinations should be given less importance; primary education should be complete in itself and not the means to further education; children should begin school at seven years or more so that they would be old enough to become productive when they finished; students should become self-confident, co-operative, creative and critical in their thinking, not mere robots to be ordered about. What the new policy did not attempt to change is the pyramid structure of education and its relationship to every individual's position in production relations.

The 'Musoma Resolutions' passed in 1974 by the National Executive Committee of TANU were important for the implementation of Education for Self-Reliance. By 1977 all seven year old children were to be enrolled in Standard I.

The university would only recruit people with Form VI or other academic credentials who had worked at least two years after National Service. Education and work were to be combined: students at school were to work, so that the schools would become places of productive activity, factories and villages were to become also places of study for workers and peasants. Productive work in school was meant to cover some of the schooling costs, to ensure that Tanzanian youth developed a correct attitude to manual labour as future peasants and workers, and to destroy the intellectual and petty bourgeois arrogance of students in higher education institutions. Less attention was to be given to examinations and more to day-to-day school work. Secondary schools were to expand in order to provide more places for primary school leavers. This expansion was to be effected along the lines of UPE 1977, i.e. by relying on local resources and untrained teachers if necessary.

The implementation of *Education for Self-Reliance* since 1967 has led to many changes in secondary education. To begin with, the Education Act of 1969 was important in 'nationalizing' all assisted schools formerly run by voluntary agencies. It reinforced the powers of the Ministry of National Education over all aspects of the school system, including hiring and firing of teachers, closure of schools, control over curriculum and selection procedures, etc. The Act therefore furthered the process of centralized control over the school system. Heads of public and technical secondary schools and Colleges of National Education were rapidly Tanzanianized in 1967 and 1968.

In 1971 the former reliance on Cambridge Syndicate of Form IV and Form VI examinations was dropped and National Examinations were established. Efforts were made to ensure that content was more local. Nevertheless the form of the examinations remained 'bookish', testing memory rather than problem solving ability and creative thought. Practical components of science examinations have been increasingly difficult to implement because of the lack of apparatus in many schools. Needless to say, unequal allocation to secondary schools of books and qualified teachers, apparatus and basic equipment, has meant unequal education. Girls' schools and schools outside of Dar es Salaam have suffered particularly from lack of such resources.

In all public secondary schools students engage in meaningful productive activities. To a varying extent, they participate in decision-making about their own work. However, manual work remains separated from the potentially meaningful 'mental' learning which could have been built into self-reliance activities.[8] Contrary to the policy, self-reliance activities are timetabled separately from 'academic' subjects and remain separate spheres of activity. The sole possible exception may be the practical sessions related to secondary diversification biases to be discussed below.

3. Secondary schools today

(i) Structure and curriculum

The formal administrative structure of secondary schools is shown in Figure 4.1. The role relationships in the secondary school are an important mechanism for socializing students (and teachers) to adapt to particular kinds of situational demand typical in this case of the authoritarian and hierarchical structures of administration and control.[9]

The structure of the school organization is like a pyramid, with Ministry of National Education bureaucrats at the top and students at the bottom, though in terms of daily face to face relationships the Ministry is usually not experienced as a part of the school structure. Both students and teachers relate directly to the Head as the 'boss' of the school, even though the Heads are very much the intermediaries of the Ministry. Heads differ with respect to the degree to which they welcome democratic procedures in the school. They have *de jure* power and control over the subjects to be taught by each teacher, which forms he is assigned to, non-teaching duties of teachers, punishment of students, etc. Underneath the Heads are Second Masters or Mistresses, or Assistant Heads, who carry many of the Head's responsibilities and some of his/her authority. Boarding Masters in boarding schools and House Masters in boarding and day schools derive their functions from the organization of students into separate 'houses' by residence or into pools of forms in day schools. The 'houses' are the basis for 'duties' such as cleaning the school, classrooms and grounds, providing services to teachers, and for some sports and other activities.

Teachers belong to different departments according to the subjects they teach, and each department has its own head. In some schools the arts and science teachers are separate groups. This has partly been caused by differential salaries, science teachers receiving a slightly higher income. Science teachers often take 'break' separately in their own 'offices', usually the laboratory preparation rooms. Students also tend to rank science teachers and science subjects higher,

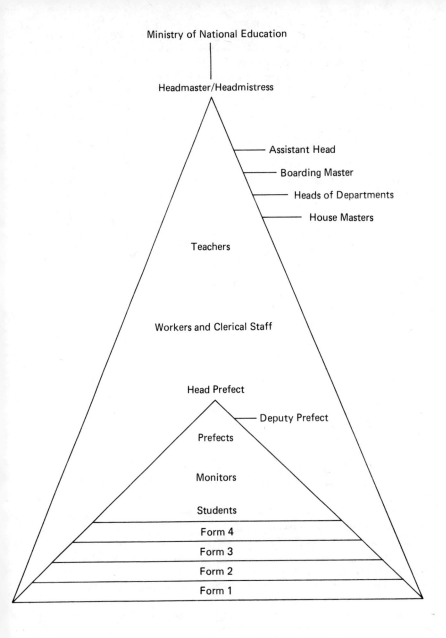

Figure 4.1

Secondary School Structure, 1976

calling them 'tough' and their positions more remunerative in terms of future prospects. This tendency is mitigated in schools where arts and science teachers are more 'united' and co-operative.

Stratification among teachers is also based on academic background (whether university graduate, diploma holder, up-graded Education Officer III, etc.), seniority, sex, and 'who is married to whom'. Ethnic origin and marital status also lead to systematic patterns of social relationships which interact with those based on the above factors. The seating pattern in staff rooms is one indication of such divisions. Students perceive the stratification among teachers, especially where it has been allowed to develop into rigid relationships of prestige and domination. It affects teacher-student relationships in the school and classroom.

According to normative expectations, teachers are meant to have almost absolute power over students, visible in methods of reward or punishment, evaluation, relationship to the subject matter, etc. This power and control is nevertheless relative. As in any social relationship, the teacher must be aware of student demands and needs and balance them with his own as well as with the situational demands he himself has to meet. This dialectical process between teacher and student is experienced when a teacher tries to develop teaching methods and modes of organization in line with 'Education for Self-Reliance' objectives. It is often the students who object to more creative, problem-solving and co-operative approaches to instruction, on the grounds that they will not have time to finish the syllabus and do well in final examinations.

The ultimate symbol of teachers' authority is the cane. According to a Ministerial directive, only the Headmaster and a teacher delegated by the Headmaster have the authority to beat students with a cane. Nevertheless, in several schools all teachers can be found wielding the stick. Reliance on flogging, symbolic of the relationship between oppressor and oppressed, was established during the German period of colonization. It is perhaps indicative of the present direction of events in Tanzania that corporal punishment has been given 'new life' in the schools today.

In most schools the supporting staff comprising manual workers, messengers, cooks and clerical staff are not considered part of the school organization as such but rather as servants of teachers and pupils. They are in a marginal position. In most schools, supporting staff do not attend staff meetings or parties nor do they join teachers in the staff room during break. This organization of work, where both teachers and students 'boss' the workers around, has a dynamic of its own and represents a significant model of behaviour to students. Friction between teachers and students and supporting staff contributes to problems over school maintenance, food, typing and duplication of teaching materials and school tests.

A set of hierarchical relationships among the students themselves links them to the overall structure of the school. Of particular significance is the prefect system originating from the British colonial education system. The powers of the Head Prefect or Head Boy are a reflection of the Headmaster's or Headmistress's own powers. Where the Headmaster is dictatorial in his/her relationship with teachers and students, he/she tends to bypass teachers and communicates decisions directly to the Head Prefect who then dictates to his fellow students, like a foreman in a factory, what has been dictated to him and ensures, together with the other prefects, that school rules are enforced. In schools where active student councils assuming some basic decision-making powers have developed, the prefect system and its relationship to the Headmaster or Headmistress is redefined.

By Ministerial Directive student councils should function in all schools. In fact most private schools do not have them or else they do not meet. In public schools the councils vary as to function and 'legitimacy' in the eyes of the students. In the majority of schools the members of the student council are prefects, which may interfere with its designated role as an organ representing the views of the students. Moreover, student council leaders are often automatically TANU Youth League leaders. However, where the Headmaster or Headmistress has encouraged some form of truly democratic student participation in decision making, councils have become meaningful institutions providing students with a voice and in some cases limited control over specific aspects of their lives at school. Discipline committees decide on the nature of student actions and what kind of discipline, if any, should be meted out. Self-reliance committees decide what kind of productive activities to engage in, where to dispose of the produce and what to do with the proceeds. Ultimately, of course, such councils still mask the reality, which is that the Headmaster or Headmistress has ultimate authority in the school, so that he/she has the option of ignoring student ideas or opposing them.

Secondary school students take as many as thirteen subjects, with different coursework dependent on streaming by ability as well as on the bias of the school. In accordance with the 'vocational diversification programme' each secondary school specializes in either agriculture, domestic science, commerce or technical subjects, though there are four combined agriculture/commerce schools. Forms I and II function as junior secondary schools, in that streaming into Forms III and IV depends on student performance in earlier years, measured by school tests and classroom work as perceived by the respective subject teachers. There are no sophisticated testing devices nor counselling apparatuses. In practice, therefore, a major function of Forms I and II curricula is selection.

All students take the following subjects throughout the four years of lower secondary schooling: political education (2 periods), history (3), mathematics (6–7), Swahili (4), English (5), biology (4), culture (3), religion (2). In Forms III and IV they also take instruction in teaching in order to contribute later to the UPE 1977 programme. In addition, they take 15 to 17 periods a week in their respective biases. Physics, chemistry, foreign languages, geography and integrated physical science are allocated, depending on performance and the bias to which a student is attached. All commerce bias students take integrated science except for a few selected by ability to enter the physics/chemistry combination. The integrated course does not fulfill requirements for entering science subjects at Form V and VI level.

In most schools, the most 'able' students are actively sought for chemistry/physics course combinations, the combination with the greatest chance of selection for higher education. The least 'able' students are placed into the literature stream, depending on their particular bias, or on the equipment and staff of the school. Conflict over streaming has arisen between students and teachers, and even among teachers, with students struggling to get into the science stream. The major exceptions are well-equipped and staffed technical schools (very few), where technical studies lead to Dar es Salaam Technical College and possibilities of joining the Engineering Faculty at the university.

In practice, the secondary diversification programme thus far does not enable all students to become productive immediately after they leave school, even if the skills taught in the biases could be absorbed productively in the economy. A sizeable but diminishing number of secondary school students still receive specialized coursework geared towards further education and professional training, with a minimum of bias coursework. Moreover, many primary school students and their parents are unaware of the bias programme and the differential outcomes the different biases have with respect to employment and further education. With the exception of those who have knowledgeable parents to guide them, Standard VII students select the school they would like to enter, if 'passed', with little or no briefing on the significance of the choice they are making. According to the latest Ministerial Directives, there will be seven Domestic Science, 26 Commerce, 35 Agriculture, and 16 Technical schools, four of which are combined Agriculture/Commercial.

Courses are divided into 45 minute periods, which are often clustered into double, triple, even quadruple periods for laboratory practicals and language/literature classes in particular. Every minute of the day is scheduled for. All courses follow a set syllabus; all culminate in the Form IV Examination. There are two school terms, at the end of which school tests are conducted for each subject. In the past, schools kept their own records of school tests, term projects and regular classroom work. In line with 'Musoma Resolutions' however, records of these activities will be kept on the Examinations Council headquarters and used to evaluate student performance together with performance in the National Form IV and Form VI Examinations.

Until now, the National Examinations have had a powerful backwash effect, and it will be important to see whether the new system of assessment will ignore this situation. Teachers strive to complete the syllabus, never mind at what speed and at what cost to students' understanding. Inspectors judge teachers partly by their ability to get through the syllabus. As Form IV examinations may draw from any of the four years, a lot of time is spent on revision in Form IV, if the syllabus has already been covered. Teacher efforts to explore new ground or to follow student interests and devote more time to certain subjects are discouraged by the sheer pressure of 'keeping up'. Teachers who do not toe the line of the syllabus are subject to scolding from fellow teachers and department heads and to hostility from students.

The organization and content of the syllabi have aroused much comment from teachers. They are overcrowded. Too many topics are covered in too short a time, with little connection between them. Under such pressure teachers find rote memory teaching, on the surface, the most 'effective' way, especially since the National Form IV Examinations measure rote memory rather than original thinking or creative problem-solving. One very common teaching method is the 'copy-copy' one: the teacher copies notes or words from a text book or notebook on the blackboard; students copy these notes into their own notebooks; on school tests and Form IV examinations they 'copy' these notes on the paper from their memories. Another common method combines lecture, copy-copy and question-answer. The teacher revises notes from the previous lessons in a ten-minute question-answer session, in order to ascertain how much has been remembered. Then he gives a fifteen-minute verbal presentation. Students do not pay very much attention at this stage. But when the teacher puts notes based on his lecture on the board for another fifteen minutes, he has the students' complete attention as they fill their notebooks. If there is time at the end, the teacher goes into another question-answer routine to see if the students have understood or remembered what they have seen and heard in the lesson. In science laboratory lessons, a demonstration usually takes the place of the verbal presentation, or else occurs alongside it, together with notes and question-answer. Because of limited apparatus, students do not usually have the opportunity to engage in experiments themselves.

These methods are typical of the 'banking' approach to teaching, where the teacher controls the content of the lesson and perceives his work to be filling up the heads of his students with his own knowledge, disregarding whatever knowledge they may have, and also disregarding their ability to investigate knowledge on their own.[10] Teachers themselves have always been taught this way, right up through the university or Colleges of National Education. And as discussed above, the need to finish the syllabus and the very structure of the syllabus almost compel teachers to behave in this way. Teaching methods can be radically altered in line with national education objectives, but the curriculum, teaching materials and textbooks, as well as evaluation devices like the National Examinations, must also be changed to reinforce the correct instructional strategies and to provide appropriate learning outcomes.

(ii) Access to secondary education

In 1974 there were 136 secondary schools, 83 public and 53 private. Their regional distribution is given in Table 4.9. The pattern of uneven development established during the colonial period has been perpetuated and is enhanced by the growth of private schools in areas already well endowed with public secondary schools.

Girls have historically had limited access to post-primary education. Approximately 27 per cent of the Form I places available, and 14 per cent of those in Form VI, are taken by girls. The ratio of boys to girls is fixed by the number of places actually available. There are 44 boys schools, 18 girls schools and 18 co-educational schools in the public school system; and 21 boys schools, five girls schools and 18 co-educational schools in the private school system.[11]

Table 4.9 (overleaf)
Source: Amri et al. *Regional Inequalities in Access to Education in Tanzania.* Dar es Salaam: University of Dar es Salaam (1976). Paper presented to Department of Education Seminar, (1976) Table 1A, p. 9
*Data for Secondary Schools adopted from Ministry of National Education, Technical Secondary Statistics, July 1974.
**Population data drawn from 1967 Census.

Table 4.9

Regional Distribution of Education Resources (1974)

Regions	Prim. Sch. (1965–73 av.)	Pub. Sec. Schools*	Private Sec. Schools*	Total Sec. Schools*	% of Mainland Total*	Pop. in % of Tot. M'land Pop.**
Arusha	182	3	3	6	4.2	0.5
Pwani	188	3	0	3	2.1	6.4
Dar es Salaam	188	9	6	15	10.8	5.8
Dodoma	222	5	1	6	4.2	5.6
Iringa	202	7	2	9	6.5	3.8
Kigoma	140	1	1	2	1.4	5.3
Kilimanjaro	367	9	15	24	18.0	5.3
Mtwara	303	5	0	5	3.6	
Lindi	—	1	2	3	2.1	8.5
Mara	193	3	3	6	4.2	4.4
Mbeya	287	4	1	5	3.6	7.9
Rukwa	—	1	1	2	1.4	5.6
Morogoro	250	4	4	3	5.7	8.6
Mwanza	311	6	2	8	5.7	3.2
Ruvuma	172	3	2	5	3.6	7.3
Shinyanga	201	2	1	3	2.1	3.7
Singida	183	2	1	3	2.1	4.6
Tabora	188	5	2	7	5.0	6.3
Tanga	318	5	2	7	5.0	5.3
W. Lake	303	5	4	9	10.8	100.0
Total	4198	83	53	136	100.0	

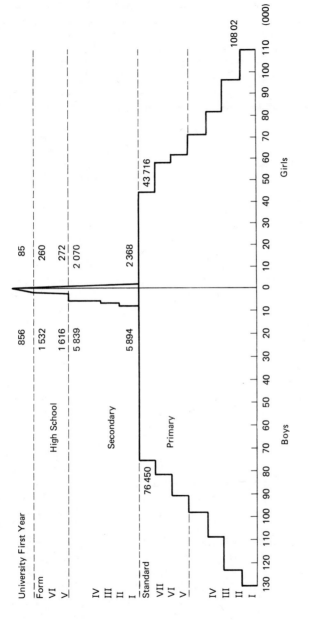

Figure 4.2

Tanzania Educational Pyramid, Public Schools 1974

Source: Ministry of National Education, Statistics.

As Figure 4.2 shows, the distorted shape of the educational pyramid has been perpetuated and become even more pronounced through primary expansion and the corresponding restriction of expansion at post-primary levels. Performance on the four papers of the Standard VII Examination (English, Swahili, Mathematics and General Knowledge) remains the major selection device for entry into Form I.

In an investigation in 1974 of seven secondary schools[11] drawn from several regions in the country, it was found that a relatively low proportion of parents were full time peasants compared with the national population.[12] According to the 1967 Census, 90.2 per cent of the total labour force are peasant producers, 4.3 per cent are numerate manual workers and craftsmen, 3.4 per cent are employed in clerical, sales and service jobs and 1.5 per cent are professionals or administrators. As Table 4.10 shows, however, only 38.2 per cent of the students' fathers were full-time peasants. Of the 43.4 per cent who were wage earners, the majority were in what could be called petty bourgeois or bureaucratic positions. Only 27 per cent of the wage earners were workers. Although 1.5 per cent of the total labour force are in professional and administrative posts, 11.7 per cent of our parent sample were found in such positions, eight times the national figure.

No major differences were found between public and private secondary school parents. However, further information is needed about the kind of financial assistance students may receive from relatives. Most peasant households depend on salaried relatives for financial expenditures, especially if they are paying the average annual school fees for private schools which range between Tshs 1 000 and Tshs 1 500.

Private schools are being used to get children through the 'back doors' into the public school system, which complicates the function of private schools with respect to access. In the last three years or so, urban public day schools have experienced an enormous inflow of students from private secondary schools, up to one third of total Form III enrolments consisting of such students. These are mainly children of 'big people', and they do not take vacant places. Instead, schools have been forced to create new streams for such students, or to squeeze 60 students into classrooms despite the 35–40 maximum prescribed. Headmasters and Headmistresses are obliged to 'receive' such students.

(iii) Motivation outcomes
What motivates a child to conform to the norms of the school and classroom? The student is placed in a set of situations with a relatively consistent pattern of role relationships and specific demands related to these relationships. In order to physically remain in the school certain rules must be followed. In order to be 'successful' or 'acceptable', the student must satisfy demands for study, do homework, pay attention to the teacher, etc. Student behaviour will depend in part on whether or not he/she identifies the goals of the school with personal goals. If the student does not 'care' about passing examinations and doing well in school, or has 'given up', many of the sanctions in the school will be ineffective.

Punishment, rather than reward, is the most depended-upon reinforcement. Caning, physical labour, and of course, suspension or expulsion represent some of the negative reinforcements relied upon. Discipline in practice is understood by teachers to be conformity to the role relationships defined by the hierarchical

Table 4.10

Occupations of Fathers (Including Guardians) of Secondary School Pupils Expressed as Percentages (1974)

	Total Public Schools (A, B, C, D)	Total Private Schools (E, F, G)	Total Per cent
Peasant only	42.6	35.2	38.2
Wage-earner	45.8	41.8	43.4
Trade	9.5	15.0	12.7
Self-employment	1.6	7.0	4.8
Other	0.5	1.1	0.9
Total	100.0	100.1	100.0
Total Number of parents in sample	190	273	463
No response	7	10	17

Source: Amri et al, Dar es Salaam: University of Dar es Salaam (1976).
Regional Inequalities in Access to Education in Tanzania.
A = Girls' Day School (Public)
B = Boys' Boarding School (Public)
C = Co-educational Day School (Public)
D = Co-educational Day School (Public)
E = Co-educational Day School (Private)
F = Co-educational Day School (Private)
G = Co-educational Day School (Private)

organization of the school and classroom. The authority of the teacher is central to these relationships, one symbol being standing to attention when the teacher enters the room, another being the well-known rule of not speaking until spoken to. Hence, by definition, conformity means subordination.

The system of external evaluation, be it positive or negative, orients the student to work in relationship to external demands and to be motivated by *extrinsic* factors. But Tanzania aims at creating a socialist society in which the worker is freed from alienation and expected to become *intrinsically* involved in his work, endeavouring to do as well as possible for his fellow workers, for his work unit, for his people. Whilst incentives may be attached to such behaviour, the internalization of values such as co-operation, plus basic self-confidence and a positive attitude to problem-solving, are equally important. In a socialist school system, fellow students should, therefore, take the primary role in creating and enforcing rules, thus laying the foundation for worker control in the factory or peasant control in the agricultural collective. Tanzania's present system of schooling operates against her socialist goals.

4. Conclusion
The aim of the 'Education for Self-Reliance' policy was to create an education

system which would serve the interests of the peasants and workers of Tanzania. Investigation of secondary schools indicates that achievement of this end requires immediate attention to be given to changing certain fundamental aspects of the education system. These include the pryamid structure of the school system, which deliberately restricts access to secondary and higher education (and therefore knowledge) to a very few, who tend increasingly to be children of the bureaucracy and petty bourgeoisie. Another is the hierarchical and authoritarian structure of role relationships in the school and classroom which reinforces alienation of students in line with a capitalist mode of work organization instead of the socialist one TANU intends to create. The form and content of syllabi and examinations are a third aspect. Recent trends towards vocationalization of curricula are of special concern. Will Tanzanians acquire the basic principles of science and technology necessary for economic development, or will they be restricted to *basic skills training* in farming, crafts, mechanics, etc. in order to produce more efficiently and productively, goods for the world-wide capitalist market? Tanzanians must be critical and politically aware of the implications of so-called education reforms like 'basic education' and 'vocationalization'.[13] The *basis* of a socialist and self-reliant economy *cannot* be basket-weaving, carpentry or hoe agriculture. Industrialization of all sectors, utilization of local energies and skills, and release of the people's creative and critical energies are necessary.

Of the many implications for education, the following are especially relevant to this paper's focus: 1) emphasis on science and technology for all students, from primary upwards; 2) increasing access to primary, secondary and higher education for workers and peasants, as well as for a rapidly expanding number of children in order to create workers and peasants capable of mastering nature and taking command of production; 3) a quota system based on class background for entry to secondary and higher education, in order to ensure equal access for all and also to create a committed leadership whose roots are of the workers and peasants; 4) radical alteration of teaching methods and organization of role relationships in school and classroom in line with socialism, together with changed curricula which focus on the meaningful learning of basic principles of subject matter.[14]

Notes

1 President Nyerere, J K 'Speech to the Mass Rally in Lourenço Marques, Mozambique—31st August 1975' in: *We Are Brothers United in a Common Struggle* Lourenço Marques, Mozambique: Empresa moderna S.A.R.L. (1975)
2 For analysis of problems of underdevelopment and class formation in Tanzania, see Shivji, I *Class Struggles in Tanzania* Dar es Salaam: Tanzania Publishing House (1976); Tschannerl, G 'Periphery Capitalist Development—A Case Study of the Tanzanian Economy' *Utafiti* (1976), No. 1, pp. 5–46; Rweyemamu, J F *Underdevelopment and Industrialization in Tanzania* Nairobi: Oxford University Press (1973). For discussion of certain aspects of appropriate industrial strategies see Thomas, C *Dependency and Transformation* New York: Monthly Review Press, (1974), and Rweyemamu, J F 'The Formulation of an Industrial Strategy for Tanzania' *Uhandisi* 3 (September 1976) No. 1, pp. 5—14
3 Muze, M S *Development of Secondary Education in Tanzania Mainland* Dar es Salaam: University of Dar es Salaam, Department of Education (1976) pp. 2, 3–4 (mimeo.). To be published in *Education Department Reader*
4 See Note 3
5 Kurtz, L S *An African Education* Brooklyn: Pageant-Poseidon Ltd. (1972) p. 135

6 See Mbilinyi, M 'Problems of Unequal Access to Primary School' in: *Who Goes to School in East Africa? Access to Schooling and the Nature of the School Process* edited by M Mbilinyi Dar es Salaam: University of Dar es Salaam, Department of Education (1976) (manuscript, mimeo.)

7 But see Mbilinyi, M 'Peasants Education in Tanzania' *African Review* (forthcoming) for analysis of the growing illegitimacy of the Standard VII Examination as the selection device for Form I, especially as perceived by peasants.

8 For a detailed discussion of implications of 'Education is Work' for implementation in schools, see Mmari, G *Agizo la Utekelezaji wa Elimu ya Kujitegemea Kazi Kuwa ni Sehemu ya Elimu Mashuleni* Dar es Salaam: University of Dar es Salaam (May 1975) Paper prepared for a seminar of the Ministry of National Education.

9 Much of the presentation here and elsewhere in the paper is based on the findings of the Secondary School Research Project in which the author and student colleagues have been engaged for three years. It involved both herself and student researchers teaching in secondary schools and investigating different aspects of teaching methods and the social organization of the school and classroom. See Mbilinyi, M et al. 'Secondary Education in Tanzania: Agent of Cultural Imperialism?' in *Who Goes to School in East Africa?* (see Note 6)

10 Freire, P *Pedagogy of the Oppressed* New York: Herder and Herder (1970)

11 Ministry of National Education *List of Secondary and Secondary Technical Schools, 1974, by Regions* Dar es Salaam: Directorate of Sectoral Planning (1975)

12 In this particular sample there were four public schools, one girls' day, one boys' boarding, two co-educational day with hostels, and three private schools; all co-educational day schools, two of which were formerly Asian schools run on a commercial basis and one of which is managed by a religious association. The schools are situated in Moshi, Arusha, Morogoro and Dar es Salaam.

13 For further discussion of the opposition between socialist and capitalist education, see Breeden, J *Papers in Education and Development* Dar es Salaam: University of Dar es Salaam (July 1975) No. 1, pp. 23–33

14 For further discussion and documentation of the role of imperialist agencies in education reform in Third World countries generally, as well as Tanzania in particular, see Mbilinyi, M (Note 7) and Mosha, H J *Policy Planning and Administration of Educational Innovations in Tanzania* Dar es Salaam: University of Dar es Salaam (1976) (M.A. dissertation in education)

4.4 Evaluating a Student's Progress
M S Muze

Introduction

In 1971 the Ministry of National Education provided guide lines for what was termed 'New Methods of Evaluating Students' Progress'. Directives emanating therefrom were a result of recommendations made by the heads of secondary schools at a meeting convened in June, 1971, following a government ruling that all secondary school examinations originating from outside Tanzania were to be replaced by 'national examinations'. At that meeting it was agreed that the above mentioned guidelines be introduced to ascertain to what extent the scope of our education, its purpose, and our national goals are being achieved.

It is now about five years since the letter containing the directives was issued, but it seems that many teachers (or schools) have yet to employ the new methods of evaluating students' progress effectively. The aim of this study is to review the Ministry's directives and to express the author's personal opinion on a few of the points involved.

1. Methods of evaluating students' progress

The methods suggested can be categorized as follows:

(a) Evaluating a student's daily progress in class through exercises and tests.
(b) Evaluating a student's progress by means of National Examinations.
(c) Evaluating a student's daily progress through observing his behaviour/attitude and his devotion to duty.

(a) Daily Progress

Daily progress should be evaluated through:

(1) Constant exercises
(2) Tests
(3) Projects

(1) Exercises: The teacher is expected to keep records of the marks obtained by each student in the exercises. These may be quizzes, or other forms of exercise taking a single period or two, or more periods in one or two days. What is important is that these exercises should be done regularly in order to assist the students in developing the habit of reading constantly as against the practice of studying seriously only when National Examinations approach. More exercises should be set on a subject taught in many periods per week than on one taught in a few. The following formula should be applied to determine the minimum number of exercises for each subject:

$$E = \frac{W \times P}{12}$$

where

E = number of exercises per term.
W = Number of weeks per term.
P = number of periods per week.

The Constant 12 has been chosen because it has been found recommendable for a teacher to set, on an average, at least one exercise for every 12 periods. To give two examples: In a term covering 24 weeks, Political Education is taught in 2 periods per week, and Mathematics in 8 periods per week. Applying the above formula the following number of exercises should be set during that term by the teachers of these two subjects:

Political Education: $\qquad E = \dfrac{24 \times 2}{12} = 4$

Mathematics: $\qquad E = \dfrac{24 \times 8}{12} = 16$

On the same basis, teachers of Swahili, Physics, Chemistry and Biology ought to set not less than 8 exercises, and History and Geography teachers not less than 6.

This formula would make it possible to differentiate between long and short terms, and the number of exercises would be dependent on the number of subjects taught in school. In Forms V and VI it is suggested that 16 be the constant number.

At the end of the term, the teacher would be expected to work out the average mark for each student's exercises. If a student failed to do an exercise without having a reasonable excuse he should be given a zero mark for it.

(2) Tests: Tests differ from exercises in that they examine the students on many subjects, taught for perhaps a period of three months or a full term, at a time. In practice this would require students to be notified of impending examinations so that they could prepare for them. One or more tests should be conducted each term. At the end of each term, the teacher should work out the average of the marks for all the tests that each student had sat for.

(3) Projects: Projects should be assigned early in order to give the students enough time to do the necessary research. A project could be undertaken by a single student, or by a group of students. The results should be submitted to the teacher towards the end of the term or year and be marked by him. Two requirements are involved in this method. First, teachers who are teaching the same class ought to consult each other as to when students should submit their projects. This would avoid situations where students might be required to submit seven or nine projects at the same time. If nine subjects are taught in a single class, one way of distributing project work over the year would be to assign three projects in the first term, three on vacations and the remaining three in the second term. There is also a possibility of having projects which combine two or three related subjects, e.g. Elementary Mathematics with Additional Mathematics, History with Political Education, etc.

Second, project work requires careful preparatory planning. It is important that teachers should assign projects that have been well thought out both in terms of aims and methods, so that they may be of benefit to the students, the school and the Nation. The Ministry stressed that these projects, 'apart from making students familiar with researching methods would contribute to economic development, the development of culture, politics and the like.'

Marks: The Ministry suggested that exercises should carry 40 per cent of the total marks in a subject, tests should carry 30 per cent and projects the remaining 30 per cent. Experiments made in some schools have, however, shown that some problems arise from this apportionment of marks in that, owing to the frequent transfers of teachers, some students may be assigned no project work. One suggestion is that the apportionment of marks should depend upon the weight of the project as the teacher sees it, and that of the remaining percentage, one half should be for exercises and the other half for tests. For example, if, after assessing the weight of a project in relation to the other testing instruments in the same subject, the teacher decides that the project should carry 20 per cent of the total marks, then exercises and tests would each have to carry 40 per cent. This suggestion has been made in consideration of the difficulty of designing every project so that it would warrant 30 per cent of the marks (see Appendix A).

At the end of the year the marks obtained in the first term should be added to those obtained in the second term and an average of the two found. At the end of the four-year (from Form I to Form IV), or two-year (from Form V to Form VI), period of study, the average of the marks obtained in those periods should be calculated for every subject.

(b) National Examinations
In the past, and probably even today, National Examinations held at the end of Form IV or VI have been given the greater weight. Considering the stage of development our country has reached, there is still a need for National Examinations, but they should be assigned a weight of one third of the total evaluation.

(c) Behaviour/Attitude and Devotion to Duty
Records should be kept on the students' attitudes and behaviour. The importance of this third section of student evaluation is emphasized in the Ministry's letter. To quote:

'Two things are involved in this: First, teachers should realize that the outcome of this evaluation of character carries the same weight as the other types of evaluation. Therefore, in the same way as they work to teach students in other subjects so that they may pass their examinations well, it is the teachers' responsibility to work still harder to teach them good behaviour so as to enable them to do well in these examinations. Second, students should be informed in detail, right from the beginning, of the importance of good behaviour in life, and that the assessment of this aspect of training carries the same weight as academic subjects. The teacher has ample opportunity of observing the students' character and behaviour. He/she could observe them in class, at play, on the farms, at work, in the fields, in the dormitory, in the kitchen etc. Wherever students engage in activities, opportunities exist of assessing their character. It is, however, of utmost importance that the teacher be honest in his assessing. He must also know the students well enough to be able to assess them correctly.'[1]

It is expected that several teachers will co-operate in making the final assessment (see Appendix B).

2. Final selection
An important requirement is that the entire record of a student over the whole period he is in school be kept together. These records should be used in the final

Ministry of National Education Student Record Sheet

COURSE................. CLASS................. TUTOR................. YEAR.................

SUBJECT.................

DATE	NAME OF THE STUDENT	1. EXERCISES															2. TESTS				3. PROJECT					
		1	2	3	4	5	6	7	8	9	10	11	12	TOTAL	AVERAGE %	J1	J2	TOTAL	AVERAGE %	%	EXERCISE %	TEST %	PROJECT %	TOTAL %	ADJUSTMENT

Appendix A

117

selection for further studies, training or employment, as they will provide a great deal of information on a student's aptitude and suitability for any particular career.

There is no need to average the marks obtained in the three categories of student evaluation. A student scoring an 'E' in one of the three categories or a 'D' in two of them, should not be considered for any kind of selection and should perhaps not be awarded any certificate.

Note

1. Ministry of National Education, EDS. SI/1/400(6.9.74) (reference number).

Appendix B

Record Sheet on Behaviour, Attitude and Devotion to Duty

	Grade*	Average Grade	Remarks
(i) In the Classroom:			
1. Attends classes punctually.			
2. Performs duties satisfactorily.			
3. Works well with others regardless of their status or rank.			
4. Departs only when duties are completed or work period ends.			
(ii) General Character:			
5. Assumes responsibilities when given leadership.			
6. Shows respect for his fellow students, staff and the general public.			
7. Willingly obeys orders and follows instructions when required.			
8. Cares for personal cleanliness.			
9. Cares for public property.			
10. Is trustworthy.			
11. Is hardworking and skilful.			
12. Is sought by others for advice.			
(iii) National Building:			
13. Positively responds to nation-building activities both at school and outside.			
14. Accepts reasonable demands even though disliking them.			
15. Inspires others to follow him/her.			
16. Voluntarily leads others in completing a task.			
(iv) Other Matters:			
17. Participates in games and sports.			
18. Participates in cultural activites.			

*Grade: A = Very Good, B = Good, C = Average, D = Weak, E = Poor.

4.5 Teacher Training in Tanzania
G R V Mmari

1. The colonial system

The training of teachers has been one of the main features of the education system in Tanzania since the days of colonial rule, when teacher training had acquired the same characteristics as the rest of the colonial system. It was organized along racial lines and trained teachers for the separate racial systems. It was also organized along religious lines, since several teacher training institutions were established by the different missionary voluntary organizations. Teachers trained in these institutions were expected to be loyal to the colonial masters and to propagate the colonial ideology. Those in mission schools were in addition expected to carry the banner of Christianity in the communities the schools were built in. If there were any shortcomings in the colonial system then teachers and teacher training institutions played their part in upholding them. If, on the other hand, there were any groups dissatisfied with the situation, then teachers and teacher training institutions did play their part in planting the seeds of revolution.

During the colonial period, mechanisms were instituted to monitor the quality of teacher training for African schools. These included the African Teachers Examinations Board[1] which controlled the examinations for prospective teachers and the training syllabi. The racial overtones are evident in the name of the Board. On assuming broader functions, it was renamed the Teacher Training Advisory Board. It was, of course, concerned only with teachers for primary schools, since pre-independence Tanzania had no institution of higher learning for training secondary school teachers. That cadre was trained outside the country at Makerere in Uganda, until the University College, Dar es Salaam established a Department of Education after independence.

While the colinial government was not committed to development of Tanzania in the sense understood today, it did attempt to introduce innovations to help improve the quality of teachers suitable for maintaining the system. One of these innovations came after the Binns Commission's[3] recommendation that British-type institutes of education should be established in east and central Africa. These institutes were just becoming known in the metropolitan country itself, having been proposed by a British Commission led by Mr McNair[4] as a way of raising the quality of teachers in Britain. Their functions included the initial education and training of teachers; advanced study and research in education in co-operation with university departments of education; services to practising teachers, including conferences, refresher courses, library facilities and publication of results of research and professional study. Because it was not possible to establish such an institute in pre-independence Tanzania, an alternative suggestion was made to expand one of the existing teachers' colleges to become a Central Teacher Training College.[5] Originally this was located in central Tanzania at Mpwapwa, but later moved to Dar es Salaam. One has to look at programmes before and after independence to appreciate the strides Tanzania has made in its efforts to train teachers for a country with socialist aspirations.

2. After independence

With independence it became quite clear that no revolutionary change could be carried through successfully without a committed teaching profession. At the same time, it was not possible to produce a revolutionary teaching cadre without training institutions geared to this new role. It is against this type of background that one must understand the aims of teacher education[6] in post-independence Tanzania. These have been stated as follows:

(i)   To educate student-teachers in the true meaning of the Tanzanian concept of ujamaa.
(ii) To train students to be dedicated and capable teachers with an understanding of, and care for, the children placed in their charge.
(iii) To deepen the students' own general education.

It is not accidental that *content* is placed last and *ideology* first. For a people who have been exploited, humiliated and ignored for so long, education is for liberation and thus a political question. If there was to be any difference between teacher training during the colonial period and that after independence, this had to be very clearly articulated in the political philosophy forming the basis of the training. It is important to note that the student teachers are being educated to understand not any brand of socialism, but the Tanzanian concept. Once the ideological perspective has been set right, then *how* to teach and *what* to teach will follow.

There are books and articles in learned journals which discuss at length the role of education in development. Some of them treat the subject as if it were above politics and 'propaganda'. Tanzania subscribes to the notion that there is no such thing as value-free education. Though in some countries the underlying principle is advertised in large banners and in others it is disguised in subtle ways, it is always the same: the dominant class dictates its terms through education, with the teacher acting as the catalyst.

The training of teachers in Tanzania at the university level is based on the same philosophy as that underlying the training of teachers for primary schools as undertaken by Colleges of National Education. According to the University Act[7] establishing UDSM, two specific objectives are:

To preserve, transmit and enhance knowledge for the benefit of the people of Tanzania in accordance with the principles of socialism accepted by the people of Tanzania.

To prepare students to work with the people of Tanzania for the benefit of the nation.

In the Colleges of National Education, it is accepted that the training of teachers will cover five main areas. These are:

National Service, which emphasizes military training and nation-building projects.

Political education, which emphasizes the understanding of the political ideology of ujamaa.

National education, which comprises principles of education, educational psychology, school organization, adult education, youth leadership, research projects.

Academic subjects and how to teach them.
Nation-building projects in the community round the College.

Since it is important to produce competent teachers who are sound both in body and in mind, the policy governing admission to colleges requires that prospective trainees have an adequate academic background, a sound character, physical fitness and a good all-round background. In case of doubt, an interview may be necessary.

Tanzania trains teachers of different types to teach at different levels of the educational system. There are the certificate teachers who have had either the full seven-year primary school education plus teacher training *or* a full additional four year secondary school education plus teacher training. Both types of teacher are posted to teach in primary schools. Then there are Diploma teachers who have had an equivalent of six years of secondary education plus one year of teacher training. These Diploma teachers are trained to teach secondary school academic subjects or vocational ones like business education, agriculture, domestic science (home economics) and technical subjects. The third type of teacher is the university-trained teacher who is expected to teach at all levels of the six-year secondary programme. Some of the outstanding ones are retained to teach at the university. The different between this type of teacher and the Diploma teacher is that the former has had a more profound academic preparation and is therefore expected to teach higher classes in the secondary school. The fourth type is the teacher for the handicapped—the blind, the deaf and the dumb. This training is specialized, and advanced training in these areas is obtained overseas.

A new corps of teachers which has come to the scene recently consists of untrained or crash-trained teachers for the UPE programme. Efforts are being made to give this group formal pedagogical training so that they can do a more satisfactory job. There are three types of teacher in this group. The first comprises primary school leavers who will teach in class three and class four with the help of head teachers. After one year, they proceed to Grade C colleges where they take a year's course before they graduate as qualified teachers. The second type comprises pupils in the upper classes of primary schools who are expected to teach their fellow pupils in classes three and four. This is regarded as a stop-gap measure while the nation grapples with the problem of training sufficient numbers for UPE. Teachers of the third type are Form V and VI secondary school pupils who are taught methods of teaching while at school and are expected to teach in classes five and six in neighbouring primary schools.

Certain features characterize the teacher training programme in Tanzania. Until the recent crash programme to achieve UPE by 1977 was introduced, Tanzania had a reputation for having a very high percentage of trained teachers in primary schools, relative to other African countries.[9] In 1967, for example, all teachers in government and assisted schools were trained. The only untrained teachers were to be found in unassisted and in private schools. After the announcement that UPE had to be achieved by 1977, the percentage of trained teachers went down as a result of an influx of untrained and half-trained teachers into primary schools, especially in the rural areas.

The second feature of teacher training in Tanzania is the combination of academic and professional training, in a sequential order. Table 4.11 shows this pattern of training.

Table 4.11

Teacher Training Pattern in Tanzania

Teacher's Grade*	Primary Schooling (years)	Secondary Schooling (years)	Teacher Education (years)	Total (years)
C	7(8)***	—	2	9(10)
B**	8	2	2	12
A	7(8)	4	2	13(14)
Diploma (EO III)	7(8)	6	1	14(15)
EO IIB	7(8)	6	2	15(16)
B.A.(ED.), B.SC. (ED.)	7(8)	6	3	16(17)
PGD (Post-graduate Diploma of Education)	7(8)	6	3 + 1	17(18)

Source: Auger, G A (ed.), (see Note 2) p.67, expanded by writer

*   Designations have been changing over the years, e.g., Grade B used to be Grade I and Grade C used to be Grade II. EO III is today's Assistant Education Officer etc. It is therefore necessary to pay attention to the number of years rather than to the designation at the end of the course.[10]

**   There are no more Grade B teachers by training. In their place one finds Grade B teachers by promotion on merit from Grade C.

***   Figures in parenthesis refer to the period before primary education was shortened from eight to seven years, which was done in the mid-sixties by phases taking a few regions at a time; now all schools are seven-year primary schools.

The third feature is the high teacher/student ratio in the school system at the primary level. In 1961, this was 1:45.5, i.e. each teacher taught an average of 45.5 pupils. The inevitable result was that teachers were not able to pay sufficient attention to each child, with consequent impact on the quality of teaching and teaching methods. In this respect matters have not improved. In 1976 the ratio was 1:53.3.

The fourth feature of teacher training is the quality of the trained teachers. In 1961, 82.1 per cent of all teachers in the primary schools were either Grade B or C while 13.2 per cent were Grade A. Four per cent were untrained and 0.7 per cent were graduates. The last group taught in special schools for children of expatriates and officials of Tanzanian origin. In order to raise this quality, the government instituted certain programmes. Plans to increase and upgrade the education of teachers at all levels were made under the First Five-Year Plan. They included the following:

Discontinuation of the training of Grade B teachers as soon as the intake then in training had completed their course. (See Table 4.11 for definition of their training). This was due to the plans of post-independence Tanzania to extend all secondary schools from Form II (Standard X) of the colonial period to Form IV, which is co-terminal with School Certificate Examinations (Cambridge Examinations at Ordinary Level).[11]

Phasing out of the training of Grade C teachers before the expiry of the Five-Year Plan. (See Table 4.11 for definition).

Up-grading of large numbers of Grade C teachers to Grade B and from Grade B to Grade A.

Instituting for a selected group of Grade A teachers a two-year course at Dar es Salaam College of National Education leading to a higher diploma.

It is to be noted that many of these plans were later abandoned as the pace of development increased and other political and economic factors came to the fore.

The fifth feature of the teacher training programme was the Diploma of Education course for holders of the Higher School Certificate, i.e. students with a six-year secondary education. According to plans laid down for the course it was supposed to last two years, but practical problems necessitated shortening it later to one year. Each batch of fresh intakes was expected to be 20 strong. Before long it became evident that not only was the duration rather long but the numbers being trained were too small to meet the needs of the nation.

Apart from the formal teacher training courses lasting for a year or more, another type of course was introduced for those who had already been teaching for some years. This might be termed retraining or in-service training. It took many forms: short seminars, workshops, correspondence courses and residential courses.

While the quality of primary school teaching depends on the quality of teacher training, the latter depends on the quality of the teacher trainers. Although it is not always possible to gauge the quality of a teacher trainer one useful index is his academic background. The following tables show the trend in Tanzania.

Table 4.12

(a) Staffing Teacher Training Colleges (Tanzanians), 1961–1974

Year	Graduates	Diploma Holders	Grade A	Others	Total
1961	1	2	48	40	91
1964	8	19	25	148	200
1965	21	35	9	18	83
1974	129	224	47	24	424

(b) Staffing Teacher Training Colleges (Expatriates), 1961–1974

Year	Graduates		Diploma Holders	Grade A	Others	Total
	Trained	Untrained				
1961	21	3	9	27	—	60
1965	38	62	8	6	21	135
1974	10	1	3	1	—	15

Source: Ministry of National Education *Statistical Handbook 1961–1974* Dar es Salaam: Ministry of National Education, 1974 (Swahili, mimeo.)

There were untrained teacher trainers every year except for 1966, 1970 and 1971. The number of expatriate teacher trainers has been on the decline in general, but a new upward trend for teachers of special subjects, e.g. English language tutors, technical subject tutors, etc., is shown in recent reports.

3. Innovations in teacher education
In response to the people's demand for more school places for their children, and the national need for better quality education, greater relevance and practical orientation of the school curricula, several innovations have been introduced. The most prominent one is the shortening of the training period. Courses which used to last two years now last one year, or even less. Whether or not this has been detrimental to the professional performance of new teachers is yet to be determined.

While teacher training for the primary school cadre was shortened by a year, that at the university was compressed within the existing degree structure to produce the concurrent degree programme. This makes it possible for students to graduate within the three years required for completing the non-education programme, by taking education çourses alongside the academic subjects. Teaching practice is done during the long vacations, after the first and the second year.

At the other end of the spectrum is the untrained teacher who has been encouraged (although not for long) to teach without having attended courses in methodology and pedagogy in a formal institution. Between the two extremes are teachers who acquire their skills as they go along through such means as correspondence courses, teachers training by radio and training on the job with the help of experienced teachers. Some teachers go to training colleges after a spell in the National Service or after attachment to TAPA, which runs its own schools.[12] Such teachers have experience in working with youth and bring to the colleges a certain background knowledge which contributes to their effective training.

By far the most important innovation is the experiment to produce hundreds of teachers in response to the call for UPE; the related training programme has been briefly referred to in the article on primary education in this book.

4. The teacher in the community
Teacher training in Tanzania has had to take into account the qualitative as well as the quantitative needs of the nation. As regards quality, the nation expects

professionally trained teachers who have specific skills to impart to the young. The type of skills required are those which will enable the recipient to be self-reliant and productive. The nation also expects the teacher training institutions to produce enlightened and informed citizens who know their nation's policies and programmes. Since there is a declared policy to aim for, this means that ujamaa must not only be understood by teachers but also practised by them. The training institutions will have to be in the frontline in producing this type of teacher and in setting an example for others to follow.

Members of the community and the larger society have voiced criticism of the poor quality of teaching and of teachers. A recent study[13] reported dissatisfaction in society with teachers' behaviour, in particular their lack of discipline, an important component of quality. There were complaints against teachers who embarked on private business during school hours, or did not go to work early thus setting a bad example to the children they taught; teachers who drank one too many for efficiency and good discipline. These complaints, if true and widespread, lead the community to lose faith in the teachers of the young generation. Society expects teachers to set an example, to be a model of good citizenship and moulders of the youth. When they fail to live up to this expectation, their image in society deteriorates.

However, not all observations made in the survey were critical. Sympathy was also expressed, especially in regard to the amount of work and responsibilities assigned to teachers. The following list was produced:

Teachers teach both children and adults;
Teachers act as cultural leaders;
Teachers organize the TANU Youth League, the youth wing of the political party;
Teachers engage in functional literacy projects;
Teachers occupy leadership positions in the party branches and its affiliates, like UWT, NUTA, and DYL ;
Teachers are involved in nation-building activities;
Teachers are involved in public holiday activities.

The list is formidable, and the sympathetic observers point out that with such a wide range of roles to play, a teacher gets so exhausted that he is unable to be effective in any of them. Those who were interviewed recommended that:

The number of teachers should be increased;
Other bodies should be required to take the load off the teachers' shoulders;
Teachers should assume a co-ordinating role with regard to adult education programmes;
Teacher training institutions and tutors in them should be given greater responsibilities over students in training and those already trained;
Substitute teaching should be introduced to alleviate crisis situations;
The number of inspectors should be increased and they should be made mobile so that they can travel quickly and easily to and from schools. They should be consultants and give help where it is needed and should monitor trouble spots early.

The survey also pointed out that there are areas where the community itself is to blame for the diminishing quality of teacher performance. It was noted that the relationship between teachers and community leaders left much to be desired. The latter tended to order the former about or ridicule them in public or interfere with their work. These factors made teachers unhappy and led to loss of interest in their work resulting in poor performance. Lack of housing is another matter in which the community could be held responsible for low motivation among teachers, and so is their relatively low pay. It has been argued, however, that compared with the per capita income in the nation, teachers are not too badly off.

While the question of quality has received much public attention, that of quantity has also exercised the minds of those responsible for education. Taking into account national needs and output from training institutions, it is obvious that without the revolutionary methods of teacher training employed, it would be impossible to achieve any of the goals set by the nation. Table 4.13 corroborates this statement.

While the needs for teaching staff can be expressed in terms of numbers, the capability of the nation to meet them must be gauged in monetary terms. For every teacher engaged, the means must be found to pay for his house, his remuneration, his teaching materials etc. These costs have to be met by the community. Table 4.14 indicates the implications for the tax-payer and the community concerned.

Table 4.13

Teaching Staff Projections, 1974–1980*

Year	Primary		Secondary		Teachers' Colleges		Total	
	Output	Shortage	Output	Shortage	Output	Shortage	Output**	Shortag
1974	3578	3047	128	502	75	149	3781	3 3698
1975	3578	2450	128	418	74	107	3780	2 975
1976	3578	1727	128	324	75	79	3781	2130
1977	3578	1209	128	216	74	30	3780	1455
1978	3578	766	128	119	75	3	3781	888
1979	3578	355	128	14	74	29	3780	398
1980	3580	—	128	—	75	—	3783	—

Source: Figures are extracted from working papers for the Third Five-Year Plan, 1975–76 and 1979–80, as drafted by planners in the Ministry of National Education.

*   Final figures will appear in the official document to be issued before the official launching of the plan, which was postponed due to financial difficulties.

**   The output figures are, at best, approximate to the real needs since they are subject to changes in enrolment and demographic patterns.

***   The shortages are expressed in terms of citizen staff since the target is self-sufficiency in manpower, not only in teaching, but in all sectors of public enterprises.

Table 4.14

Costs of Primary Education, 1975/76–1979/80 (in Tsh)

Year	Teachers' Quarters*	Teachers' Salaries**	Teaching Materials	New Classrooms***	Total
1975–76	79 060 000/=	242 232 000/=	191 997 733/=	103 500 000/=	398 780 933/=
1976–77	52 340 000/=	375 408 000/=	121 751 990/=	72 320 000/=	283 952 790/=
1977–78	84 700 007/=	258 756 000/=	148 281 762/=	105 940 000/=	364 797 362/=
1978–79	104 666 000/=	363 228 000/=	261 986 274/=	132 100 000/=	535 069 074/=
1979–80	46 780 000/=	451 428 000/=	278 997 345/=	131 280 000/=	501 300 145/=
Total	545 140 000/=	3 675 400 000/=	1 691 105 200/=	1 1002 115 104/=	2 083 900 304/=

Source: Figures from Third Five-Year Plan working papers. Totals may not be very accurate. Self-help being an important element in the estimates, the figures given are on the low side especially for teachers' quarters, teaching materials and new classrooms.

*   Teachers' quarters are estimated at a very modest 20000/= each.

**   Teachers' salaries are calculated at 14400/= p.a. for Grade C and A teachers, i.e. an aggregate of one Grade C and one Grade A teacher.

*** Each new classroom is estimated to cost 20000/=.

To rich countries these figures may not be very impressive, but when it is considered that the educational budget accounts for a sizeable chunk of the Tanzanian national budget, then education is clearly an expensive business.

5. The university and teacher training

The university has been involved in teacher training for over ten years, continuing a policy established during the colonial period. When higher education was introduced in East Africa[14] and centred at Makerere in Uganda, teacher training was one of the main preoccupations of the university. In the 1920s through the late 1940s, Makerere trained secondary school teachers for East and Central Africa. When Makerere attained University College status (under special relationship with London University), teacher training took two forms: training of non-graduate and of graduate teachers. Graduate teachers did their B.A. or B.Sc. degree work first and then spent an extra year studying pedagogy to obtain a Diploma in Education. Non-graduates took a two-year teacher training programme after an initial two years of academic work at the University College.

The University College of Dar es Salaam decided to adopt a concurrent degree and teacher training programme. In practice this means that on graduation the student is ready to begin teaching. The pattern of courses at the university is as follows:

Concurrent B.A./Education programme:

First Year   Education courses, four units
    Non-Education courses, ten units
Second Year   Education courses, two units
    Non-Education courses, ten units
Third Year   Education courses, two units
    Non-Education courses, ten units

At the end of first and second years, students spend six weeks doing teaching practice in different schools/colleges in the country.

The education courses are run by the Department of Education, which is an integral part of the Faculty of Arts and Social Science. Courses in non-education areas are taken in either the Faculty of Arts and Social Science departments or the Faculty of Science departments. Courses in Education cover a wide range, as follows:

First Year   Theory, History and Practice of Education, Sociology and Psychology of Education, Teaching Practice
Second Year   Curriculum Development, Educational Measurement, School Organization and *one* of:
    Teaching Methods in Secondary School subjects
    Teaching and Planning in Adult Education *plus* Teaching

Practice. Third Year   One course each from (a) and (b):
    (a) Philosophy of Education
    Sociology of Education
    Adult Education

Contemporary Education in East Africa
Psychology of Human Development and School Learning
Social Psychology of Learning
Economics of Education
(b) Educational Administration and School Organization
Test Construction and Evaluation
Research Methods in Education
Library Education
Art Education
Audio-Visual Education
Physical Education
Music Education
Drama in Education (Theatre Arts)
Primary Swahili Literacy Skills

The new graduates are posted as secondary school teachers or college tutors (teacher trainers) or as planners of adult education. Some get posted to other training institutions such as the College of Business Education, the Institute of Development Management, the Dar es Salaam School of Accountancy, etc. In the past, a few education graduates have been assigned to administrative posts immediately upon graduation as principals of colleges, student advisers in Foreign Service and so on.

Realizing the need to train non-education graduates who wish to teach, and in response to the demand for teachers with differing competencies, the Department of Education has recently introduced the Post-graduate Diploma in Education for candidates from different academic and professional backgrounds.

To increase the depth and breadth of knowledge of those involved in education, the university offers courses for the M.A. in Education. This is a one-year course which covers such areas as Foundations, Curriculum Development, Policy Planning and Administration, Research Methods and Independent Study leading to an M.A. thesis. There are candidates who take the M.A. Education by thesis and the Ph.D. Education by dissertation. Other Faculties conduct studies in their specialized fields.

6. The position in 1975/6
Before looking into the prospects for teachers and teacher training in Tanzania, some facts and figures on the current positions are given in Tables 4.15 and 4.16.

Table 4.15

Total Number of Teachers, 1975/76

Primary Schools	28 783
Secondary Schools	1 947
College of National Education	612
University	434

Table 4.16

Total Enrolments by Educational Levels 1975/76

Primary Schools	1 532 953
Secondary Schools	38 327
Colleges of National Education	9 080
Universities: Dar es Salaam (Tanzania)	2 644
Makerere (Uganda)	89
Nairobi (Kenya)	125
Overseas	907
Total	1 584 125

Source: Elinewinga, I N *Budget Speech, Ministry of National Education Estimates for 1976/77* Dar es Salaam, 1976

7. The future of teacher training

It is becoming abundantly clear that there must be serious planning for new methods of training teachers in Tanzania. Small numbers of high-quality teachers will have to give way to large numbers of average-quality teachers, if the demand for teaching personnel arising from such needs as UPE is to be met. Besides, the emphasis on practical education in schools calls for a new type of teacher who can teach practical skills alongside academic disciplines. It may not be possible to produce an adequate supply of this type of teacher immediately, but re-training of those already in service might help. The possibility of employing untrained teachers who possess practical skills is being looked into, and schools are encouraged to make full use of skills available in the community.

Multi-media methods in teacher training are another approach for the immediate future. The radio is being used to train and retrain teachers; correspondence courses are mounted for teachers in training in the schools; newspapers have occasional articles useful for teachers.

In-service training, seminars, workshops, weekend professional meetings are going to feature more and more prominently in the future. Teachers, tutors, principals, headmasters, classroom teachers are all involved in a nationwide retraining exercise set afoot by the Party and government. Some attend political education classes, some mathematics workshops, others chemistry seminars etc. lasting between a day and a year.

Training of future teachers in secondary schools has already started and may become the main method of training teachers in the future. Alongside their academic and practical work, boys and girls in secondary schools are introduced to pedagogy and can thus be useful to their communites as teachers immediately upon completion of their secondary education.

These are just a few of the ways in which the problem is being tackled. With the political will of the leadership and determination of the people, it will be possible to produce a teaching force of the size and type required by the people. For the only valid criterion is whether or not the provision meets the people's demands. Ideas about 'international standards' still linger on, but the will to set up relevant national ones will triumph.

Notes

1 Cf. Cameron, J and Dodd, W A *Society, Schools and Progress in Tanzania*, p. 187 Bibl. 64
2 See Auger, G A (ed.) *Institute of Education and Department of Education Handbook, 1968* Dar es Salaam: University College (1968) p. 60
3 See Castle, E B 'A Proposal for Institutes of Education in East Africa' in: *Report of the Conference on Institutes of Education, Mombasa, Kenya, January 27–30, 1964*, edited by A J Lewis and L V Lieb
4 See Note 3, p. 2
5 See Note 3, p. 13
6 See Ministry of National Education *Programme Grade 'A' Teacher Education*, p. 2 Bibl. 126
7 See The United Republic of Tanzania *The University of Dar es Salaam Act, 1970* Bibl. 179
8 See Note 6, pp. 6–15
9 See Note 2, p. 67
10 As designations have changed again in 1976, it is difficult to be consistent in their use. The present designation of teachers at the primary level are: Teacher Grade IIb, Teacher Grade IIc, Teacher Grade IId, Teacher Grade IIIa, Teacher Grade IIIb, Teacher Grade IIIc; see Elinewinga, I N *Budget Speech, Ministry of National Education Estimates for 1976/77* Dar es Salaam, June 1976
11 Up to independence, classes were designated Standards I, II, etc. up to Standard XII which also coincided with the number of years a pupil had normally been in school, e.g., Standard X meant that he was in his tenth year of studies. After independence, the term 'Forms' was introduced to distinguish between classes in primary and in secondary schools. Thus primary school classes were called Standards I–VII and secondary school classes Forms I–VI.
12 TAPA is one of the affiliates of TANU and runs primary, secondary and craft schools.
13 The Report on the survey by the National Advisory Board on Education has not yet been made public at the time of writing. These are general statements from the working papers. Some observations have appeared in the Readers Forums in the newspapers—*Daily News* (government newspaper), *Uhuru* (Party newspaper), *Kiongozi* (Catholic Church newspaper), *Mfanyakazi* (Swahili word for worker) and *Sunday News*, which appear weekly. Admittedly, this covers mainly the literate and vocal section of society.
14 Makerere was founded in 1922, University College Dar es Salaam in 1961, the University of East Africa in 1963, the University of Dar es Salaam in 1970.

Chapter 5 The Non-formal and Formal Sector in Education and Training of Adults

I Basic Education in Adult Education

5.1 The Decision-making Machinery of Adult Education in Tanzania
Y D M Bwatwa

1. The beginnings

Historically, adult education in Tanzania can be traced back to the colonial era; but at that time it was nobody's particular responsibility. For a while it was supposed to be one of the functions of the Social Welfare Department. R W Blaxland, Social Welfare Organizer in Tanganyika, stated:

'Social welfare centres had been constructed before my appointment as social welfare organiser because the government was afraid that there might be trouble after the demobilization of the army among the soldiers who were used to canteen facilities.'[1]

At the time of independence, only a few Tanzanian adults had had higher education. The task of organizing adult education was, therefore, assumed by the TANU party under the leadership of its President, Mwalimu Julius K Nyerere, as one of its tools for developing the country. The decision-making machinery of adult education has thus been part of the TANU machinery, which has changed continually since 1954. The vital importance of adult education for the development of Tanzania was officially recognized in the First Five-Year Plan and further emphasized in the 'Arusha Declaration', the Second Five-Year Plan and the TANU guidelines and resolutions. All of these are products of the TANU decision-making machinery.

2. The First Five-Year Plan (1964–1969)

This plan embodied TANU's policy, to be implemented by the government and its institutions. It was President Nyerere, the architect of Tanzanian ideology, who emphasized the importance of adult education.

In his Presidential address to Parliament on May 12th 1965, Mwalimu Nyerere said:

'The purpose of government expenditure on education in the coming years must be to equip Tanganyika with the skills and the knowledge which is needed if the development of the country is to be achieved . . . first we must educate adults. Our children will not have an impact on our economic development for five, ten or even twenty years.'

This appeal by the President to the members of Parliament to implement the education of adults in Tanzania has been instrumental in producing progressive decisions, furthering the development of the country.

3. The 'Arusha Declaration'

TANU has been committed to building socialism and self-reliance since early 1962, but to achieve this goal it became necessary to overcome ignorance and encourage adult education. In order to enable the people to understand and implement the national policy they had to be taught to read and to write, as well as to develop and use their intelligence and knowledge. For these purposes TANU opened Kivukoni College, providing adult education at all levels. In 1967 President Nyerere announced the 'Arusha Declaration', which had been approved by the TANU National Executive Council, the decision-making machinery of Tanzania since the formation of the party in 1954. In this declaration TANU stated:

'The second condition of development is the use of intelligence. Unintelligent hard work would not bring the same good results as the two combined. Using a big hoe instead of a small one; using a plough pulled by oxen instead of an ordinary hoe; the use of fertilizers; the use of insecticides; knowing the right crop for a particular season or soil; choosing good seeds for planting; knowing the right time for planting, weeding, etc.; all these things show the use of knowledge and intelligence.'[2]

All of these things are adult education. In addition to the National Executive Committee, President Nyerere and other TANU leaders have acted as decision-makers either through guidelines, directives or speeches. For instance in his speech on the 'Arusha Declaration', the President said:

'People cannot participate in developing their country as free citizens if they are ignorant of their rights and obligations and of the policies of their own country. Nor can ignorant people learn from their fellow-men or from their past and

133

correct and adapt their plans accordingly. The gap of knowledge between the developed and developing nations is always widening and Tanzanians would be left behind in this technological age if they did not wake up and embrace adult education as a tool in their own development. There is a further danger that ignorant people could become slaves of their environment or systems in their organizations which they could control for their own benefit only if they were knowledgeable.'[3]

In that period, implementation of adult education in Tanzania was widened and specific decision-making powers were vested in responsible leaders or institutions.

4. The Second Five-Year Plan (1969–1974)

The strategies for implementing adult education in the rural areas of the country were first spelt out in the Second Five-Year Plan:

'The main emphasis in adult education in this plan period will be on rural development. It will include simple training in agricultural techniques and craftsmanship, health education, housecraft, simple economics and accounting, and education in politics and the responsibilities of the citizen. In rural areas, virtually the whole of this work will be conducted in Swahili. Literacy will be included in response to popular demand, as people become aware of its functional importance.'[4]

The Second Five-Year Plan named various institutions that were involved in the process of implementing adult education:

'The characteristic feature of adult education is that various organizations participate. Among them are government departments, TANU, UWT, the co-operative movement and the churches. Part of the work to be done is the co-ordination and encouragement of existing activities and another part is the promotion of new activities.'[5]

Decisions concerning adult education at the grassroots were made the responsibility of community leaders and community centres:

'The general principle is to place the main organizing responsibility on the primary school. The school will then become a community educational centre, at which the provision of primary education is only one function. A school so conceived will increasingly become a focal point for the total educational needs of the community, rather than serving as a somewhat detached institution for the education of children. The general responsibility for adult education activities of the centre will rest with the headmaster. It will be the duty of the headmaster to ascertain community needs, to identify suitable instructors and to arrange classes. Each headmaster would have at his disposal a small grant for equipment and materials.'[6]

The president of TANU transferred the duties of adult education from the Ministry of Regional Administration and Rural Development to the Ministry of National Education. During the period 1969–1973, a Directorate of Adult Education was created. It had four sections:

1. Design and Co-ordination Section
2. Functional Literacy Section
3. Workers' Education Section
4. Inspection and Evaluation Section.

At this juncture the decision-making machinery was expanded through the establishment of the National Adult Education Committee, a subcommittee of the National Advisory Committee on Education (NACE). Its function is to advise the Minister on policy matters pertaining to adult education. The membership of NACE was drawn from TANU, NUTA, UWT, TAPA, TYL, CUT, IAE, Voluntary Agencies and other Ministries involved in adult education.

5. The new era

To promote the development of adult education in Tanzania the TANU Central Comittee decided to make 1970 an Adult Education year. On December 3rd 1969, President Nyerere announced the new era to the nation and explained the philosophy and aims of adult education. He called on the people to realize the importance of adult education, emphasized the need for careful planning of programmes, and challenged all educated Tanzanians to participate fully in carrying them out:

'For a long time we have been saying that we must educate the adults of Tanzania. I myself have pointed out that we can not wait until our educated children are grown up before we get economic and social development; it is the task of those who are already full grown citizens of our country to begin this work.'[7]

In 1969, 62 administrative officers attended a residential training course in the history, philosophy, methodology and organization of adult education at Kivukoni. The following year their number increased to 71. These administrators became the decision-makers in their districts and organized seminars for teachers of adult education in their respective areas. This was followed by a national mobilization campaign to implement adult education programmes at all levels. Funds for this purpose were allocated as shown in Table 5.1.

In 1971, President Nyerere called on six districts in Tanzania to do their utmost to eradicate illiteracy by December 9th 1971. He stated:

'We have done quite well recently, especially as we have used experience gained in earlier campaigns, so that the learning is more interesting and relevant to adults. Thus, in the first nine months of this year, almost 200 000 people were attending literacy classes . . . everywhere in the country, make further efforts. *But in six districts* I am asking that a very special effort should be made so as to eradicate illiteracy completely. These districts are Ukerewe, Mafia, Masasi, Pare, Kilimanjaro and Dar es Salaam. In these districts I hope that every citizen will be able to read and write by 9th December, 1971. That would really be an achievement to be proud of!'[8]

Following this speech, party and government officials went into action organizing the campaign in these six districts. Mass mobilization was carried out, and a large number of literate persons, stimulated by the President's directive,

Table 5.1

Government Expenditure on Adult Education in Tanzania 1969–74

Year	Estimates	Approved Estimates	Actual Expenditure*
1969–70	—	—	2 457 495/ =
1970–71	9 960 500/ =	—	7 828 908/ =
1971–72	—	11 071 800/ =	11 009 001/ =
1972–73	18 732 700/ =	7 258 200/ =	—
1973–74	20 185 400/ =	—	—

Source: Directorate of Adult Education, *1971 Annual Report*. Dar es Salaam: Ministry of National Education.
*Figures do not include external funds.
/ = Tanzanian shillings
Missing figures not available

were utilized in the adult education programmes. Adult education committees were set up and helped to register illiterates. The results are shown in Table 5.2.

6. TANU resolutions and directives
(i) Resolutions
In 1971 President Nyerere presented the results of development in Tanzania to the TANU Biennial Conference, a decision-making body of the party. He stressed the importance of adult education as a life-long learning process bound up with living and working:

'Just as working is a part of education, so learning is a necessary part of working . . .. But learning must become an integral part of working and people must learn as and where they work . . .. It is therefore essential that we should stop trying to divide up life into sections, one of which is for education and another, longer one of which is for work with occasional time off for 'courses'. In a country dedicated to change we must accept that education and working are both parts of living and should continue from birth until we die.'[9]

The conference then decided that all literate persons must participate in the adult education programmes as part of their work. But Resolution No. 22 directed that plans be made to wipe out illiteracy in Tanzania within the next four years. At the fifteenth session on September 18th–26th 1971, the TANU Annual Conference, another important element in the decision-making machinery, adopted the following resolutions on adult education:

Clause 20:
The Annual Conference bears in mind the important role that adult education plays in the development of man, ujamaa and democracy. Therefore it congratulates the government and all those who have made adult education a success since the Party President appealed to the entire nation to participate.

Table 5.2

Results of Literacy Campaign in Six Districts, 1971

District	Total Population	Illiterates January, 1971	Number Registered During Campaign		Total M/F Registered	Success of Campaign (Percentages)
Mafia	16 748 (Based on 1967 census)	8 545 (known)	M	3499	8599	100
			F	5100		
Kilimanjaro	473 832 (Based on 1967 census)	46 510	M	17692	45466	97
			F	27774		
Pare	149 635 (Based on 1967 census)	24 121	M	8888	24121	100
			F	15233		
D'Salaam	600 000 (Presidential Speech)	100 000 (estimated)	M	12834	28306	28.3
			F	15472		
Masasi	227 858 (Based on vaccination records)	51 973	M	20775	45364	89
			F	24589		
Ukerewe	109 277 (Based on 1967 census)	36 000	M	11992	35843	99.6
			F	23851		

Source: Directorate of Adult Education, *1971 Annual Report* Dar es Salaam: Ministry of National Education

M: Male

F: Female

Clause 21:

The Conference has been very much impressed by the efforts made by the people of Mafia which enabled them to wipe out illiteracy completely before December 1971 as a response to the President's appeal.

The Conference congratulates and gives special acknowledgements to all Mafia residents for that success and calls upon all leaders and people all over the country to learn the methods used. Moreover, the Conference appeals to all literate Tanzanians, especially workers, to participate in adult education programmes. The Conference also directs that from now on education should be part of work at all places of work, and plans for implementing this directive should be made.

Clause 22:

The Conference acknowledges that the great success which has been realized in the field of adult education recently is a product of the revolutionary methods which have been used; therefore it urges the government to take necessary steps for changing the methods now in use in primary schools and find ways and means of reaching our target for Universal Primary Education.'[10]

(ii) TANU directives

In 1970 and 1973, the TANU President and Vice-President respectively issued directives to the effect that the heads of all national, regional and parastatal institutions were to form councils to deal with continuous education of adults, and that one hour per day should be set aside by all public or private establishments for continuing adult education for every worker.

In 1974, the National Executive Committee passed a resolution changing the regulations for University entrance. Unless otherwise stated, only adults with work experience were to be admitted. At the same sitting the TANU NEC decided to revolutionize the education system by pushing the target date for Universal Primary Education forward to 1977. The guidelines issued stressed the following objectives of UPE:

De-emphasis of examinations and more weight to be given to the overall performance of students including (1) agricultural (2) other self-reliance work. The many new schools needed to reach the target will have to be built on a self-help basis, minimizing material support from the government.

Any type of building may be used as classrooms and standards of buildings are suspended.

Teachers will be recruited in the villages, in Umoja wa Wanawake Tanzania (The Women's Organization) and in the community. Co-operative societies must contribute money to pay them.

Untrained teachers will only be given seminars and short courses before starting the work.

Teaching materials cannot be provided in normal quantity and quality.

As only main guidelines were issued, without detailed instructions on their implementation, fulfilment of these objectives involves local or community decision-making machinery—the grassroots.

7. Some results achieved by the decision-making machinery

The decision-makers for adult education in Tanzania have attempted to involve the educated as well as the 5.86 million (cumulative figure) illiterates, of whom 2.56 million or 44 per cent were males and 3.30 million or 56 per cent were females. The enrolment of illiterates in adult classes has been rising steadily, as shown in Table 5.3.

Table 5.3

Enrolment of Illiterates in Tanzania 1971–75

Year	Enrolment
1971	908 351
1972	1 508 204
1973	2 989 910
1974	3 303 103
1975	5 184 982

Source: Ministry of National Education *Annual Reports on Adult Education (1971–75)* Dar es Salaam: Ministry of National Education.

Nation-wide literacy tests were held in 1975. The tentative results presented in Tables 5.4 and 5.5 show that the decision-making machinery has been able to achieve substantial progress towards eliminating illiteracy in Tanzania.[11]

Table 5.4*

Results of the Nation-Wide Literacy Tests, 1975

Level	Males	Females	Total
III	548 287	578 906	1 127 193
IV	405 457	376 361	781 818
Total Number of Successful Literates	953 744	955 267	1 909 011

Source: Mbakile, E P R *The National Literacy Campaign: A Summary of Results of the Nation-Wide Literacy Tests*, p. 34 Bibl. 158
*The figures are tentative.

Table 5.5

The Illiteracy Rate in 1975*

Males	Females	Total
34%	44%	39%

Source: Mbakile, E P R *The National Literacy Campaign: A Summary of Results of the Nation-Wide Literacy Tests* p. 35 Bibl. 158
*Estimated percentages.

8. The future of decision-making

The basis of the decision-making machinery for adult education in Tanzania has been a political one involving the grassroots in the process. Very soon, the two political parties, TANU and Afro-Shirazi, will be joined into one strong liberation party. And it is to be hoped that decision-making on adult education will then be still more effective than it has been before.

By careful planning, TANU, with the clear objectives of ujamaa and self-reliance, has been able to help, direct and promote adult education through national campaigns. Tanzania's political ideology and its decision-making machinery provide a strong driving force for the promotion of adult education. The decisions taken have made adult education work-oriented. They have enabled the people to acquire knowledge and relevant skills and to apply this knowledge and these skills to the problems existing in their environment. The people have been made participants in discussing party issues and implementing self-reliance projects. These innovations will be lasting ones. Thanks to TANU's decision-making machinery, adult education in Tanzania has assumed a unique position. It has grown from a non-development process in colonial times to a sophisticated national work-oriented programme based on a strong political foundation.

Notes

1 Blaxland, R W 'Mass Education in Tanganyika' *Overseas Education* 22 (January 1951) No. 2, p. 52
2 Nyerere, J K *Ujamaa—Essays on Socialism* Dar es Salaam: Oxford University Press (1968) p. 31
3 Ministry of National Education, Adult Education Division 'The National Policy of Adult Education in Tanzania' in *Comparative Adult Education* by I Sallnäs, pp. 24–25
4 The United Republic of Tanzania *Tanzania Second Five-Year Plan for Economic and Social Development* . . ., p. 157 Bibl. 18
5 See Note 4
6 See Note 4
7 Nyerere, J K *Freedom and Development* London: Oxford University Press (1973) pp. 137–138
8 Nyerere, J K 'Annual Presidental Speech to the Nation' in: *The 1971 Literacy Campaign Study* by L Budd et al., p. 6 Bibl. 151
9 See Note 3
10 *Resolutions of the 15th TANU Biennal Conference* Dar es Salaam: National Printing Company, 1973
11 For more information on illiteracy and the literacy campaign in Tanzania see the article by S Malya 'Literacy—A Work-Oriented Adult Literacy Pilot Project and a National Campaign', pp. 141–152 of this book.

5.2 Literacy—a Work-oriented Adult Literacy Pilot Project and a National Campaign
S Malya

Introduction

For the past five years (1970–1975) there has been a literacy campaign that is a component part of a bigger concerted effort by Tanzanians to liberate themselves. This campaign is to be seen as a mass movement which forms the backbone of the entire adult education endeavour whereby TANU, the Government and the Peoples of Tanzania are bent on bringing about economic and social justice by means of rural transformation, self-reliance (this does not mean self-sufficiency), and eradication of poverty and ignorance through enlightenment and hard work.

1. Adult literacy prior to 1969

It is true that in the years prior to 1969 there were attempts to attack illiteracy as a stumbling block to development. But it is equally true that these efforts were on the whole ill-defined and shortsighted. The teaching of literacy to adults was usually conducted as though adult literacy was an end in itself. There was no real plan to integrate it with adults' daily work. Adult literacy was handled more or less in the same fashion as the teaching of the three Rs to school children.

This way of teaching adult literacy was further characterized by a lack of distinct philosphy that took into account Tanzania's real situation. There was no purposeful co-ordination, no curriculum. There also existed a serious shortage of trained personnel and teaching materials. There was no provision for follow-up reading materials and no evaluation. Consequently this 'traditional' way of teaching adult literacy was generally ineffective. A more tangible and practical approach had to be sought, defined in clear-cut terms and implemented.

2. An aspect of the general census of 1967: interpretation of its implications for literacy

One of the results of the general census of 1967 was the identification of the number of illiterate adults in mainland Tanzania.[1] It was noted that out of 13 million people in the country, over seven million were adults (i.e. over 15 years of age), both men and women, and that about 75 per cent of them were illiterate. This meant that there were over 5 250 000 adults who were unable to read or write. It was these adults who formed the productive sector of the population. In order to enlist their participation in reconstruction and development, they had to be made conscious of the need for change. To enable them to be aware of this need there had to be a dialogue between them and the agents of change on what it was that had to be changed. It was at this point that adult literacy was recognized as an essential medium of the dialogue on development and change.

It was further noted that out of six million youths, about three million were of school age. Yet half of these, that is over 1.5 million youths, did not go to school at all, either because schools did not exist near their homes or, where schools did exist, there was apathy towards schooling. This meant that in addition to the

5.25 million adults, there were 1.5 million youths who were going to become adults without knowing how to read and write.

It was noted, moreover, that over 90 per cent of the total population lived and worked in the countryside and that the rate of illiteracy in the rural areas as compared to that in urban areas was overwhelming. The implication of this was that any serious attempts to eradicate illiteracy had to be focused largely on the rural areas.

It was noted further that owing to the lack of follow-up materials, previous efforts to attack illiteracy had been somewhat wasted because about 60 per cent of the adults who had become literate were relapsing into illiteracy. The implication of this was that in future attempts to combat illiteracy, sound steps would have to be taken for the provision of follow-up reading materials at the same time as the efforts to teach literacy were being conducted.

Finally, it was noted that the incidence of illiteracy was some 10 per cent higher among women than it was among men. Since women are our homemakers, this was an important observation. For homes are microcosms of a bigger community, the nation. Hence the urgent need to give special attention to attacking illiteracy among women and prepare relevant reading materials capable of inducing them to continue reading and avoid relapsing into illiteracy. The number of women being so large and their role being so vital, it would be hopeless to expect to transform the society without their participation. It is difficult to think of a better place to begin combating illiteracy than in the home, but this will not be possible if parents themselves, especially mothers, are illiterate.

So this was the overall picture regarding the incidence, of illiteracy in Tanzania that emerged from the census of 1967. A sad picture, indeed, and it was felt that something had to be done.

No other statement points out the ethics upon which Tanzania is going to be constructed as a nation more lucidly than does the 'Arusha Declaration'. In it, one of the principal aims and objectives of TANU is given as:

'To see that the government mobilizes all resources of this country towards the elimination of poverty, ignorance, and disease.'[2]

This is an important development regarding the literacy drive in Tanzania. TANU has never been afraid to enlighten the citizens of Tanzania. It would be this party that would direct the government on what to do, and not vice versa.

Indeed TANU has taken literacy as one of its major responsibilities. It realized that it could enlighten the masses only marginally if they were illiterate. The first important step therefore was to make them literate. Thus as soon as TANU recognized the need for literate citizens in the construction of the nation, adult literacy ceased to be a mere task to be done. Henceforth combating illiteracy became a political issue which no government institution could dare to ignore.

Apart from giving the problem of illiteracy a political significance and drive, the 'Arusha Declaration' also provided a well-defined philosophy based on mass participation; for it is from the masses—the peasants and the workers—that TANU acknowledges its existence and power. As regards the direction education was to take, this philosophy was further expounded in the document 'Education for Self-Reliance'.

In sum, it is reasoned in the document that in order to avoid exploitation of man by man there ought to be equal educational opportunities for all. There is no room for elitist education. And all stages of education, starting from the primary stage, must be geared towards the requirements of the community where most of the citizens live. But it is not realistic to talk of equal opportunities for education in a situation in which the majority of the people are illiterate while a few have many years of formal schooling. In the policy of socialism and rural development the masses are expected to participate fully. But their chances to do this are severely limited by the fact that they are illiterate. Hence the importance of the literacy campaign as a key to mass mobilization. After the 'Arusha Declaration' and 'Education for Self-Reliance', the handling of the literacy problem in Tanzania entered a new phase and became integrated, more and more, in the national development plans.

In the First Five-Year Development Plan, adult education is recognized officially as crucial if the plan is to succeed, for, as President Nyerere observed on introducing it, it is the adults and not the children who will have an immediate impact on the country's development. With the shift in emphasis to rural reconstruction the need to co-ordinate various bodies engaged in adult education is stressed and, as an initial step in organizing adult education in the country, a major responsibility is placed on primary schools, while increased importance is attached to the training of adult educators.

3. A work-oriented adult literacy pilot project

In 1968–69 Tanzania was one of 12 countries participating in the Unesco/UNDA Experimental World Literacy Programme. The Tanzanian project, a five-year programme initiated in Mwanza, was planned for illiterate peasant farmers and established around Lake Victoria in four pilot districts for a number of reasons: the area was one of the most important economic zones in the country, producing cotton and coffee as major cash crops and foreign exchange earners, as well rice, bananas, and tea; other activities included fishing and cattle-keeping; the zone was the most densely populated area in Tanzania; it has a well-established educational infrastructure, a good number of extension personnel, and two large well-established co-operative movements for cotton and coffee growers. Illiteracy was thought to be one of the major bottle-necks in the process of introducing or enhancing socio-economic changes, in particular the diffusion of agricultural innovations. Groups of illiterate farmers were therefore to undergo programmes of instruction which would closely link literacy to vocational skills in improved farming.

This functional literacy pilot project had probably been by far the most well defined, intensive and organized attempt towards the work-oriented approach in adult education in Tanzania. According to the operational plan, the specific objectives of the project were:

'to teach illiterate men and women basic reading and writing, and to solve simple problems of arithmetic, utilizing as basic vocabularies the words used in agricultural and industrial practices;
to help them to apply the new knowledge and skills to solve their basic economic, social and cultural problems;

to prepare them for a more efficient participation in the development of their village, region and country;

to integrate the adult literacy and adult education programmes with the general agricultural and industrial development of the country.;

to provide the necessary and adequate reading materials, impart the knowledge of community and personal hygiene, nutrition, child-care and home economics, which will help to improve family and community life, provide opportunity for a continuing education and avoid relapse into illiteracy.'[3]

Teaching and learning materials used in the project included primers on:

Cotton-growing	(Primer I and Primer II)
Banana-growing	(Primer I and Primer II)
Rice-growing	(Primer I and Primer II)
Fishing techniques	(Primer I and Primer II)
Cattle-rearing	(Primer I and Primer II)
Home economics	(Primer I and Primer II)
Political education	(Primer I and Primer II)
Tobacco-growing	(Primer I)
Maize-Growing	(Primer I)

Each of these primers was accompanied by teachers' guides and practical demonstration guides. In addition, rural newspapers as well as teachers' newsletters were prepared and circulated within the four districts. A network of rural libraries and radio groups was also established. The purpose of all these things was to create literacy surroundings in the four districts on an experimental basis.

Assessment of project results

The project results were to be discussed in relation to the purpose, objectives and major activities of the project.

The project achieved, to a large degree, the main purpose assigned to it, namely, to assist the Government of Tanzania in organizing and implementing a work-oriented adult literacy pilot project, closely linked to vocational training, particularly in agriculture. The Government of Tanzania decided in 1971, before the project came to an end, to launch a campaign to eradicate illiteracy throughout the country by 1975. In this campaign, which was accorded national priority in terms of financial and manpower resources, the government decided to adopt:

'the functional literacy approach piloted by the project;

the project's system and procedure for the selection of both primary school teachers and voluntary teachers as functional literacy teachers;

the project's programmes and decentralized system for training such teachers by selecting and training;

the administrative field structure developed and tested during the expansion phase of the project;

an extensive programme of follow-up to provide reading materials for new literates through such measures as the establishment of rural libraries and the preparation and distribution of rural newspapers along the lines developed by the project;

the project's assistance in establishing writers' workshops throughout the country, similar to those used in the pilot projects, for preparing work-oriented literacy materials produced by the project in additional areas of the country;
the introduction of functional literacy as a subject into the teaching programmes of the university colleges of national education and agriculture training institutes;
the continuation of interministerial co-operation and co-ordination at the national level as practised in the pilot project.'[4]

Despite these successes, the project's operations met with some failures and problems: evaluation failures; lack of a coherent in-service training scheme for all categories of literacy teachers; weaknesses in the field supervisory machinery; inadequate teaching materials for literacy classes and field demonstrations; lack of sufficient competent personnel to conduct agricultural demonstrations to ensure that a proper functional approach was maintained; breakdowns in production and distribution of rural newspapers; lack of proper reading materials for rural libraries.

Some of these problems were bound to happen considering that work-oriented adult literacy and its evaluation were innovations without precedent in the country where they were being applied, and that the life-span of the project did not allow for proper consolidation work to be done.

Although the original goals fixed for the evaluation of the Experimental World Literacy Programme were not completely met by the project, a limited scientific and experimental approach was devised and put into operation resulting in preliminary findings and hypotheses for further studies. Subject to the availability and analysis of more data, as well as the limitations placed upon the evaluation exercises, preliminary findings (which should be taken with caution) indicated the following:

'A positive response among the learners was observable, particularly to the practical aspects of the programme. This was manifested more clearly in the implementation of some of the recommended production-increasing agricultural practices.
The standard of living of participants appeared to be positively affected by the programme's impact, particularly that part represented by health and nutrition, although less clearly by housing conditions and consumption.
A trend towards the shaping of attitudes concerning education and economic improvement appeared to be taking place.
The acquisition of technical information on questions concerning some agricultural, health and nutrition practices appeared to be taking place.
Some participants did manage to acquire certain levels of literacy skills particularly in the fields of arithmetic and reading, less so in the field of writing. However, the project's operational objective of bringing its participants to the level of four years of primary schooling could in most cases not be achieved. The majority of participants who showed measurable literacy skills attained the level of two years of primary schooling.'[5]

Other factors affected the project results, as revealed by the following evaluation findings:

'indication that the training of approximately two years was not enough for the majority of the participants in any programme to become functionally literate; indication that the training cycle was affected by high drop-out rates and drop-in rates, shorter life of classes in months and sessions, relatively low attendance rates and time utilization;
indication that although the majority of participants in most programmes were women, it was they who dropped out more often then men;
indication that individual deficiency in the knowledge of the Swahili language acts as a stumbling block in the learning process.'

Although motivational studies which could have given, among other things, some indications for behaviour and performance of literacy classes were not attempted, a number of socio-economic and cultural factors do emerge to account for most of the class instability. Such factors include: social and cultural obligations, domestic problems, ill-health, scarcity of basic necessities, adverse weather conditions, farm-oriented activities, poor leadership at the grassroots level, and the physical and social environment surrounding the classes, particularly when teaching is in progress. Any or a combination of these factors could impair the stability and progress of the teaching and learning processes.[6]

4. The national literacy campaign

By 1970, the adult education movement in Tanzania had taken a definite direction under the guidance of TANU. While addressing the nation on the eve of the new year, President Nyerere reiterated one of the TANU vows: 'I shall educate myself to the best of my ability and use my education for the benefit of all.' He then proceeded to designate 1970 Adult Education Year in the country and stressed the three broad objectives of adult education as (1) to shake Tanzanians out of their resignation and make them realize what they can do for their community and for themselves; (2) to provide people with the skills necessary to bring about change in their environment; (3) to foster nation-wide understanding of the policies of socialism and self-reliance.

From that year, the organization of life-long education on a national level began. A Directorate of Adult Education was established within the Ministry of National Education, thus giving adult education a status equal to all other forms of education such as Primary, Secondary, Technical or Teacher Training. This Directorate had the responsibility of co-ordinating adult education activities in each district through a network of primary schools which had to be used as adult education centres, apart from catering for schooling needs of the young.

Indicating the preoccupation with adult education, the President again took literacy as the theme of his message to the nation on the eve of the new year 1971. After pointing out the achievement made in 1970 in appointing and training adult education officers in each district, he made the point that if illiterates are not to be exploited by those who know how to read and write, and if each adult citizen is to play a complete role in development, then the high incidence of illiteracy in the country had to be removed. So to begin with, six districts had been selected for intensified literacy campaigns and assigned the duty of ensuring that illiteracy disappeared by December 9th 1971, the tenth anniversary of independence.

146

With the experience gained from this campaign and from the feedback received from the Literacy Project in Mwanza, the Party, at its Biennial Conference in 1971, resolved that the entire nation had to work for total eradication of illiteracy by the end of 1975. All governmental, parastatal and voluntary organizations had to mobilize their resources and ensure that within four years from 1971 every adult Tanzanian would be able to read and write.

In order to have an effective literacy campaign on a national level that would lead to the wiping out of illiteracy by the end of 1975, a number of organizational steps were taken by the Ministry of National Education. In the first place, a National Advisory Committee on Adult Education was formed. Similar committees were formed at regional, district, division, ward and cell levels. Even individual functional literacy classes established their own adult education committees. From the grassroot level, for example, the ten-cell leader is a key person in the whole system. Under this type of leadership, it was expected that it would be possible to identify adult literacy problems at all levels up to the national level and involve all institutions.

Another step was that of appointing Adult Education Officers, otherwise designated Regional Adult Education Co-ordinators. They were charged with the responsibility of organizing and co-ordinating all adult education activities in their respective regions. It was also part of their duty to widen educational opportunities for adults, especially in the rural areas. To assist them, District Adult Education Officers were appointed to every district.

Thirdly, there was training of permanent teams of trainers at the national, regional, district, divisional and ward levels. The tasks of these teams were, first, to instruct those who were going to handle the actual teaching of the three Rs to illiterate adults in the methodology of teaching functional literacy. In other words, these teams formed corps of trainers for functional literacy teachers at the various levels. Their second duty was to sit on the adult education committees at their respective levels so that, in collaboration with other leaders on that level, they could advise on what should be done and who should be involved.

Fourthly, as far as possible, the teaching of functional literacy in various regions was conducted in accordance with adults' needs in their day-to-day lives in those regions. Primers and other teaching materials for this purpose had been developed by the Literacy Project and reproduced on a large scale by the Ministry of National Education.

Fifthly, intensive publicity was carried out throughout the country on the need to be literate. So wide and effective has the campaign been that adult literacy is often taken to be all there is to adult education! By the end of 1971, over 1 500 000 adults had enrolled in the Ministry of National Education centres alone.

Evaluation of the progress showed that up to October 1974, 3 180 000 adults had enrolled in adult literacy classes. That is to say, about 63 per cent of illiterate adults in 1967 had shown a willingness to expose themselves to the literacy process.

To mobilize over three million adults to enrol in adult literacy classes is, however, far from being a guarantee that the adults will actually attend, given the well-known problem of drop-outs. Even less certain is whether the adults who have enrolled and attended will eventually become literate. Several

Table 5.6

Performance up to October 1974

Region	Percentage of population enrolled*	Region	Percentage of population enrolled*
Arusha	15	Ruvuma	63
Dar es Salaam	33	Tanga	65
Kigoma	37	Lindi	67
Tabora	37	Rukwa	67
Iringa	53	Mara	70
Shinyanga	57	Mtwara	75
Pwani	58	Dodoma	78
Mbeya	60	Morogoro	92
Kilimanjaro	61	Singida	95
Mwanza	63	West Lake	100(?)

*Out of adults who were registered as illiterates in 1967.

problems have been identified as having caused partial enrolment. They include: weak participation by leaders, especially at the grassroot level; lack of trained literacy teachers (currently there is a squad of about 100000 teachers from primary schools, and volunteers); insufficient teaching materials; poor transport facilities; implementation of other national projects; vacant adult education officer posts, especially from the district level downwards; and priority given to such important occupations as farming and population movements, mostly to planned villages.

5. Nation-wide literacy tests
The following definitions have been given of literacy in the Tanzanian context:

'A person is literate if he is able to read and write letters within the family, is able to locate streets, buildings, etc., to observe danger warnings in the streets and at work, to follow simple directions in many everyday situations, to read a newspaper to keep up with current happenings and to obtain information, to keep records, to read "how to do it yourself" books, little books on better living, better foods, better ways of farming, etc.

An individual is literate when he has acquired the essential knowledge and skills which enable him to engage in all those activities in which literacy is required for effective functioning in his group and community and whose attainment in reading, writing and arithmetic makes it possible for him to continue to use these skills towards his own and his community's development.

Adult literacy, an essential element in overall development, must be closely related to economic and social development priorities and to present and future manpower needs. All efforts should therefore tend towards functional literacy. Rather than an end in itself literacy should be regarded as a way of preparing man for a social, civic and economic role that goes beyond the limits of rudimentary literacy training, consisting merely in the teaching of reading and writing. The very process of learning to read and write should be made an opportunity for acquiring information that can immediately be used to improve living standards; reading and writing should lead not only to elementary general knowledge but to training for work, increased productivity, a greater participation in civic life and a better understanding of the surrounding world, and should immediately open the way to basic human culture.'[7]

On August 12th 1975, nation-wide literacy tests were administered. Primary schools were closed so as to allow teachers and the premises of primary schools throughout the country to be available for this exercise. Following the overall results of the literacy tests it is possible to categorize people who participated in the national literacy campaign, thus:

'Level I: A participant who has enrolled but must have attended two-thirds of the literacy sessions in any one year of literacy activities.

Level II: A participant who qualified for Level I above, but who also has successfully passed one or both tests for the following sub-levels:
Sub-level (i):
A person who is able to recognize words and/or symbols, writes letters of the syllables, writes numbers and/or arithmetic signs including mental calculations.
Sub-level (ii):
A person who is able to read a short, simple meaningful sentence, is able to write a simple short sentence and can add and subtract one-figure numbers.

Level III: A person who qualified for Level II above, but who also has successfully passed one or both tests for the following sub-levels:
Sub-level (i):
A person who is able to read a short, simple meaningful sentence, is able to write a simple short sentence and can add and subtract two-figure numbers.
Sub-level (ii):
A person who possesses mastery over symbols in their written form, or is able to encode and decode written messages. Such a person should be able to perform the following: be able to read fluently a simple text with understanding (the text itself being based on common syllables and vocabularies in the functional primers and according to the most frequent syllables and vocabularies used in the Swahili language). He should also be able to write a simple short message or passage, add and subtract three-figure numbers, multiply two-figure numbers, and divide by one figure.

Level IV: A person who continuously used the acquired literacy skills. Such a person should have qualified in Level III above, but also should be able to read and write messages; to read a newspaper (for example, *Uhuru*, *Ukulima Wa Kisasa*, etc.) to keep up with current happenings and obtain information; to read "how to do it yourself" books, little books on better living, better food, better ways of farming, etc.; and to keep records and solve simple arithmetic problems. He should also be able to keep a simple book of accounts on income and expenditure.' [Note] 8

Hence people who passed Level IV in reading, writing and arithmetic are literacy graduates, while those who passed only Level III are functionally literate adults.

The results of the Literacy Campaign can be gauged from Tables 5.7 and 5.8. Data provided by the campaign and the nation-wide literacy tests in August 1975 revealed that the cumulative figure of illiterates had been somewhat higher than was shown by the census in 1967, namely about 5.9 million, out of which more than five million had enrolled in literacy classes.

Table 5.7

Numbers of Illiterates and Enrolments According to Sex, Prior to August 1975

Sex	Illiterates	Enrolments
Males	2 561 221 (44%)	2 287 921 (44%)
Females	3 299 216 (56%)	2 897 061 (56%)
Total	5 860 437 (100%)	5 184 982 (100%)

Source: Mbakile, E P R *The National Literacy Campaign . . . p. 18 Bibl. 158*

On their performance in the nation-wide tests, an estimated 1.9 million adults can be called literacy graduates or functionally literate adults according to the above definition.[9] The estimated figures for the other levels are shown in Table 5.8.

Table 5.8

The Estimated Illiterate Population According to the National Definition of Literacy as of August 1975

	Males	Females	Total
Did not Enrol	297 200	378 255	675 455
Below Level I	211 945	343 895	555 840
At Level I	361 407	521 888	883 295
At Level II	760 825	1 023 658	1 784 483
Total	1 631 377	2 267 696	3 899 073

Source: Mbakile, E P R *The National Literacy Campaign . . . p. 35 Bibl. 158*

Thus in 1967, Tanzania had an estimated illiteracy rate of about 75 per cent. In 1975, after a hard struggle through the national literacy campaign it had been possible to reduce the illiteracy rate to 39 per cent and to have many people at levels II and I who may become literate within a few years if the concerted effort is continued.

6. Post-literacy literature and writers

Who will be the readers of prospective writers in Tanzania? At present, certainly those adults who fall within Levels III or IV. In the early stages of the literacy campaign the adult participant's main concern was learning to read, to write and to count. Now the adult learner is concerned with reading as a tool for learning to live better.

Considering a writer as a potentially powerful adult educator, there are four themes from which topics for books could be chosen, given the circumstances of a country like Tanzania. A writer has to be clear in his own mind as to which areas deserve emphasis: whether or not his material will be oriented towards practical subjects, towards pleasure, towards information or towards solving problems.

It seems clear that, for a writer to play a useful function as an adult educator in Tanzania, he would have to consider the following priority themes in the order they are presented:

(a) Work-oriented literature: Since a big proportion of adults who qualify as new literates are peasants, herdsmen, fisherman, workers or housewives, writers ought to direct their attention to literature that will enable a peasant to select better seeds and take better care of the soil on which he toils. A herdsman will be looking for literature that will help him tackle problems related to destroying vermin, producing more and better milk and meat. A worker in an industry will be interested in such literature as will enable him to understand the nature of profit and loss, safety at his place of work, punctuality, electricity and spare parts of the machinery he uses. Similarly, a housewife will be interested in post-literacy material that will help her raise her family, feed it, keep it clean and healthy.

(b) Crafts and technology-oriented literature: There is room for literature that will assist adults to have more meaningful control over their environment. For instance, how to build better and permanent houses, how to make and maintain simple tools like hoes and ploughs, how to construct tools. Associated with these skills are crafts such as brick-making, tailoring, carpentry, masonry, tin-smithery and pottery.

(c) Information-oriented literature: Then there is a need for literature that will make the newly literate adult a broad-minded individual. He will be living in an ujamaa village, for example. He will need information related to the policy of ujamaa. He will need to read and understand national policies of socialism, self-reliance and co-operation. Since he will be a producer and consumer of goods he will need to have information on money, industries, markets and how these are related to neighbouring countries as well as the world at large. It is here that such subjects as political education, geography, history and economics become relevant to a newly literate adult.

(d) Pleasure-oriented literature: The fourth area is reading for pleasure. It is an area to which the majority of writers in Tanzania have addressed themselves,

with the result that out of about 700 book titles, more than three-quarters are either novels or stories. While there is no intention to play down the importance of this type of literature, especially in promoting our culture, it would seem that for newly-literate adults it has a rather subsidiary significance. An adult in our country will first of all look for literature that will enable him do something better than he did before.

According to the Director of Adult Education in the Ministry of National Education, by 1974 the following steps had been taken to provide for follow-up reading materials:[10]

Over half a million books have been despatched to the regions to establish rural libraries. Ultimately each of the 1 760 wards is to have a library.

A book-production unit has been established, and through it some three million 'graded follow-up books' are so far under preparation.

Thanks to the IAE, 15 different titles in the 'Juhudi Series' have been produced. Every region has formed its own book-production committee consisting of six members. These committees are charged with the responsibility of ensuring that books suitable and relevant to the regions are produced. A number of manuscripts prepared by these committees are being studied for production into books.

As a direct result of the literacy campaign, writers of books for the newly literate Tanzanian have a rapidly expanding market. For those who have specialized knowledge on 'how to do' something, there is no limit on how many books they could write, provided that they are aware of the audience for whom they are writing and the problem they wish to see solved.

Notes

1 See Egero, E and Henin, R A (eds.) *The Population of Tanzania. An analysis of the 1967 population census* Bibl. 6

2 *The Arusha Declaration and TANU's Policy on Socialism and Self-Reliance* Dar es Salaam: TANU, Publicity Section (1967) p. 2 (e)

3 UNDP, Special Fund *Plan of Operation*, p. 3

4 Mbakile, E P R *The National Literacy Campaign* . . ., p. 10 Bibl. 158

5 See Note 4, pp. 10–11

6 See Note 4, p. 11

7 Mbakile, E P R *Radio Education Programmes as a Support to Literacy Methods: The Experiences in Tanzania*, pp. 3–4 Bibl. 159

8 See Note 7, pp. 5–6

9 For a few more results see the article by Bwatwa, Y D M 'The Decision-Making Machinery of Adult Education in Tanzania', pp. 132–140 of this book

10 'Adult Education Lessons Geared to Production', 'Face the People' Interview with E. Kibira *Sunday News* (15.12.1974.)

5.3 Literacy and Development: What is Missing in the Jigsaw Puzzle?

Y O Kassam

The basic proposition in the concept and programme of functional literacy revolves on the fact that if literacy has a potential role to play in generating development, then its impact can be greatly enhanced if it is made functional by relating it directly to the major economic activity of a given community, and to the national priorities of economic development. The crux of a functional literacy programme, in other words, is the simultaneous integration of literacy skills and vocational training on a selective and intensive basis.

The theory and hypothesis behind the concept of functional literacy sound very appealing and convincing. But do the evaluations of the functional literacy projects in different countries show any evidence that the functional literacy approach is an effective method of generating socio-economic development? As far as the evaluation of the Tanzanian functional literacy project[1] is concerned, the evidence on such a question is very shaky. For example, the 1971 cotton programme of the Tanzanian project has shown that out of the 13 indicators of socio-economic development which were actually measured and whose results were reported in definite and precise terms, only four, or about 30 per cent, revealed a significant positive change at 0.01 level. These four indicators were: use of modern equipment and practices, nutrition habits, agricultural knowledge and quantitative knowledge. Eight indicators, or about 69 per cent, revealed an insignificant positive net change, these being possession of durable goods, consumption, health practices, interest in education, level of socio-economic aspiration, participation in economic organizations, participation in social and civic organizations, and health and nutrition knowledge. One indicator, namely housing conditions, showed no positive net change at all. One may conclude, therefore, that the evaluation results do not indicate a definite and substantial improvement in the socio-economic life of the participants involved, but only a few small tentative trends of change and improvement.

Some of the most important and crucial indicators, such as production, productivity and income, were not measured because they were found to be of enormous complexity. The project treated the indicator relating to the use of modern equipment and practices as a 'proxy' measure of productivity, but such an exercise leaves much room for speculation.

On the attainment of literacy itself, if was found that apart from some proficiency in arithmetic, the participants' performance was on the whole poor. Furthermore, the majority of the participants who had shown some measurable literacy skills had attained a Standard II level of literacy and not Standard IV level which was the operational objective of the project. The revelation of the generally low attainment in literacy challenges the hypothesis of the 'built-in motivation' of a functional literacy programme whereby it is argued that since the subject matter of the primer is directly related to the occupation of the learners, the need to become literate takes on a meaning and a purpose. The evaluation of the project did, however, come up with a most interesting finding, namely that participants tended to do better on vocational skills even with low performance on literacy.

It should be noted that the evaluation of the Tanzanian functional literacy project has to contend with a lot of problems and constraints. And in any case, it would probably seem quite reasonable to argue that the impact of a given educational programme on economic growth and social change is a long-term proposition. Substantial and discernible changes could more realistically be measured over time, and inducing change among rural peasant communities has not proved easy anywhere.

Although the evaluation results of the functional literacy project in Tanzania have been rather discouraging, the fight against illiteracy should and must continue. For there is no doubt that given a literate population, development can be greatly accelerated. Besides, literacy is a human right irrespective of its relationship to development. On the other hand, it is a myth to think that a person who is illiterate is not capable of learning a host of useful things, or that he is not capable of achieving his own development and of contributing to national development. However, in talking about the causal relationship between literacy and development, a number of other important factors and variables tend to be overlooked. In other words, the eradication of illiteracy per se is not necessarily an automatic instrument of bringing about development. The questions to ask are: What are the various 'interrelationships' that weave around literacy and development? What are the other factors and variables that go hand in hand in the jigsaw puzzle of literacy and development? Let me summarize the possible answers to these questions in the following way:

(i) Notwithstanding the 'built-in motivation' of the functional literacy approach, the rural peasants, first and foremost, need political mobilization and the awakening of critical awareness of their environment. In the words of President Nyerere, the first objective of adult education in Tanzania is 'to shake Tanzanians out of a resignation to the kind of life they have lived for centuries past.'[2] The psycho-social approach in literacy teaching as advocated by Paulo Freire[3] very much reflects the point made by President Nyerere. Freire argues for the need to engage the illiterate adults in the process of 'conscientization' which can change their pessimistic and fatalistic perspective on reality and enable them to acquire a 'critical' vision of their environment and an awareness of their capacity and means to change this environment. It would seem, therefore, that without this preliminary mobilization and raising of the people's conciousness, literacy, be it 'functional' or of any other kind, cannot make its desired impact on their development.

(ii) Teaching adults how to improve and increase their agricultural produce through functional literacy cannot be fully effective if the peasants cannot financially afford to adopt the recommended agricultural practices, e.g., the use of fertilizers and insecticides. Furthermore, they tend to lose the incentive to produce more if the price offered for their products is very low while at the same time their buying power is considerably reduced by heavy inflation.

(iii) The peasants' efforts at increased agricultural productivity are hampered if their basic health and nutrition conditions remain poor.

(iv) Many developing countries are trapped in the vicious circle of economic dependence on the industrialized and capitalist countries. Such dependence makes it difficult for the developing countries to build a 'self-centred' economy which could generate adequate surplus, and which in turn could be invested in producer goods in order to generate more surplus. In the absence of a self-centred economy, literacy, and for that matter education in general, does not really contribute to the development of the majority of the people. Consequently, to use a common phrase, the poor countries are becoming poorer and the rich countries continue to become richer. India is a classic example illustrating the fact that education alone cannot bring the desired development for the majority of the people in an economy that is 'outward-looking', i.e. not self-centred. For, on the one hand, India has mass illiteracy and, on the other hand, and paradoxically, it faces the problem of a surplus of very highly educated people who cannot be absorbed into its own economy. To conclude, while some development can take place without literacy, literacy does not automatically bring about development. Under certain conditions, however, literacy can greatly accelerate development. In other words, the causal relationship between literacy and development is not so simple and linear as some people tend to assume. The relationship is multi-dimensional and therefore depends on the interplay of a number of other factors and forces. Some of these factors or pieces in the jigsaw puzzle of literacy and development have been outlined above. But, of course, this list of factors is not exhaustive. Rather than make global generalizations on the relationship between literacy and development, there is probably a need to analyze such a relationship in the total context of a given country's political, economic, social and cultural forces.

Notes

1 UNDP/Unesco *Work-Oriented Adult Literacy, Pilot Project Lake Regions of Tanzania, Final Evaluation Report, 1968–1972* Mwanza (May 1973)
2 Nyerere, J K 'Adult Education Year' in: *Freedom and Development* p. 137. Bibl. 12
3 See Freire, P *Pedagogy of the Oppressed* New York: Herder and Herder (1970)

5.4 'Chakula ni Uhai'—a Radio Study Group Campaign in Mass Adult Education
B A P Mahai, H Hinzen and A K Joachim

Major educational attempts to free Tanzanian society from poverty, disease and ignorance have been made in the form of mass education campaigns with the use of radio, printed materials and study groups combined as interrelated parts of a single effort. Most important examples are the 'Mtu ni Afya' (Man is Health) and the 'Chakula ni Uhai' (Food is Life) campaigns; both involved millions of adults.

After some smaller pilot projects[1] dealing with political, economic and historical contents, the health education campaign, 'Mtu ni Afya', a radio study group campaign, was the first to reach the masses in the rural areas. That is to say: it reached the target group, farmers of both sexes and of all ages, in almost all villages.[2]

As a follow-up to the health education campaign, 'Chakula ni Uhai' again took health as one subject but combined it with two other closely related problems: food production and food consumption. All three are part of the vicious circle of poor nutrition, poor health, poor work, low productivity. Of course, this is a simplified view ignoring other factors which contribute to or hinder agricultural production and a healthy life; for a deeper analysis the whole range of historical, political, social, economic and cultural factors in their relation to development should be taken into consideration.

In the present study, a more descriptive presentation with some critical comments and recommendations concentrating on the campaign itself has been chosen. Though these mass campaigns have their drawbacks, which will be discussed in the later part of the paper, they have achieved noticeable successes and there is every reason to believe that given more thought and proper planning they can be greatly improved.

1. Elements of radio study group campaigns
In its search for appropriate materials and methods to provide educational opportunities for the rural masses, Tanzania made use of the radio which, being spread widely all over the country, is relatively easily accessible and can transmit useful knowledge to the illiterates as well. The discussion group method, where the people sit together, discuss their affairs, decide on how to improve their living conditions, and an action-oriented component, to take action as a group or individually, are other important elements.

The radio study group method requires:
building up a national co-ordination committee;
writing of study materials;
preparation of radio programmes;
training group advisers;
setting up regional, district, and divisional teams for supervision;
organizing groups;
creating a system of formative, decentralized evaluation.

2. The case of 'Chakula ni Uhai'

The campaign had the following main objectives:

to inform adults on diseases caused by malnutrition, to convince them of the necessity of a balanced diet and teach them how to prepare it;

to encourage peasants and workers to increase and diversify food production in order to make Tanzania self-reliant in food supplies;

to encourage decisions and actions on the basis of self-reliance following the participation of all group members in discussion.[3]

A National Co-ordination Committee was formed 18 months before the official launching of the campaign.[4] It had members drawn from various Ministries and other bodies concerned with the provision of adult education: the Ministries of National Education, Agriculture and Health, the University of Dar es Salaam Faculty of Medicine, Kivukoni College, TANU, IAE, and others. It was supported by a Material Working Committee which dealt with co-ordination and planning, the preparation of study materials, publicity, and the development of a formative evaluation from the initial stage to the last stage of the programme.

The National Co-ordination Committee, whose centre was the IAE, had some troubles performing its functions. In particular, it was difficult to get all the members together whenever a meeting was convened. This was due to problems of communication and other commitments at the time of meetings. Another problem, caused by frequent changes of representatives from ministries or parastatals, was that of continuity in planning and organizing.

The National Co-ordination Committee divided the campaign into three stages. The first stage was the preparatory and publicity phase, in which the study materials were written, the radio started publicizing the campaign through songs, a signature tune, announcements on the content and the methodology of the campaign, and the group leaders were trained. The second stage, officially launched by President Nyerere on June 2nd and ending on September 29th 1975, was the implementation phase of the campaign. Study group members met to listen to the radio for 15 minutes, then read the relevant chapter in the book. Then they started discussing the given information in relation to their own experiences, and finally agreed on possible solutions. The third phase was that of establishing follow-up programmes, writing reports on the problems faced and solutions found by the study groups. These reports were written at district, regional, and national levels. During the final phase, reports from the various regions were broadcast so as to inform the public of the degree to which the campaign had been successfully implemented. The duration was from October 1975 to March 1976.

The *written materials* produced were to guide the study groups in attaining knowledge about improved methods of agriculture, about diseases like kwashiorkor and marasmus, about nutritional habits of eating and preparing a balanced diet to combat the malnutrition affecting many parts of the country. These printed materials had to be written in simple Swahili and in short sentences so as to make them easy to read. The books were accompanied by attractive pictures and diagrams relevant and related to the environment of the target population. According to the feed-back from the participants, most parts of the textbooks were found to be comprehensible and educational, but there were criticisms that some sections had contained too many technical terms which had sometimes not been translated into simple Swahili and were difficult to understand.

The initially-estimated number of study group members was 1.5 to two million; exactly 1.5 million books were printed and distributed. Thus, in many parts of the country, not every participant of a group received a book. In some regions the books only arrived weeks after the launching of the campaign, leaving the groups without study materials. Where this coincided with a bad reception of the radio programme, the groups could not work properly.

The 15-minute *radio programme*, on the air on Mondays and repeated on Wednesdays, combined some repetition with new information on the campaign content; in addition there were announcements about the campaign, music, and interviews with participants and organizers. On the whole the radio programme was liked by the participants who called it informative and educative, and stated that it had a motivating effect. But in many places groups did not have radios, and in some areas the reception was bad at the time the programme was transmitted.

The *training of study group advisers* prior to the official launching of the campaign was another element in the planning of the campaign. A training system in stages was developed at national, zonal, regional, district, and divisional levels, and started five months before the beginning of the second phase of the campaign. In those training seminars the history and objectives of the campaign, the content of the textbook, group leadership and other matters related to the campaign were taught. According to the reports from the districts and regions, and to observations made by the members of the evaluation section, the major problem in conducting these seminars was that instead of having three days for training, especially needed at the lower levels, in many cases the seminars on the divisional level lasted only one day because the funds had been almost entirely spent at the district level. This was apparently not enough for proper training, and quite a few of the problems in the groups were due to this lack of training.

The study group advisers were to be supported by *visiting teams* from the respective divisions and districts. The members of these teams were drawn from the Ministries of Agriculture, Health, and National Education, from UWT, TANU and others agencies involved in the training seminars for the study group advisers. During the campaign they had to visit the groups in their areas to provide additional motivation and much-needed help in running the study groups. Lastly these teams were to write a joint report evaluating the effectiveness of the campaign at their respective levels.

From the reports obtained, and some crosschecking by the evaluation section it is obvious that many study groups were not visited by these teams during the campaign period or after, so that these groups were left without any assistance. In some cases this was due to either lack of transport or commitments in other projects, e.g., the national literacy examinations or the election campaign. Experience has indicated that, where a study group was visited and given further help, the output was greater than in study groups that were not visited throughout the whole campaign.

As far as the *study groups* are concerned, reports have shown that the initial plan to have eight to fifteen members in each group was not adhered to. Some groups had 30 or even 60 members. One reason was that many of the groups were literacy classes—not surprisingly, since about 80 per cent of the adults in Tanzania were then in literacy classes—and it was felt difficult to separate members who had been used to each other for a long period. This obviously had an impact on the discussion style in the groups; often enough participation in the discussion was rather limited, and the group adviser actually become a teacher. In some places the group advisers did not appear to have control of the group discussion method as anticipated; some of them seemed to be simply dictating without caring about participatory procedures in putting and answering questions related to the given topic. In addition, most women if mixed with men tended to be shy, and so men dominated the discussions for many reasons, some of which are historical and traditional.

In spite of these difficulties the groups took steps to improve their living conditions by starting thousands of *projects*. Many groups cleared land for gardens and starting growing vegetables like lettuce, cabbage, and tomatoes. In many places participants decided to undertake poultry-keeping projects in order to get eggs and meat. Both types of project will supply the people with the protein and vitamins urgently needed for a balanced diet. In parts where it is difficult to get sugar, people started bee-keeping. Many day-care centres for children and canteens for workers were opened, or are at planning stage. Most of these projects are running on a self-help basis to intensify and integrate the concept of self-reliance.

In addition to these directly visible projects, *knowledge* of diseases like marasmus and how to prevent them, of the necessity of having a balanced diet and how to prepare it, was improved. The realization of the aim to make Tanzania self-reliant in food crops and to further enhance the production of cash crops was urged in 'Chakula ni Uhai', and is hoped to be another side-effect. But only the future will show how far the achievements are continuous; a follow-up in one way or another is definitely necessary.

In order to cross-check the information obtained from the districts and regions, to assist the evaluation section in doing some additional research of its own on special problems, and to *build in formative evaluation* that could be used to improve the programme while the campaign was in progress, a well-designed evaluation format was developed. It was jointly produced by many REOs (AE) and DEOs (AE) several months before the official launching of the campaign. Several different evaluation instruments such as attendance registers, question-naires on food habits, and a knowledge-gain test have provided the evaluators with most important details on the implementation of the campaign and its problems as well as on the participants themselves. They are now being further analyzed. Problems were caused by lack of materials, and in some places also by insufficient technical know-how on evaluation methods, due to a lack of proper training. The decentralized system of evaluation involved many people from the ward up to the national level in accordance with the aim that all those who plan, organize, implement, and participate in a project should also be the evaluators of their own programmes. On the national level a report is now being prepared which will combine the results from all districts with the separate findings made by the evaluation section.

3. Concluding remarks

Finally, it may be appropriate to draw attention to a few general problems and questions. What will be the future for radio study group campaigns in Tanzania? One of the findings that must be closely looked into is the necessity to integrate the planning, financing, and manpower requirements of such mass adult education activities with the yearly plans of the regions and districts. In addition there is a need for integration with other major activities. For instance, 'Chakula ni Uhai' interfered with the national literacy examinations, the election campaign, and the villagization programme; launching it a few months later would have solved that problem.

Or should Tanzania in the future have regional or district campaigns in order to come even closer to the differing needs of the various parts of the country? Or should we start off with a nation-wide programme and then, after some weeks, diversify it regionally, putting emphasis on specific problems? Or should we in the near future concentrate on follow-up projects that are closely related to the content of 'Mtu ni Afya' and 'Chakula ni Uhai', such as poultry, fishing, or garden projects with a built-in educational element? How can we strengthen the educational element in other campaigns like the villagization programme, the cotton-growing programme, and how can the IAE come still closer to the people living in the rural areas and thus render them an even better service?

4. Suggestions for radio study group campaigns in other countries

Without a doubt, as a result of the experiences gained in five radio study group campaigns, each of which aimed to reflect the overall Tanzanian policy on adult education more fully than the preceding one, some elements in these campaigns are now rather unique to the Tanzanian context. However, there are also valuable findings open to generalization.

Earlier in this article, seven elements of the campaign format were stressed as being, in the authors' view, the most important for Tanzania. In the following, some tentative suggestions are put forward for those who may be thinking of introducing radio study group campaigns for adult education in their own countries.

In respect to the overall adult education policy, it may be useful if the campaign is supported by:
a policy statement relating adult education clearly to the overall national goals;
a clearly defined target group—for most African countries, the masses living in the rural areas;
an identification of their educational needs:
an administrative structure for providing adult education programmes from national down to village level.

For radio study group campaigns, it may be advizable:
to start with small pilot schemes in order to develop local manpower for administration, book-production, radio-programming, training, and so on, for later mass campaigns;
to start planning long—maybe a year—before the first programme is to be broadcast, in order to allow for contact to be made with various bodies that should be involved in the preparation (materials, radio programmes, training) and implementation (organization, supervision);

to produce materials related as closely as possible to the needs, cultural background, and aims of the campaign (e.g., simple language, large letters, pictures, music, both educative and entertaining);

to publicize the forthcoming campaign rather early (posters, radio spots) to get, if possible, some early feedback;

to make use, as far as possible, of local resources regarding manpower (adult educators, community development staff, extension workers) and materials;

to train group advisers intensively in group leadership to enable them to stimulate lively discussions in the groups, preferably directed towards practical implementation of the newly acquired knowledge;

to prepare a systematic follow-up;

to build in formative evaluation, so that there will be a chance of improving the programme while it is running, and of receiving at the end a summative report containing useful details before starting a new campaign.

Notes

1 Cf. Kassam, Y O 'Towards Mass Adult Education in Tanzania: The Rationale for Radio Study Group Campaigns', pp. 79–84 Bibl. 153; Mlekwa, V M *Mass Education and Functional Literacy Programmes in Tanzania*, pp. 3–9 Bibl. 160
2 See Hall, B L and Zikambona, C *Mtu ni Afya* Bibl. 152
3 For further details see Mahai, B A P; Haule, G S; Timotheo, E K; Joachim, A K *Chakula ni Uhai* Bibl. 155
4 Cf. Mahai, B A P; Timotheo, E K; Haule, G S; Makene, J K; Bibangamba, J G *The First Follow-up Formative Evaluation Report of the Preparation of the 'Food is Life' Campaign* (December 1974–May 1975), and by the same authors, *The Second Follow-up Formative Evaluation Report of the 'Food is Life' Campaign* (June 12th–July 21st 1975) Dar es Salaam: Institute of Adult Education, Research and Planning Department (1975) (mimeo.)

5.5 Some Observations on Adult Education in Tanzania
M von Freyhold

Evaluation research on the impact of adult education programmes in Tanzania has been rather scarce and handicapped by close links between the evaluators and the planners of these programmes. As a result, very little is known about the needs and objectives of adult learners and the way in which adult education programmes tie in with these, rather than with the needs and objectives the planners might have had. A number of somewhat unsystematic observations made by the author as a volunteer adult-education teacher, and in the course of research dealing with rural development, may therefore contribute towards a better understanding of the reality of adult education in Tanzania. Perhaps they will also stimulate researchers to look more carefully into some of the obvious problems that arise from the present system.

1. Adult education in urban ward in Dar es Salaam

The adult-education station in the ward had been started in 1970 with a vigorous campaign of recruitment initiated by the party branch. By 1971 there was one main station and four sub-stations running classes in different parts of the area. Classes lasting for 1.5 hours each were held twice a day, in the afternoon and in the evening, six times a week. There were three courses: Beginners I, Beginners II and Advanced.

The teaching staff was composed of low-level clerical workers, domestic servants, an independent tailor, two housewives and some unemployed youths, altogether about 18 people for the five stations. Remuneration for holding one course was 30 Tsh per month, but payments were often irregular and sometimes did not arrive for several months. Sometimes there were disagreements over the remuneration. When, for instance, teachers and learners decided that classes should continue during the month of Ramadan, the teachers were later told by the District Office that they should have closed the classes and that they would receive no payment. The money was of some importance to the teachers. When they were told in 1973 that two sub-stations would have to be closed down because attendance there did not justify the teachers' remuneration, teachers were obviously not prepared to continue without payment. On the other hand, many of the teachers who arrived after an 8 hours' day of work somewhere else had a considerable commitment to the task, and at least two risked their jobs by refusing to do overtime for their employer at times when they would have missed their classes. Particularly the older teachers had a genuine understanding for the learners and treated them with respect, patience and interest in their progress. They knew without being told, that adults could not be ordered around and that it was important to praise a good performance but never criticize a failure. When a young school leaver joined the team and started to use primary school methods on the learners he was soon told that he would not be allowed to hold classes by himself and would have to assist other teachers until he had learned the appropriate style.

The afternoon classes were mainly attended by women, mostly housewives, a few domestic servants and some barmaids. The men who came in the evenings came from all kinds of unskilled and semi-skilled occupations. Attendance was poor. A class of 60-80 registered members was usually attended by about ten to fifteen people. This was partly due to the fact that some of those who had registered had yielded to party pressure but had no motivation to get involved, while others had come to attend two or three times and then decided that the course was too boring and success unlikely. No efforts were made to visit those who had dropped out and to hear their reasons.

Learning was unattractive due to the methods used. Learners spent their time repeating the lessons in the book, after the teacher. The teacher first read the lesson to the class, then the class repeated in chorus and then each individual learner repeated it to the teacher. In the end the teacher wrote some words on the blackboard, read them to the class, the class repeated them and then copied them into their notebooks. The books in use included a general literacy primer which was quite well constructed as far as the gradual introduction of new words was concerned. It contained mildly amusing stories which were, however, of limited relevance to the experiences and thoughts of urban residents. The second book was a nutrition primer admonishing people to eat sufficient proteins and vitamins without explaining how this could be done on the limited budgets available to most of the women who read it. The third was a political primer which was rather unpopular because too many complicated words were introduced too rapidly, and because the text was completely abstract with no reference whatsoever to any direct experience of the readers. After 1972 a few primers on agriculture and fishery were added which were also of limited interest to readers, most of whom were not engaged in agriculture at all.

Whatever the contents and merits of these books, there was no discussion about them, and the tedious repetition of the texts soon blocked any ideas the readers might have gained from them. The teachers had no guidelines or training which would have helped them to use other methods. After almost three years of operation the station had its first and only seminar on teaching methods conducted by a person sent from the IAE. Most of the time of this seminar was taken up by lectures on visual aids (for which the teachers had no materials) and on home economics.

The advanced course was attended by people who had learned how to read in some other context and wanted to maintain this ability. For many this was the only opportunity of doing so that they knew. No efforts were made to introduce them to newspapers and library facilities, and to enable them to become more independent of organized classroom teaching. Nor was there any provision for those who wished to pursue further education after the advanced course, since all other courses offered within the adult education system started at a higher level.

For a country officially committed to development by the people and for the people there was surprisingly little interest in using adult education as a base for communal action. Most of the women who attended the classes did not suffer so much from illiteracy but from complete dependence on poorly paid husbands and from their inability to contribute towards the maintenance of the children. Almost all of them were longing for some productive work and usually their husbands would have had no objection if they had found some work. Some of the men who came to the classes were also unemployed. The adult education station, with its links to the party branch on the one hand and the ten-cell leaders on the other, would have been well placed to articulate such needs and to collaborate with other agencies in setting up small neighbourhood factories (somewhat along the lines of the Chinese model), in which women could have used newly acquired knowledge to contribute towards their own development and the development of the country as a whole. The only timid attempt in that direction was the opening of a sewing class.

2. 'Mtu ni Afya' campaign

This country-wide campaign for preventive medicine and sanitation was conducted by the IAE in 1973. 'Mtu ni Afya' means 'man is health', a slogan which sounded meaningless or absurd to most of those who heard it for the first time. Some thought it was a printing mistake. Unlike previous campaigns, such as 'Wakati wa Furaha' which only reached a few places, 'Mtu ni Afya' did manage to get a wide coverage. In urban areas, ten-cell leaders were instructed to assemble the members of their cell and to select someone as a teacher who was trained in a brief introductory course. Adults within the ten-cell were expected to attend sessions twice a week, listen to the radio and read the text. As non-attenders were threatened by heavy fines, most people assembled for the first few sessions until discipline was relaxed. After the broadcast and the reading there were supposed to be discussions, and the groups were expected to make decisions on what they could do to combat diseases in their area. In practice, there were almost no discussions and no communal action since measures for sanitation were believed to be the task of the local authorities. 'Mtu ni Afya' was accepted as a slogan to be raised whenever the garbage collectors or the cars emptying the pit latrines or the health inspectors of markets did not provide services according to schedule. Issues which would have required the voluntary action of individuals or groups received very little attention.

In the rural districts the main problem was the lack of co-ordination between the national campaign and the activities of local departments concerned with health and community development. In Moshi district, for instance, locally proposed schemes for the introduction of improved latrines, water protection and mosquito eradication had to be shelved due to the lack of funds for some of the materials needed, while the national campaign continued to reiterate the need for sanitation in the same abstract manner as the numerous health campaigns previously conducted by district officials had done.

The one scheme in Moshi district which was a success was a special scheme in an ujamaa village dealing with only one illness, bilharzia, which the residents had identified as a major problem, and for whose eradication they were provided with all the necessary material. The lesson to be drawn from this and a number of other examples is that health campaigns are most successful when they are based on investigations identifying a particular local problem, when they deal with one disease at a time, when they mobilize people who have already learned to co-operate in some other context and when they not only provide health education, but also access to the materials or facilities necessary for action. A general nation-wide campaign conducted from the centre which does not involve either the local experts or the local population in the planning, and which provides only words and not drugs and construction materials, is unlikely to be of much use to the people to whom it is addressed.

3. Literacy programmes in ujamaa villages

As long as literacy is taught in a conventional manner using frontal instruction and texts prepared by some remote specialist, the learning process cannot generate any motivation by itself but is dependent on the motivation the learners derive from other experiences. Although those who can read and write in the village are respected for their skill and can apply it in dealing with government officials and co-operatives, in recording local history and in reading the few written materials that may reach the village, literacy is not considered a necessity for rural life. Most peasants still believe that education is important mainly for those who want to get a job in town, not for those who have buried such ambitions. When a literacy campaign started, many attended for a few sessions, but when they found that it would take them a long time to become literate they usually decided that it was not worth the trouble. The most advanced ujamaa villages were able to counteract this attitude by making it clear to the members that literacy was necessary for meaningful democratic participation in all village affairs, and that it was also part of a more cultured life which the villagers endeavoured to create for themselves.

Following from this understanding, the village community exerted pressure on all its members to educate themselves. At Ngamu Ujamaa Village in Singida, for instance, the duties of a village member included seven hours of communal work per day and two hours of adult education. At Mbambara Ujamaa Village in Tanga, classes were closed during the main agricultural season, but during the rest of the year everybody was expected to participate in adult education programmes.

Yet, even where education had become a collective task, villagers rarely managed to keep up educational programmes long enough to benefit the members. The morale of these more committed villages was constantly threatened by a social and economic environment inimical to communal progress. When prices fell, when a village was unable to market its crops, when essential assistance was denied and when bureaucratic measures from outside weakened the village leadership, educational endeavours were usually among the first activities to be discontinued, since they were based on the hope for a better future but had no organic link to village development.

The few villages that had started with a high level of political awareness had usually taken the initiative in beginning an educational programme themselves and had asked for text-books or assistance if these were available. In most other villages, where adult education was started by government staff, the planning of educational programmes often remained completely outside the control of the villagers.

Where educational campaigns were launched under official auspices, the different people who had to co-operate in implementing them at the local level tended to view them as part of the power struggle going on in the village. The opportunity to 'give' something to the learners—at least in the early stages of a campaign when learners were still interested—or the chance to pose to the outside world in front of a group of people doing what the nation wanted—were seen as tactical advantages gained by one side or the other, by government staff of the village leadership or by certain factions within the village. Educational programmes thus came to be seen not as a way of giving the ordinary villagers more power but as a way of exercising power over them. Most campaigns did not survive the struggle over the question of who should have this power.

4. The planning of functional literacy programmes

The idea of making literacy 'work-oriented' by writing primers on the production of various crops is based on the assumption that people will be more motivated to learn how to read and write when they learn something useful to themselves while doing so. Whether it is correct to motivate people to seek education for the sake of immediate material gains instead of making them aware of the role of education for their cultural and social self-development may be a matter of philosophical principle, but if peasants are addressed as producers then they should at least be addressed as producers who enjoy the right to make choices between crops and techniques according to their means and their own understanding. Functional literacy primers in Tanzania uncritically praise whatever crop they deal with and equally uncritically repeat the advice given by extension agents on the methods of growing these crops. In the primer on cotton, for instance, peasants are told that cotton can make them wealthier, though they know that maize or rice growers are better paid for their labour. Similarly, the primer exhorts peasants to plant early and weed early, though peasants know that they have to look after their food plots first. It also encourages them to use fertilizers when peasants fear that the costs of the fertilizer might be higher than the gains in yield. Such fears and considerations need to be discussed openly before peasants can make a rational choice.

After a visit by Paulo Freire to Tanzania there were some discussions on whether it would be advisable to make the primers more 'problem-posing' and open. In the end this suggestion was turned down. The planners argued that: 'If we allow peasants to criticize the advice of the extension agent, we undermine his authority'. Nor should there be any discussion on the choice of crops: 'If peasants begin to discuss whether they want to grow cotton or not they might decide against it, and if they produce no cotton where are we going to get our foreign exchange from?' As long as peasants in Tanzania have reason to suspect that most of the foreign exchange they earn for the country is used to produce or to import consumer goods for other classes, it may indeed be difficult to convince them that it is in their interest to produce an export crop which has a relatively low price. Maybe peasants would still continue to grow cotton because it is drought-resistant or easy to market and maybe they would find some of their reservations against the extension advice unwarranted. An education, however, which carefully avoids giving the learners an opportunity of articulating these experiences and is satisified with communicating to them the wishes and opinions of those who rule over them, cannot be helpful in realizing the aspirations of the peasants. It will, therefore, not arouse much interest in either the educational process itself or the messages that are communicated.

Conclusion

The organizational structure in which education takes place, the methods of education used, and the content of the educational programme, determine the function which any education is designed to fulfil. Adult education may be designed to make workers or peasants more subservient and dependent or it may be designed to help them to raise their own consciousness, articulate their own interests and make their own choices. The political philosophy of the President of Tanzania sees adult education as a tool for the liberation of the masses, but the way in which adult education has actually been planned and implemented in Tanzania appears to be unrelated to this objective.

II Lower, Middle and Higher Level Manpower-Oriented Training and Education of Adults

5.6 An Integrated Approach to Technical Research and Training of Engineers, Technicians, and Craftsmen in Tanzania
P von Mitschke-Collande

Introduction

Tanzania is aiming at a self-centred economy and self-reliance in manpower development. Emphasis is given to agricultural production as a major source of the Gross National Product (GNP).

Agricultural production requires industries which can develop and manufacture the capital equipment necessary to increase the productivity of labour. Such basic metal-working and engineering industries in turn require an integrated educational system, providing future workers, technicians, engineers and managers (see Fig. 5.1) with a fairly high standard of general education, basic technical training, experience in manufacture and creativity. A strategy of industrial development thus has to consider all levels of education, and these have to be carefully co-ordinated with each other and integrated with production.[1]

1. Primary education

Primary education is of importance for all groups, but has particular significance for semi-skilled workers who constitute more than 70 per cent of the employees in agricultural and industrial production. As most of these workers will never enter further education, they require a certain standard of knowledge useful and applicable to the work they will actually perform after leaving primary school. Curricula of primary education ought to be of a 'polytechnical' nature and take into account the agricultural, technical and social needs of the country.

A concept of polytechnical education would also benefit those groups who, in contrast to workers and peasants, pass through secondary education. It would help to provide basic practical knowledge for future administrative and management staff.

2. Training of Craftsmen

Skilled workers are the most important group in production because they have to implement the production programmes provided by engineers. Therefore, craftsmen must be able to communicate with other groups, they must know engineering drawing and the basic principles of planning and work organization, and they must have sufficient knowledge of their particular craft.

Most large-scale enterprises in developing countries engage only in the 'processing' or 'assembly' type of production. It is known that in such production departments, technology and work organization have very little impact on skill development. The majority of workers operate either special-purpose equip-

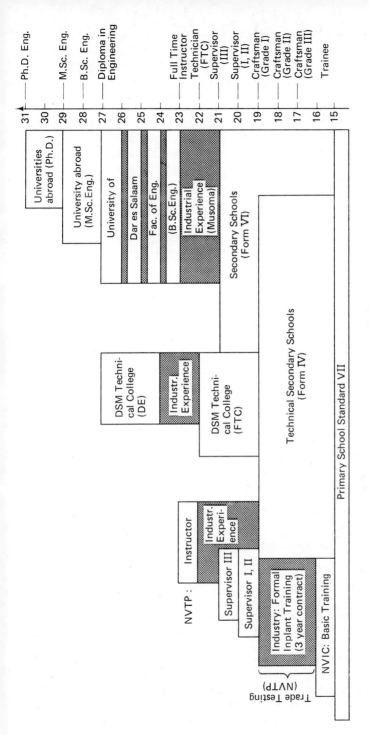

Figure 5.1

System of Formal Technical Education and Training (1975)

(For abbreviations see List of Abbreviations, p. ix of this book)

169

ment, or do 'highly-divided manual partwork', which are both of a repetitive nature. This kind of industrial work actually underdevelops skills and does not require general education or technical training, except some on-the-job training of very short duration. Centralized basic technical training such as that provided by the NVTP seems, therefore, indispensable for any indigenous industrial development. To achieve the political objective of the country, as many workers as possible should undergo this 'basic year of centralized technical training'. At present, however, the capacity of the scheme is limited to 400 apprentices per year, and major engineering crafts like tool making, foundry work etc. are not included in the programme. After the year of basic training, workers should continue with 'in-plant training' before they enter production. The most appropriate places to gain experience are the central workshops dealing with maintenance and repair work.

In the present large-scale enterprises, central workshops—if they exist—are the only places where practical engineering skills can be developed, since they are equipped with 'multi-purpose machinery' most suitable for training. They are the potential for future production of capital equipment within their particular branch. That is why all central workshops should also be 'centres for in-plant training', contributing to and recommended as part of the national training system.

After practice in central workshops craftsmen will be sufficiently experienced to join production. The general technical training will have prepared them not merely for particular operations but will enable them to practise 'job rotation', which will further increase their technical competence and motivation for qualified and efficient work. This may lead in the long run to replacement of the hierarchical work organization by self-reliant, co-operative group-work in industrial production.

The present system of annual trade-testing overemphasizes 'formal education' criteria. As a result, many workers with little qualification but much practical experience are excluded from the promotion system in use. To implement Tanzania's social development policy, greater emphasis should be given to the criteria of practical experience and individual attitudes in order to foster education and motivation.

The major obstacle to industrial development is the lack of training capacity and facilities, particularly for engineering crafts. Craftsmen are heavily under-represented compared with technicians and engineers, as can be seen in Table 5.9.

3. Training of Technicians
Technicians are usually the intermediate group between workers and engineers. Their tasks are to communicate the manufacturing programmes developed by engineers to the workers, to instruct them in technical terms, to demonstrate practically how to operate equipment and instruments, and last but not least to motivate workers for efficient manufacture. So far the Dar es Salaam Technical College (DTC) recruits all its students for the FTC-course from Form IV of Technical Secondary schools, without any industrial experience.

It seems clear that the present curriculum at the DTC needs some revision because its tendency to increase academic subjects and reduce workshop practice

Table 5.9

Technical Education and Industrial Employment Ratios

Employment and Output Ratios — Categories, Degrees and Institutions of Technical Education	Necessary Employment Ratio in a self-centred industrial Society	Employment Ratio by 1974 in Tanzania based on 28 major industries (including expatriates)	Output of Formal Technical Education in Tanzania by 1977 (Projections are based on input figures provided by Ministry of National Education DSM Technical College, National Vocational Training Programme)	
			Ratio	**No. of students**
Engineers (B.Sc. at the Faculty of Engineering, UDSM M.Sc., Ph.D. Eng. from universities abroad)	1	1	1	600
Technicians (FTC, Diploma in Engineering at the Dar es Salaam Tech. College)	5	5	2	1 200
Craftsmen (Grades II and I only at the National Vocational Training Centre)	25	13	5	3 000

Source: Directorate of Adult Education, 1971 Annual Report Dar es Salaam: Ministry of Education.

runs counter to industrial requirements. In between or after the FTC course, technicians should also spend at least one year at the central workshops in industry, and this should be the most important stage in their technical training. In fact, it would be most appropriate if technicians underwent the same training as craftsmen and got their up-grading at the DTC. They definitely require more practical knowledge and skill than academic education.

4. Education of engineers

In the education of engineers, mathematics and science are essential since they provide the theoretical tools for technical research and the development of products. But without practical experience on the shop floor as part of his education an engineer will not be able to do his job. He must have practical knowledge of materials, tools, machinery and technical processes. In particular he must know how to design a product, how to organize production and how to instruct all staff involved. A new product has to suit customers' needs, but it must also fit into the given factory set-up. Organization of production can be studied only on the shop floor; technical imagination and creativity can only result from that experience.

Engineer education, therefore, has to start with practical training in industry. The 'Musoma Declaration' stipulated a period of two years of productive work within which every Form VI secondary school leaver has the chance to gain experience according to his/her major interests—even if he/she has not yet decided on a future profession. However, this period has to be properly utilized. If these two years are not to be lost time for the students, industrial enterprises must be required to provide a minimum of training facilities and a certain standard of instruction. Once they have organized a kind of in-plant training programme for secondary school leavers they can also assist in the selection of the most suitable students for engineering courses at the university.

Such a period in industry might in the long run permit the four-year course at the Faculty of Engineering, UDSM, to be shortened. At present the first year at the Faculty of Engineering has to take account of the lack of practical experience of the majority of students, who are direct entrants from non-technical secondary schools. Fifty per cent of the first-year timetable is allocated to workshop training within the premises of the Faculty of Engineering to teach the students basic engineering skills.

After the first year of the B.Sc. Eng. course all students can opt for their departmental preferences. But at the same time the full capacity of 120 students has to fit the planned manpower development ratio of 60 civil, 40 mechanical and 20 electrical engineering students.

The annual two-month periods of industrial training are an important part of the curriculum. During their four-year course all students pass through three periods of training in production. This practice, supervised by staff members of the Faculty of Engineering, is insufficient without a proper system of in-plant training conducted by industrial instructors who could assist all institutions of technical education. The co-ordination of all these efforts requires a lot of initiative from CORI (Committee for Relations with Industry), a joint body of industrial and academic representatives which was set up to foster close co-operation between industries and institutions of technical education, particularly in regard to engineer education. Industries may make use of this forum to present their problems, specify their needs and exchange experience and information.

The Faculty of Engineering tries by various means to achieve a merger of theory and practice. In the third and fourth year, emphasis is given to 'project-type learning', in which students are expected to apply their theoretical knowledge and practical experience to designing and developing technical products and also to building prototypes.

For the 'final project' students are required to identify, on their own, a particular problem in the enterprise to which they are attached for their last industrial training period. This technical problem must be solved within the last academic year; the solution might be handed over to the enterprise as a contribution of applied research. Some companies do not yet appreciate the usefulness of such an exercise. It obviously requires time and a lot of public relations work for industrial establishments to realize, influence and utilize the potential of technical education and research. There is still a long way to go to integrate education, research and production.

In 1977 the first batch of 60 engineers left the Faculty of Engineering for industrial employment, and suitable criteria had to be established for their allocation. The Faculty of Engineering could assist the High Level Manpower Allocation Committee in this task so as to ensure the most appropriate distribution of engineers according to specialization and qualification.

We also knew that by 1977, 600 engineers trained in several countries of the world would be back in Tanzania. In this case the Engineers Registration Board had the important duty of evaluating and classifying the different international degrees and assisting in manpower allocation.

It seems that next to academic performance, industrial practice and teaching experience should be considered as most important. This applies particularly to the appointment of staff for institutions of technical education, where the emphasis should be on industrial experience and applied research rather than on the number of academic publications. Solutions for indigenous engineering problems are more important than international academic standards.

Conclusion

At present about 90 per cent of the Tanzanian industrial establishments are of the processing or assembly type. Only ten per cent are engineering works, and these are mainly concerned with repair work and spare part production.

The development of a self-centred economy thus particularly requires the establishment of a sector for the manufacture of capital equipment. Such a transformation involves a lot of investment. During the transitional period the central workshops of the major enterprises within each branch of industry could be expanded to start manufacturing equipment that can be employed in the production departments. Additional posts for engineers should be created in design departments for product and equipment modification and development. The Faculty of Engineering could assist in matters of research and technical development by offering laboratory facilities and manpower expertise.

Such an approach would make it possible to initiate a first phase of indigenous industrial development. Design departments, central workshops and systematic in-plant training programmes attached to industrial production seem to be the most appropriate counterparts of formal general and technical education. This is the only way to co-ordinate all the institutions concerned and to integrate education, research and production.

Note

1   For further reading see Barker, C E; Bhagavan, M R; von Mitschke-Collande, P; Wield, D V *Industrial Production and Transfer of Technology in Tanzania, Industrial Survey* Dar es Salaam: Institute of Development Studies, UDSM (1974/75)

5.7 Workers' Education
J J Shengena

'We in Tanganyika do not believe that mankind has yet discovered ultimate truth—in any field. We do not wish to act as if we did have such a belief. We wish to contribute to Man's development if we can, but we do not claim to have any 'solution'; our only claim is that we intend to grope forward in the dark, towards a goal so distant that even the real understanding of it is beyond us—towards, in other words, the best that Man can become.'[1]
(J K Nyerere)

The development of the Tanzanian society and the development of the workers' consciousness and job skills have always been inseparably linked.[2] The great task of building an independent nation after 1961, and particularly after the resolve taken in 1967 to build a socialist society, could clearly not be completed or even advanced without an all-round development of the working population towards acquisition both of the new national identity and ideology and of modern production techniques. A high level of education, culture, social consciousness and appropriate skills of all workers was as important for the advancement of the society as was the establishment of the required material and technical bases.

From the earliest days of the nationalist struggle, TANU has believed that man as a social being consciously organizes his social life and in so doing builds his own personality. Nothing is done as an end in itself, for every action requires the ability of man to perform it and must serve the well-being of every man. This principle necessitates a transformation of the Tanzanian society system.

A diversified and effective education policy has, therefore, to be developed. The policy directive 'Education for Self-Reliance'[3] issued in March 1967 demanded, among other changes, an egalitarian approach in the planning and the content of the educational process for the liberation of Tanzanians. Whereas on the formal education level changes began to take effect immediately, non-formal education continued to be a haphazard activity until 1970 when President Nyerere issued a policy declaration on life-long adult education,[4] followed by a circular on workers' participation in management. In 1973, these two policy papers on non-formal education were reinforced by a further policy statement on workers' education, made by the Prime Minister; all three form the basis of this article, with special emphasis on workers' education.

It is important, however, to stress from the outset that this discussion will be based on the premise that the development of workers' education is only a component of overall educational development, and as such is subject not only to co-ordination but also to subordination of the whole education system, and adult education in particular, to the historical conditions and the desired future social system in Tanzania.

1. Background information
While the very wide range of workers' education activities in Tanzania now includes all levels of the educational hierarchy, from preliteracy to postgraduate studies, the earliest ventures—which go back to pre-independence days—took the form of ad hoc activities designed to offset the consequences of restricted

access to formal education of a large sector of the working population. They also satisfied certain individual occupational needs like mobility in work or economic needs of the employing agent and the political regime. These activities were carried out in a number of ways in special institutions or in foreign countries, with the use of conventional teaching methods or innovatory practices, and by a variety of agencies, governmental and non-governmental, social or religious institutions, voluntary movements and private enterprises.

2. Developments since Independence

It hardly needs mentioning that the colonial type of workers' education was designed to adapt the few selected workers to colonial needs, e.g., support of the colonial administration at the middle manpower level. But since the attainment of national independence in the sixties, workers' education had, though still in an ad hoc manner, made some unprecedented progress, both quantitively and qualitatively, in response to the needs arising from the challenge of nationhood. Civil servants were needed to take responsible positions in the government, and so were professionals, middle-level technicians and political activists. All of them had not only to be provided with general knowledge but had also to be familiarized with the new tasks and roles in national reconstruction.

(i) Main institutions concerned with workers' education

Although a considerable number of institutions and agencies became automatically involved in organizing workers' education, or admitted a few workers in their specializations, three institutions which organized training programmes specifically for workers should be specially mentioned. They are Kivukoni College, the Institute of Adult Education (IAE), and the National Institute of Productivity (NIP). Their contributions will be briefly examined.

(a) Kivukoni College

In all new nations the process of changing old political values and attitudes has occupied a place of high priority in the activities of leaders and ruling parties. The assumption, which these politicians share with students of behavioural science, is that the political values and attitudes of the people directly and significantly affect the survival potential of the new nations and the ruling party. Thus, just before Tanzania became independent in 1961, the TANU party established Kivukoni College with the aim of preparing a few Tanzanians for leading positions in the Party, its affiliated institutions, and in the government, by giving them a general basic education in economics, political science, history, geography, administration, law, literature, modern languages, and in subjects relevant to life in Africa.[5] In his opening speech Mwalimu J K Nyerere said to the students:

'To come here as a student is to be given a wonderful opportunity, and a privilege. The responsibility is proportionately great. If a student ever tried to divorce himself from the people who indirectly sent him here he would be abusing the privilege . . .. The graduates of Kivukoni must be like the yeast in a loaf, effective because it cannot be isolated, its presence being known by the work it has done.'[6]

From its inception in 1961 to 1966 the college enrolled 794 students and conducted residential three-month and nine-month courses, of the nature described above, for workers. These courses were qualitatively slightly different from those offered in other post-secondary institutions. Since 1967, Kivukoni has been undergoing structural changes. From being independent it came under the direct supervision of the Party, and from an institution providing a general education it was transformed into an ideological one. In other words, it ceased being a general institution with a subject-centred approach and now limits itself to a particular target audience composed of Party workers, political activists and peasant leaders. In order to fulfil this new purpose, four zonal colleges were opened in the regions in 1974, and similar branches are to be opened in all the other 16 administrative regions of Tanzania mainland. In the 15 years of its existence, Kivukoni College has trained 3989 students, the majority of whom are workers of all levels.

(b) Institute of Adult Education (IAE)
Until its establishment by law as a parastatal institution in July 1975, the IAE had been part of the University of East Africa and later, when that university was dissolved in 1970 it became part of the University of Dar es Salaam. From its inception the IAE has played a prominent role in promoting workers' education in the framework of the adult education programme. Its major activities have been direct provision of continuing education, training of adult educators, research in the field of adult education and, more recently, mass education campaigns.

Continuing education has been provided by the institute through four components at different levels, as shown in Table 5.10. Firstly, through a programme of evening courses and seminars, workshops and short residential courses. The range of these activities has been wide and varied and the majority of students have been workers as all IAE facilities are located in towns. Most of the courses, seminars and workshops are designed to help the students increase productivity in their places of work, or to provide an insight into, and an understanding of, problems of development in Tanzania and the Third World in general. An important aspect of this type of continuing education is counselling for the Mature Age Scheme, whereby working adults can secure a place in any of the three Universities in East Africa without going through the formal education examination. Since one of the qualifications required for admission as a mature-age student is that the candidate must have worked for at least 3 years, it is de facto a workers' education programme. From 30 to 65 workers have been able through this programme to gain entrance to the Universities in East Africa each year.

The second component of continuing education has been the provision of a two-year part-time course for the Certificate in Law. Although the tuition of the course is primarily the responsibility of the Faculty of Law of the University of Dar es Salaam, the administrative work and the learning facilities have always been provided by the IAE. So far 341 students have completed this course, and a good number of them have been admitted for full-time degree courses. Again it has been mainly workers who were able to avail themselves of this course, but now a similar programme has been introduced in Arusha town. This, it is hoped, will establish the basis for expanding the programme to the rural population.

Table 5.10

Enrolment of New Students in the Dar es Salaam Centre of the Institute of Adult Education, 1964–1975

Year	Courses			
	Evening Courses	Certificate in Law	Diploma in AE	Correspondence Courses
1964	582	—	—	—
1965	941	—	—	—
1966	1 273	—	—	—
1967	1 387	—	—	—
1968	1 039	47	—	—
1969	700	38	23	—
1970	1 091	41	24	—
1971	1 457	37	28	—
1972	1 699	40	28	325
1973	2 010	43	30	4 909
1974	*	48	29	5 860
1975	*	47	36	6 285
Totals	12 179	341	198	17 379

Source: The Institute of Adult Education, Annual Reports (collected by author)

The third component, the diploma course in adult education, was started in 1969 for the purpose of training qualified adult educators and administrators, who are badly needed in the national literacy campaign and the workers' education programme. Most of the students of this course are required to have worked for at least three years in occupations related to adult education. Whilst the results so far have been encouraging, two main obstacles still have to be removed. The first is that those ministries and organizations which ought to send trainees to the course, send only a few or none at all. Secondly, a good number of the graduates from the diploma course are posted to jobs which have no relation to the training they have received. It is to be hoped that some solution will be found to both problems, especially now that workers' education and adult education programmes have been given priority in the national mobilization strategies.

Although education by correspondence is reviewed in detail in article 5.9 by E M Chale, it should be mentioned here as yet another component of the workers' continuing education programme. Before Tanzania established its own correspondence facilities in 1972, the majority of people who used distance learning facilities belonged to the working population. And despite the fact that the major aim of the national correspondence programme is to reach the rural population, the statistics available at the end of 1975 show that out of a cumulative enrolment of 20 000 students, about 59 per cent were workers. Thus this facility has been, and will continue to be in the foreseeable future, an appreciable aspect of workers' education in Tanzania.

(c) National Institute of Productivity (NIP)

Founded by the Government of Tanzania in 1965 with technical assistance from UNDP, NIP has developed into one of the leading management training and consulting institutes in the country, for the government and for industrial and service organizations in the private and public sectors. At the beginning, most of its work was classroom-oriented, with courses and seminars ranging from three weeks to one year, conducted in Dar es Salaam or up-country. But since 1971, there has been growing demand from clients for practical problem-solving development assistance. This has resulted in an increased amount of consultancy work which combines the application of improved management techniques with on-the-job training of clients' personnel, to accelerate their development into efficient workers. Unlike the IAE which has been offering training opportunities of a general nature, open to anybody, NIP from the outset has been a workers' institute dealing directly with management training in the classroom and on-the-job, and providing consultancy services for the government, organizations and industries. Further, it supplies at its clients' request special tailor-made programmes to meet particular training needs. As will be shown shortly, this institute has been the nucleus of a real workers' education programme since this became a Party and government policy.

From its inception in 1965 until 1975, the NIP conducted about 376 courses for 7781 participants. The grand total of consultancies during the same period was 567. Both the courses and the consultancy assignments have been able to develop and extend professional competence and increase the productivity of the expanding Tanzanian economy and services. The yearly breakdown of courses and consultancies carried out by NIP is shown in Table 5.11.

In this short appraisal of the three principal institutions concerned with workers' education, no attempt could be made to give a full description of their functions and activities which have been many and complex, since they were undertaken in the context of specific situations involving particular constellations of time, place and circumstance. The author's purpose has been merely to indicate the major areas in which these institutions contribute to the general aim of workers' education in Tanzania, that is, to provide for workers of all levels learning opportunities which will help them to understand the ideology of socialism and to become more productive and effective in their work places, and thus to reduce the education, communication and professional gap.

(ii) Workers' participation

With the expansion of the economy and services since independence, the Tanzanian salaried work force increased so rapidly that by 1972 there were 405 713 workers. As employment opportunities continued to materialize, as shown in Table 5.12, the rate of increase was expected to rise further, which necessitated re-thinking about the need to give the Tanzanian workers more opportunities to learn so that they could make socialism a reality. For history teaches that liberation of the working people from exploitation, oppression and low productivity is possible only when they learn that their own creative powers should determine their acts, and when by their deeds they contribute to the political, economic and cultural progress of humanity. In 1969 this need to enable the workers to learn was declared a policy by the President. Although his

Table 5.11

Activities of the National Institute of Productivity Between 1966 and 1975

Year	Courses	Participants	Consultancies
1966	5	83	18
1967	34	545	36
1968	41	794	166
1969	51	1026	102
1970	77	1472	26
1971	54	1092	38
1972	30	671	68
1973	28	653	41
1974	20	529	26
1975	36	916	46
Totals	376	7781	567

Source: The National Institute of Productivity, Annual Reports (collected by the author)

Table 5.12

Employment by Major Industrial Divisions 1972–1974

	Employment (Numbers)			
	1972	1973	1974	% Change 74/73
Agriculture	113843	109047	123973	+ 13.7
Mining & Quarrying	5558	5013	4762	− 5.0
Manufacturing	56389	59336	64921	+ 9.4
Public Utilities	12324	18904	16074	−15.0
Construction	51842	104777	72810	−30.5
Commerce	24777	26713	25322	− 5.2
Transport and Communication	37049	38115	45166	+18.5
Finance	6356	6515	7399	+13.6
Community Services	98575	104083	123659	+18.8
Total	405713	472503	484086	+ 2.5

Source: Dar es Salaam, The Central Statistical Bureau.

message dealt with the general aims of adult education, there is no doubt that workers' education is and ought to be an important component of any adult education programme.

The *Presidential Circular No. 1* of 1970 on workers' participation in management[7] called for the establishment of workers' councils in all parastatal enterprises employing more than ten workers. Also included in the council by virtue of their status are the general manager, heads of departments and the chairman of the Party branch in the enterprise. The main functions of the workers' councils are to advise on wages policy, planning of production, targets and quality, marketing, and training programmes and to receive and discuss the balance sheet. This was the first step towards the establishment of socialist labour relations. As such it required educating the workers to enable them to assume their new roles and understand the various operations of their enterprises, their contribution to national development and socialist industrial discipline.[8]

NIP and NUTA were assigned the work of drawing up a comprehensive workers' education programme which was to aim at reaching beyond the few individuals who sit in the workers' councils or management executive committees, to the workers on the shop floor who may be anxious and willing to break the chains of ignorance or insufficient knowledge.[9]

As a take-off stage in the implementation of the circular, a six-week training programme was arranged for 65 instructors. After finishing the course these were distributed to parastatal enterprises to teach the workers throughout the country. The content of instruction concentrated on the following areas:

The political ideology and policy of TANU (Socialism and Self-reliance)
Labour/Management Relations (including labour legislation)
Elementary Economics
Wages Policy
Workers' Trade Union
Literacy
How to read a Balance Sheet
Presidential Circular No. 1 of 1970
The structure and functions of the organization concerned.

Meanwhile, other on-the-job training programmes, vocational training and other refresher courses continued to be conducted within and outside the country with no particular commitment by the government and, as we have seen, in an unco-ordinated manner until July 1973.

(iii) Lifelong education for workers
A directive issued by the Prime Minister, Ndugu Rashid Kawawa, on July 5th 1973[10] firmly committed the state to workers' education. This circular stated in clear terms that workers' education was part and parcel of the continuing adult education programme and a lifelong process for all workers in any field or specialization, at any place of work. Its objectives were the same as those laid down in 1970 for adult education in general, that is:

to liberate Tanzanians economically, mentally and culturally;
to teach Tanzanians how to change their environment;

to make Tanzanians understand their country's policy of socialism and self-reliance.

All firms, parastatals, ministries and institutions were requested to organize well-considered and comprehensive workers' education programmes involving all their workers; to quote:

'Workers' education programmes must involve ALL WORKERS, from the illiterate worker to those who have university degrees or are at top managerial level.'[11]

The circular also included a seven-point guideline to be implemented with 'immediate effect' by every ministry, institution, parastatal and industrial enterprise. It clearly indicated the importance attached by the state to the success of the workers' education programme. The seven points of this guideline were:

(i) Any establishment employing workers must have concrete programmes for educating them in various matters, from eradicating illiteracy to technical education;

(ii) A Workers' Education Officer must be appointed who will be responsible for making programmes of education at the work place. The appointed official should be able and should have full responsibility which will enable him to execute this work;

(iii) A separate financial vote for workers' education should be budgeted;

(iv) All reports on workers' education programmes and progress reports should be forwarded to the Regional Labour Officer and the Regional Co-ordinator of Adult Education who will be required to send them to the Regional Adult Education Committee and later to the Ministries of National Education and Social Welfare;

(v) Workers' education should be conducted during normal working hours for at least one hour every day but institutions are at liberty to use any other time, both outside normal working hours and in excess of one hour per day, for workers' education activities, so long as such liberty does not reduce production and efficiency of the factory or office and is reached by consensus of workers' committees on education.

(vi) All workers must attend classes organized by their institutions as part of their duties. Any worker who fails to attend these classes without a valid reason will be regarded as absent from work and disciplinary action will be taken against him. This will also be applicable to any worker assigned to teach in these classes;

(vii) Labour officers in the Ministry of Labour will have the right to inspect the places of work to make sure that workers' education programmes exist and that they are being implemented.[12]

Further, it was believed that although a successful permanent workers' education programme has to be centrally planned and directed, it must also be a collective responsibility of all the people and their institutions. Hence elected workers' education committees were to be formed at all levels of the administrative structure. The main functions of the committees are to ensure that in their respective juridical areas workers' education plans are consistent with the national policy, and also to mobilize the workers to enrol in the classes. To give these committees the necessary executive and functional powers, the head of the institution or juridical area is the chairman of the committee while the workers' education co-ordinating officer acts as the secretary. At the national level, the National Advisory Council to the Minister for National Education must ensure that the Adult Education Committee also handles matters pertaining to workers' education.

The first Ministry to comply fully with the Prime Minister's call was the Ministry of National Education, which, being in the advantageous position of having a solid adult education infrastructure and personnel, set up a workers' education section in the Adult Education Division on July 15th 1973, and formed a workers' education committee. Implementation of workers' education then began to spread throughout the country. On May 2nd 1974 the Ministry of Labour and Social Welfare established a Workers' Education Division whose staff nucleus consisted of professionals from the workers' education section of NIP. In the regions and districts, the labour officers were also assigned the extra duty of co-ordinating workers' education in their respective areas.

As may already have been observed, the Presidential circular on workers' participation affected only parastatals and was organized by NIP and NUTA, whilst the Prime Minister's circular on workers' education affected the entire work force in Tanzania. Thus the implementation of the Prime Minister's circular posed a bigger and more complex challenge, requiring co-ordination of a large number of agents and individuals. Moreover, the national adult education programme inaugurated by the President in 1970 in which the illiterate workers participated, was in full operation. In view of these difficulties the two Ministries charged with responsibility for workers' education, i.e. the Ministry of National Education and the Ministry of Labour and Social Services, began to plan strategies and organize resources for the immediate and future programmes. The following operational objectives were formulated:

To formulate and implement government policy on workers' education in general and workers' participation in particular;
To act as co-ordinating centres of workers' education activities and of management relations concerning workers' education and participation;
To evaluate the effectiveness of the workers' education programme, to act as information and research centres for labour/management relations concerning workers' education and workers' participation;
To assist employers in planning, directing and controlling workers' training programmes at national, regional and factory level;
To propose and review standards for workers' education and provide the framework within which the scope and nature of the programme will be planned;
To design educational methods and materials for the workers' education programme;
To contribute to the preparation of national plans for workers' education and workers' participation and monitor the implementation of these plans for the purpose of identifying progress and problems.

The take-off stage for workers' education began with the organization in each of the 20 administrative regions of three-day seminars in which the objectives of the workers' education programme and the committee members' duties were explained to 1600 members of workers' education committees. Further, two-week courses on planning, identification of training needs, communication and adult learning pedagogy were organized for 460 workers' education officers. Also, available reports clearly indicate that many work places started running classes, for by September 1975 the total number of workers receiving workers' education was 60000. To have reached a figure of this magnitude within three years was an encouraging achievement which augured well for the future.

Although under the original mature-age entrant scheme some workers had managed to secure places in the universities, this has been regarded as a privilege accorded to a few, since university education had been traditionally reserved for secondary school leavers. This attitude was changed by the 'Musoma Resolution' of 1974, which stated that university education must be regarded as an extension of adult education and hence as a right for the population working already.[13] It is hoped that in the long run this approach will help to intellectualize the workers and peasants and to transform university teachers into workers and peasants. The University of Dar es Salaam began to implement the resolution in the academic year 1975 to 1976, when 2041 enrolled Tanzanian students were workers. The programme will continue to be the major entrance gate to university education.

3. Future plans
In the Five-Year Development plan drawn up for the years 1976 to 1981, the outline for the workers' education programme included:

eradication of illiteracy amongst the workers;
strengthening of the skills of workers who are literate so as to prevent their relapse into illiteracy, or ignorance of modern technological developments;
provision and reinforcement of a workers' education environment and a permanent, lifelong education;
establishment of four zonal workers' education programmes by the Ministry of Labour and Social Services.

Institutions for workers' education
Now that, following the Prime Minister's circular of 1973, education has become a national policy goal, a co-ordinated multi-disciplinary effort must be made to achieve it. All the following institutions must make still greater contributions by giving expertise, writing and reading materials, teaching, organizing and supervizing, mobilizing or increasing the number of workers in their specialized training institutions: Kivukoni college with its zonal branches, the National Union of Tanzanian Workers, the People's Development Colleges, the Co-operation Education Centre, NIP, the Tanzania Library Services, Radio Tanzania, the Institute of Development Studies, the Tanzania Examination Council, the University of Dar es Salaam, the Small-Scale Industries Development Organization, all specialized institutes, and others as the need arises.

With all the workers and their institutions thus involved in promoting workers' education, it will be necessary for the two ministries responsible for co-ordinating workers' education to establish an efficient network for lively communication, both horizontally between the various agencies and institutions and vertically between the grassroots activities (classes) and the national centres of policy- and decision-making.

Conclusion

Aware of the inseparable connections between society and education, and in consideration of the necessity of designing concrete development strategies with an historical perspective, the Party and government have decided to adopt practicable policies that will help to produce the desired 'free man' of the future. The many changes our education system has undergone since independence and the short history of workers' education outlined in this article are evidence of the determination of this nation to raise workers with a socialist outlook and morale. Considering the instructions given to factories and offices, the different seminars organized for workers and the increasing number of opportunities offered to the workers by our education institutions, all provided by the state free of charge, there is every reason to believe that with the support of the whole society, the programme of lifelong education for workers should be able to achieve the goal of increasing the knowledge, skills and capacities of the Tanzanian workers and of reinforcing their convictions and attitudes.

Notes

1 Nyerere, J K '"Groping Forward", the Opening of Kivukoni College' in *Freedom and Unity.* . . ., p. 121 Bibl. 10
2 'Workers' will throughout this paper refer to all persons employed in the public or private sector, from the highest-paid professional to the lowest-paid unskilled labourer.
3 Nyerere, J K 'Education for Self-Reliance' in *Freedom and Socialism.* . . ., by J K Nyerere, p. 290 Bibl. 11
4 See Nyerere, J K *Education Never Ends* pp. 33–37 of this book
5 For more details of the past history of Kivukoni College see Wickens, J E 'The Beginnings of Kivukoni College' *Mbio Journal* Dar es Salaam: Kivukoni Ideological College. V (1968), No. 8, pp. 3–11
6 See Note 1, p. 123
7 'Presidential Circular No. 1 of 1970, the Establishment of Workers' Councils, Executive Committees and Boards of Directors' in *Guide to Workers' Education.* . . ., edited by National Institute of Productivity, pp. 1–4 Bibl. 175
8 For a critical analysis of workers' participation in Tanzania see Mapolu, H (ed.) *Workers and Management* Bibl. 50
9 See Lusinde, J 'Address to 3rd NDC Group Managers Conference in November, 1970' in *Guide to Workers' Education.* . . ., edited by National Institute of Productivity, p. 12 Bibl. 177
10 Prime Minister and Second Vice-President's Office. *Guideline Regarding Adult Education—Workers' Education* Dar es Salaam: (1973) (mimeo.)
11 Cf. Note 10
12 Cf. Note 10
13 For this part of the 'Musoma Declaration' see *Daily News* (3.1.1975)

5.8 Post-Secondary Training and University Education
A S Meena
Introduction
Before independence, education in Tanzania was run on a racial basis.[1] For the whole forty-year period of British administration, Tanganyika did not have any institution of higher learning in the real sense. General education at this tertiary level was provided outside the country to a few Tanganyikan Africans. The main institutions available to them were Makerere College in Uganda, the Royal Technical College, Nairobi, in Kenya, and overseas universities, mostly British.

One fact illustrating the legacy of the colonial education is that before independence in 1961, the European schools took the proportionally largest share of public funds. Next came the Asian schools and finally the African schools, which received only a very small allocation per student as can be seen from Table 5.13.

Table 5.13

Net Expenditure on Education in Tanganyika Territory in 1947

Race	Estimated Population 5.5 Million (1947)				
	Total Population	Students in School	Enrolment as Percentage of Race	Government Expenditure	Expenditu per Stude
Africans	5480391	113198	2.1	£251000	£2.2
Asians	50332	9831	19.5	£51000	£5.2
Europeans	14727	958	6.5	£36000	£37.6

Source: *Annual Report of Education Department, Tanganyika* Dar es Salaam: Government Printer (1947)

So the number of people trained to man the skilled and semi-skilled jobs was small, and even at the time of independence the situation was no better. There were only 1603 Form IV pupils in Tanzanian secondary schools—as compared with 8183 in 1975—and about 2000 students in East African university colleges. Training oportunity for the middle (semi-skilled) cadre was therefore minimal since university-educated people were not available to train this group. In fact Kitchen[2] noted that in the middle of 1959 there were only 70 Tanganyikan Africans with university degrees, 20 of whom were teachers. 40 other Tanganyikan Africans were non-graduate but held Makerere College Diplomas in various fields, e.g., medicine, veterinary science, and teaching.

Colonial education, especially at tertiary level, had many weaknesses which the young state had to counteract. For example, it

encouraged wrong attitudes—'ivory tower' feeling;
promoted subservience among the indigenous people, most of whom did not have access to primary education at that time;

created human inequality;

inculcated wrong measures of social merit, e.g., people could not be employed in a specific job unless they had reached a certain educational level;

stressed foreign values resulting in neglect and contempt of local culture;

introduced irrelevant curricula, i.e. what was being taught was not related to problems of rural areas where the majority of the population lived;

created misinterpretation or abuse of 'academic freedom'.

Ways and means of solving the above-mentioned problems had to be found before any development of the country as a whole could be envisaged.

1. Higher education after independence

One of the first moves made by the newly-independent state was to introduce in 1961 a new Education Ordinance transforming the loose groups of racial educational systems from the colonial regime into a single education system.[3]

(a) Aims and objectives

Integration was an important national instrument for producing a maximum number of citizens to be trained as higher-level manpower. Another important decision the government took immediately after independence was to give priority to the expansion of secondary education and teacher training, so as to ensure a constant flow of post-secondary manpower to whatever sector(s) needed it. All major policies were governed by development plans. For example, one of the main objectives of the First Five-Year Development Plan was to train sufficient manpower of the middle and upper levels to meet the country's needs by 1980. These two levels were emphasized in order to get skilled and semi-skilled manpower to fill important posts which were either to be vacated by expatriates, or required urgent development. Consequently, training facilities for positions requiring post-secondary education, i.e. university or equivalent professional training, were created. They are shown in Table 5.14. The training period after Form VI ranged from two years, e.g., for the teacher's diploma, to five years for medical practitioners.

(b) Revision of the curriculum

Every educational level, from primary to university, was to have a fresh look into its programme and to have necessary changes made so that the content as well as the methodology would become more akin to Tanzanian aspirations. To achieve this, several panels for secondary, primary and teacher-education subjects were formed at the Institute of Education. The membership of the panels varied, but in general it comprised Ministry officials, school teachers, college tutors, university lecturers, and for some subjects, e.g., political education, politicians. The reason for bringing together people with varied experiences was to direct the content towards the national objective whilst not forgetting the psychological implication of the pupils' understanding. At the tertiary level, e.g., the University of Dar es Salaam, discussions were held in various departmental and faculty board meetings in which people from outside the university were also represented. The objective was to include in the discussion some feedback not only from personnel practising the university theories, but also from others who were closer to the people that were to be served by the curricula.

Table 5.14

Facilities for Post-Secondary Training in 1974
(For abbreviations see the List of Abbreviations, p. ix)

(a) Facilities for University Degrees and Comparable Professional Diploma Courses

Serial No.	Subject	Place	Serial No.	Subject	Place
1	Accountancy	IDM	18	Engineering, Radio	OS
2	Agriculture	UDSM	19	Engineering, Survey	UNai
3	Architecture	UNai	20	Engineering, Textile	OS
4	Arts (B.A.)	UDSM	21	Engineering, Water	UDSM
5	Busines Studies	IDM	22	Forestry	UDSM
6	Commerce	UNai	23	Geology	UDSM
7	Community Dev.	IDM	24	Law	UDSM
8	Dentistry	OS	25	Library School	UMak
9	Economics (Land & Bldg)	Unai	26	Medicine	UDSM
10	Education (Arts)	UDSM	27	Pharmacy	UDSM
11	Education (Science)	UDSM	28	Public Admin.	IDM
12	Engineering, Aircraft	OS	29	Quantity Survey	OS
13	Engineering, Chemical	OS	30	Science B.Sc.	UDSM
14	Engineering, Civil	UDSM	31	Social Work	UMak
15	Engineering, Mech.	UDSM	32	Town Planning	AI
16	Engineering, Elec.	UDSM	33	Veterinary Sc.	UNai
17	Engineering, Mining	OS	34	Art (Fine)	UMak

(b) Other Post-Form VI Level Diploma Courses

Serial No.	Subject	Place	Serial No.	Subject	Place
35	Education (various)	CNE	40	Forestry	OL
36	Agriculture	Inst.	41	Physiotherapy	OS
37	Co-operative Management	CC	42	Land Survey	AI
38	Estate Managm.	AI	43	Valuation	AI
39	Fisheries	KFI	44	Wild Life	CWM

Source: Ministry of National Education *F 6 Sel 74 Application for Higher Education, Training or Employment by Pupils Completing Form VI at Secondary Schools in Tanzania* Dar es Salaam: Ministry of National Education (1974)

An example of the outcome of such planning sessions is the teachers' programme adopted by the UDSM, which is described in detail in the article on Teacher Education (article 4.5 of this book). Its pattern is completely different from the traditional one of a three-year academic degree course followed by a post-graduate diploma course in education. This way the government not only saved time and money but the curriculum itself was more suited to Tanzania's needs than that which students pursued overseas.

(c) Localization[4] of staff

It was felt that by staffing the institutions with Tanzanians, the changes could be speeded up. Whilst non-Tanzanians continued to be employed, the policy was to phase them out gradually as more qualified Tanzanians became available. The non-Tanzanians were selected from a wide cross-section of nationalities (about 30 in the UDSM). The government paid particular attention to personnel who have a commitment to understanding and helping to solve the problems of the Third World.

(d) Integration of university staff with civil servants

Since the UDSM became a national university in 1970, no member of its staff, or for that matter, of the staff of any other institution in the country, be it a factory or the defence forces, should feel that he occupies a permanent post in his area. Where the need arises for exchanging or replacing a member of staff in the middle or upper grades with another, the President or authorized official may direct such a change to be made for the benefit of the nation. At the UDSM for instance, several professors, directors, and lecturers have been seconded to various government or national institutions. Likewise, leading civil servants such as principal secretaries and senior education and administrative officers have joined the academic or administrative staff of the university. Experiences gained by either group are passed on to the relevant group of people—students or workers.

(e) National service and political education

Form VI leavers are required by law to undergo a two-year period of compulsory National Service. One part of the period is spend in camps and another in their places of work. During the two years, not only do students receive a small allowance for meeting incidental expenses but they study political education, farming methods and military craft. This programme is intended to instil in Tanzanian Youth an awareness of their obligation to the nation by requiring them to render some service to the peasants in return for the free education they have received for fourteen years or more. Students who are to be admitted to tertiary institutions for their education are covered by this scheme.

(f) Mature students' scheme for entry to institutions of higher learning

Before the 'Musoma Resolution' was passed by the TANU NEC in 1974, Form VI leavers could join institutions of higher learning or direct employment after doing only the first six months of the National Service programme. Now those wishing to be admitted for tertiary level of professional training are required:

to have worked for at least two years (excluding the National Service period) before they are considered for further education or training;

to produce a satisfactory report from their employer and the community in which they were working regarding their suitability of character, general work performance, commitment to work etc.;

to fulfil the entrance requirements of the particular institutions, for example, at least two passes at 'advanced level' or equivalent in the case of the University of Dar es Salaam.[5]

As from the academic year 1975 to 1976, only Tanzanian mature students with practical experience have been admitted to the UDSM. In addition, non-education students, like education students in their fourth term, had to do some practical work in their respective fields, e.g., in industries, government and parastatal institutions, rural areas and so on. This practical training of people who have already been in service also originated from the Musoma deliberations and has the following advantages:

They can relate their skills directly to their course at the university or similar institution.

The training period after graduation will be reduced since they have already undergone an adequate apprenticeship.

The students will have more effective bonds with the institution which selected them to join further training, so that wastage of manpower through transfers to other sectors will be reduced.

(g) In-service programmes in political education
Political education in training institutions is given great attention in order to develop correct attitudes in leadership. The leaders of various national institutions encourage students and workers to participate in political education seminars. When they return to their places of training or work, they directly or indirectly spread the ideas to their colleagues or subordinates. Awareness of current political needs and aspirations amongst Tanzanians at every level plays an important role in the development of the nation. Even party leaders and heads of institutions sometimes attend courses at the party's ideological college at Kivukoni in order to be equipped with the necessary skills in leadership. Besides, political seminars, adult education classes and addresses by party leaders, as well as the mass media, are frequently used to educate the masses.

All the above-mentioned programmes intended to bring about rapid changes in the young state were typical for all levels of educational institution throughout Tanzania, since efficient development of the country does not depend on one educational sector alone. However, the leadership role is played by the post-secondary educated group comprising 'the middle and upper grades' personnel. They are urged to learn new things just like the people they are supposed to lead. Members of this particular group are governed by the 'Tanzanian Leadership Code' which, among other things, forbids them to build a house or houses for rent, to earn more than one salary, to hold a directorship in any privately owned enterprise, and so on. The leadership code thus prevents individuals from accumulating wealth which would ultimately contravene the socialist ideology that Tanzania is trying to build.

(h) The Tanzanian concept of 'academic freedom'
According to the Western concept prevailing in Tanzania before independence and even up to the Arusha Declaration, academic freedom was held to mean freedom from any interference with an exclusive and superior world of its own. In fact, the manifestation of this arrogance led to the expulsion of about 400 students from the then Dar es Salaam University College and other institutions in October 1966, when they defied the National Service call. The university community at that time felt that its teaching programme should not be

scrutinized by society. For instance, a university could teach and train hundreds of geographers or lawyers without reference to the nation's social and economic requirements. Universities of that type were concerned with education for education's sake. This concept, it is now understood in Tanzania, may work in highly-developed societies, though even they are facing many problems and are now beginning to change their attitudes.[6] In a poor country aspiring to build socialism through a system of a planned economy such as Tanzania, how can a university claim this kind of uncontrolled freedom?[7]

(i) Objectives and functions of the UDSM
The objectives and functions of the university were defined in the University of Dar es Salaam Act as follows:

To preserve, transmit and enhance knowledge for the benefit of the people of Tanzania in accordance with the principles of socialism accepted by the people of Tanzania.
To create through education a sense of public responsibility and to promote respect for learning and the pursuit of truth.
To prepare the students to work with the people of Tanzania for the benefit of the nation.
To assume responsibility for university education within the United Republic and to make provision for places and centres of learning, education, training and research.
To co-operate with the Government of the United Republic of Tanzania in the planned and orderly development of education in the United Republic.
To stimulate and promote intellectual and cultural development of the United Republic for the benefit of the people of Tanzania.
To conduct examinations for, and award degrees, diplomas, certificates and other university certification.[8]

(j) The UDSM as a service institution
One of the important themes in the document, 'Education for Self-Reliance' concerns the relationship between education and society, especially the relevance of university courses. The government policy statement that 'planning is to choose' does not refer to a choice between bad and good things but rather to an intelligent (relevant) choice among the greatest needs of any particular period. Therefore, the university should not only train students according to manpower requirements but must also design courses which are relevant to the society's chosen priorities.

The National High Level Manpower Allocation Committee directs each year's intake for courses of study in every institution, including courses leading to specific professions required by the state. Any surplus applicants are either allocated vacant places in other university departments, or released for other types of training or direct employment in other areas. At present, for instance, the university has been requested to train fewer history and geography teachers as there are already too many of them. In secondary schools also the emphasis is on science-based subjects in order to obtain a sufficient number of students for the various science fields.

Table 5.15

Estimated University Entry and Output, 1969–1974

Year	No. of Students Qualified to Enter		Offered Places		University Output	
	Science	Arts	Science	Arts	Science	Arts
1969–70	247	318	247	318	165	186
1970–71	456	380	436	360	192	259
1971–72	540	419	510	389	203	245
1972–73	611	425	581	395	198	286
1973–74	684	430	654	400	349	324
1969–74	2538	1972	2428	1862	1107	1300

Source: The United Republic of Tanzania *Tanzania Second Five-Year Plan for Economic and Social Development . . .*, Vol. I (1969) Bibl. 18

The heavy increase of science over arts (Table 5.15) during the Second Five-Year Development Plan reflected Tanzania's urgent need of personnel for university-level occupations which require a high standard of science and mathematics. Unfortunately, the necessity to put a large number of students through Forms V and VI Science in order to produce enough advanced level passes qualifying for university entrance resulted in a high rate of wastage. The lesson is that if proper planning does not start at school level the target will be missed.

As a service institution, UDSM has also responded to the needs of society by co-operating with the government in creating the following institutes and bureaus within the university campus:

(i) Economic Research Bureau, which undertakes research on behalf of the government in areas determined jointly by the university and the Ministry of Economics and Development Planning.

(ii) Bureau of Resource Assessment and Land Use Planning, which undertakes research in land use and planning as stipulated both by the government and the university.

(iii) Institute of Development Studies, which not only trains students to tackle the problems of National and East African development but also undertakes research on problems connected with the construction of a socialist society in Tanzania.

(iv) Institute of Kiswahili Research, which does research on and development of Swahili as the national language.

Until last year the IE and IAE were part of the university as service institutions. They are now autonomous (parastatal) institutions, but remain corporate members of other educational institutions including the UDSM.

It is impossible to enumerate all the services offered by the university community. They include, to mention only a few, contributions by both staff and students to research, computer service, setting, moderating and marking the

Table 5.16

Enrolment of Tanzanian Students for Degree Courses in the East African Universities, 1961–1974

Institution	1961–2	1962–3	1963–4	1964–5	1965–6	1966–7	1967–8	1968–9	1969–70	1970–71	1971–72	1972–73	1973–74
University of D'Salaam	7	17	34	89	261	454	711	964	1 223	1 313	1 557	1 481	1 894
Makerere University	122	102	160	144	140	159	187	204	212	180	176	200	163
Nairobi University	49	38	68	104	173	178	278	289	305	274	412	100	221
Total	178	157	262	337	574	791	1 176	1 457	1 740	1 767	2 145	1 781	2 278

Source: Sectoral Planning *Takwimu za Elimu ya Juu* (Higher Education Statistics Schedule) Dar es Salaam: Ministry of National Education (1975)

national examinations, writing syllabi, offering legal aid to those who cannot hire lawyers, technical advice from the Faculties of Science, Engineering, Medicine and Agriculture, and participation of staff in various ministerial and parastatal meetings.

(k) The achievements
From the inception of the University College of Dar es Salaam to date the government has provided the money to cover the costs of education for all students. Bursary holders have been required to work in the government service for a specified period after their studies. The enrolment of students at the UDSM and comparable institutions in the country and overseas has increased tremendously. Table 5.16 shows the enrolment of Tanzanian students for degrees at the three East African Universities since independence. In the academic year 1973–1974, 3 748 (3 370 male and 378 female) students were registered for degree and diploma courses outside Tanzania (see Table 5.17). It should be noted that the courses which were being pursued were mostly science-based.

Citizens and others shown in Table 5.18 were serving as officers in senior and middle grades on permanent terms; 7 467 places were filled by temporary staff, or left vacant.

Table 5.18 indicates how Tanzania has succeeded in the objective of localizing the middle and senior positions in national institutions by means of all this training at post-secondary level, the end products of which are middle (mostly diploma holders) and upper grades (graduates and equivalent professional qualifications).

Today, Tanzanian senior and middle-level manpower are also found in many other offices throughout the country. There are now for example, Tanzanian aircraft captains, consultant engineers, university professors, medical consultants, chartered accountants, lawyers etc. These and other highly-qualified personnel were undreamed of 15 years ago.

(l) The constraints
Despite the aforesaid achievements, some problems still impede the smooth development of the plans and their implementation. The following is a brief description of some of these problems, with possible suggestions for alleviating them.

(i) Failure rate, especially among science students
The main purpose of Forms V and VI is to prepare students to enter universities or equivalent professional institutions. The failure rate, which is estimated at 25 per cent for science students, greatly increases the cost of educating each successful student. This trend has been fairly persistent. In 1967, for example, the scheduled yearly input of Tanzanian students into Science Faculties of the University Colleges of East Africa and elsewhere was 296. But only 254 Form VI science students actually passed the examination and 217 entered universities, leaving a shortfall of 79. In 1968 only 247 out of 490 Form VI science students, or 50 per cent, passed.[9] Today, all non-specialized administrative posts have been localized, but those requiring long experience after extensive training in scientific skills for which a strong mathematics or science background is needed

Table 5.17

Tanzanian Degree and Non-Degree Students Studying Outside the Country, 1973/74

Course	Males	Females	Total
1. Accountancy	245	18	263
2. Administration	13	—	13
3. Agriculture	272	38	310
4. Architecture	50	2	52
5. Arts	524	82	606
6. Commerce	35	6	41
7. Economics	18	3	21
8. Education	513	86	599
9. Engineering	424	3	427
10. Forestry	39	—	39
11. Horticulture	1	—	1
12. Lands	59	—	59
13. Law	95	11	106
14. Management	11	—	11
15. Marine Technology	2	—	2
16. Medicine	548	36	584
17. Music	3	—	3
18. Nursing	2	23	25
19. Religion	20	4	24
20. Science	365	48	413
21. Social Studies	9	3	12
22. Veterinary	83	3	86
23. Various Others	39	12	51
Total	3370	378	3748

Source: Sectoral Planning *Takwimu za Elimu ya Juu* (Higher Education Statistics Schedule) Dar es Salaam: Ministry of National Education (1975)

are still unoccupied. If no solution is found to this problem, obviously the targets cannot be reached. The government has, therefore, revised the yearly intake into Form IV science and is prepared slightly to raise the number of students to be trained beyond Form IV in order to allow for wastage.

A complementary strategy is to combine the academic course with vocational training, (cf. B.Sc. (Ed) and B.A. (Ed) programmes) so that the unsuccessful students may also be employable. In this connection the Ministry of National Education has already worked out some plans, known as diversification/vocationalization in secondary school education, to make all Forms IV or V leavers specialize, in addition to academic subjects, in one vocational subject, e.g., teaching, agriculture, technical trades, domestic science or commercial subjects.

Table 5.18

Progress in Localization of the Public Service Achieved Since Independence

Year (December)	Citizens	Others	Total	Percentage of Citizens
1961	1 170	3 282	4 452	26.3
1962	1 821	2 902	4 723	38.5
1963	2 469	2 580	5 049	48.9
1964	3 083	2 306	5 389	57.2
1965	3 951	2 011	5 962	66.3
1966	4 364	1 898	6 262	69.7
1967	4 937	1 817	6 754	73.1
1968	6 208	1 619	7 827	79.3
1969	6 123	1 351	7 474	81.9
1970	8 042	1 377	9 419	85.6
1971	9 708	1 015	10 723	90.5
1972	11 988	745	12 733	94.1

Source: The Manpower Planning Division *Annual Report to the President* Dar es Salaam: Ministry of Economic Affairs and Development Planning (1972)

(ii) Financial instability

Inflation of prices, e.g., of consumer goods, fuel, etc., and failure of cash crops due to crop pests, insufficient rainfall, etc., have tended to affect the financial position of the country. This has in turn made it impossible for some of the government plans to be fulfilled. There have been cases where government projects had to be postponed or cancelled because of such constraints.

(iii) Unequal representation of women in education and employment

The participation of women, not only in higher education and training but also in public service, has been disappointingly low (see Table 5.17). The government is concerned about this and is investigating the causes in order to be able to fulfil the Party's objective of giving fair and equal opportunity to all citizens irrespective of colour, sex or religion. In many instances, priority access to higher education and employment has been given to women. It is gratifying to note that several women in Tanzania are members of Parliament or of the East African Legislative Assembly, Area Commissioners, Area Secretaries, etc. In the present 1975 to 1980 Parliament Tanzania has, for the first time, two women cabinet ministers. This and the increase in the number of other senior women officers will raise the morale of women not only in Tanzania but in other parts of the world as well.

(iv) Misallocation of manpower

Very often there have been instances where staff in the middle and senior grades in the public service were placed in jobs for which they were not specifically trained. This is not done deliberately but results from an urgent need to fill temporarily a vacancy created by the departure of a substantive officer. The temporary measure then ends up by being a permanent one. When this situation occurs, output and efficiency tend to be low because the young officers feel frustrated about the irrelevance of their education and field practice to the job they are doing. However, the Ministry of Manpower Development, together with the institutions where such anomalies have been found, are aware of this situation and steps are being taken to rectify it. Furthermore, the institutions of higher learning, for example the University of Dar es Salaam, now refrain from over-specialization in one particular area and have designed 'multi-subject streams' in which students are able to train in broad areas of their future careers.

(v) Lack of academic legitimacy and authenticity
The UDSM, the highest institution of higher learning in the country, is 15 years old, but still seems to be without legitimacy and authenticity in respect of academic standing. It is continuing to invite external examiners from as far away as Europe or America to assess the preformance of students in some of its courses. One wonders whether it is really necessary to strain the country's meagre resources by incurring the expenses involved in bringing foreign academics to judge the quality of the curricula Tanzania has decided to adopt.

(vi) Shortage of manpower
The lack of manpower for the specialized fields necessitates the employment of aliens, who might tend to negate the Tanzanian effort. To avoid this possibility, Tanzania has attempted to appoint citizens as heads of all institutions in the country. Provided these are not 'dictated' to by the so-called 'foreign experts' this is a good move. Furthermore, these experts are screened through a system of interviews, reliable referees, etc., and they are recruited from many nationalities. All these precautions should ensure that people sympathetic to the aspirations of the country and its philosophy of non-alignment are selected.

(vii) Failure to recognize the academic standing of experienced students
In an attempt to maintain the high standards expected by distinguished scholars officiating as external examiners in various subjects, the university has failed to accommodate the mature students who had special training prior to their entry to university. Besides having many years of field experience, a considerable number of such students had been trained for two to four years in Diploma courses, e.g., in education, agriculture, medicine, or engineering. If these same students had gone to Canada or the U.S.A., their advanced standing would have been recognized and their studies shortened by a year or more. Such recognition would not only have saved public funds but the students would have gone back to work with their employers much earlier.

(viii) Problem of 'ivory tower' or 'elitism'
Their scanty number leaves students that get an opportunity to acquire post-secondary training with a feeling that they are a very special group, an elite. Such class distinction has no place in Tanzanian socialist philosophy. The government has tried its best to subject this group to national service programmes, mature students' entry scheme, productive labour, etc., in order to minimize the elitist tendency. Unfortunately, attitudinal factors such as academic gowns, use of a (colonial) foreign language instead of the national

language (Swahili) as the medium of instruction, degrees, etc., are still exclusive to this group. Moreover, they tend to create an attitude that 'colonial things' were good and anything Tanzanian is 'second class'. As long as these factors are allowed to persist it will be difficult to convince this special class that it must come down from its 'ivory tower'.

Conclusion

Despite the aforementioned problems, post-secondary training, particularly university education, has played a very important role in the development of Tanzania. This has been due to the wise leadership which all along has been able to identify many of the problems of underdevelopment which Tanzania inherited from the colonial masters. The economic development plans have been the key to our educational achievements. The creation last October of a separate Ministry of Manpower Development by the President is another step to enhance the training efforts. It is hoped that the new ministry, which has already achieved notable successes, will be able to co-ordinate effectively the educational and training efforts made by the ministries concerned. There are indications that as a result the nation will be able to succeed in its objective of self-sufficiency in manpower by 1980.

Notes

1 This account is confined to Tanzania mainland; in fact before 1968 higher education was not a Union matter.
2 See Kitchen, H (ed.) *The Educated African—A Country-by-Country Survey of Educational Development in Africa* London: Heinemann (1962)
3 See *Education Ordinance No. 37 of 1961, An Ordinance to Make Provison for Single Education System in Tanzania* pp. 256–274
4 Localization is the term used in Tanzania for replacement of expatriate staff by Tanzanian citizens.
5 TANU, *Proceedings of the NEC Meetings held at Musoma, November* (1974) Dar es Salaam: TANU Headquarters (mimeo)
6 Cf. Faure, E et al. *Learning To Be. The World of Education Today and Tomorrow* Paris: Unesco/London: Harrap (1972) p. 17
7 Cf. Nyerere, J K *Relevance and Dar es Salaam University* See article 2.3 of this book
8 The United Republic of Tanzania: *The University of Dar es Salaam Act, 1970* Bibl. 179
9 See Eliufoo, S *The Role of the University College, Dar es Salaam in a Socialist Tanzania* Speech delivered by the Minister for Education. Dar es Salaam: University College (1967) (mimeo)

5.9 Correspondence Education in Tanzania
E M Chale

In Tanzania, as in most British ex-colonial countries, correspondence education was initially provided by overseas-based colleges and later by indigenous institutions. While it might be interesting to compare the two types of institution, this paper will limit discussion to the indigenous type, in order to focus on experience that is unique in Tanzania. A critical look will be taken at the history, objectives, tutorial experiences and future plans of correspondence education in Tanzania.

1. Historical background

Indigenous correspondence education activities in Tanzania began in 1964 with the establishment of the Moshi Co-operative Education Centre (CEC), which was designed to cater for the rural population. The considerable experience gained with the CEC indicated 'that in a large country like Tanzania, correspondence instruction provides a relatively cheap means of instruction for a very large student body'.[1]

This conviction led in the late sixties to recommendations for setting up a comprehensive correspondence institution, on which this paper will concentrate. The recommendations were made by the National Advisory Committee on Adult Education in co-operation with certain ministries and institutions, notably the Ministries of National Education, Regional Administration and Rural Development, Economic Affairs and Development Planning, Agriculture, Food and Co-operatives on the one hand, and the Kivukoni College, IAE, the University of Dar es Salaam, and the TANU party on the other. As a result of these recommendations, technical and financial assistance was sought from international organizations, notably Unesco and the Swedish International Development Authority (SIDA), and a Plan of Operation for a Five-Year Pilot Project was drawn up.

The project started operating officially on November 25th 1970, with the signing of a Tanzanian/Swedish aid agreement for the establishment of the National Correspondence Institution (NCI) to be attached to the IAE, then part of the University of Dar es Salaam.[2]

2. Philosophy, objectives and range of courses

In general, it could be argued that the indigenous correspondence education system in Tanzania, as in the rest of the developing countries, was established because of the need to restructure the existing Western-oriented education systems so as to develop a system suited to the specific needs of the country. Overseas-based colleges in Tanzania invariably provided their students with foreign-based curricula[3], and it was felt that an indigenous college would be more capable of relating its course materials to the students' immediate background. Creation of new curricula is thus one of the arguments.

Another reason for Tanzania's keen interest in correspondence education has been the necessity to expand educational opportunities in response to pressure from the public since the early 1960s. It may be mentioned at this point that this natural interest coincided with the recent interest taken by world organizations like Unesco, UNDP, UNECA and SIDA in non-formal mass education. That explains why in its initial years the Tanzania NCI was not financed from the public budget. Besides, the demand for education had risen to such an extent that it could not have been met by the 25 per cent of the national budget spent on it.

The most important consideration in establishing correspondence education has, however, been to help the country build an egalitarian society based on the principles of Socialism (Ujamaa) and Self-Reliance (Kujitegemea). Within this egalitarian society every citizen had to have equal educational opportunities regardless of age, sex, marital status, family size, place of residence, economic background, social position and similar external barriers. Every student has the right to make the most of himself. The country is not socialist yet, and because of economic constraints her educational planning, particularly at post-primary level, has been implemented 'only to the extent justified by the manpower requirements of the economy for development'.[4] It is for this reason that President Julius Nyerere had to appeal: 'Our sights must be on the majority'.[5]

This purview indicates that there is a clear harmony between the broad philosophy of correspondence education in the world and Tanzanian policies, as expressed not only in political rhetoric but also in practice. Before the inauguration of the NCI, for example, the Second Five-Year Plan of 1969 outlined the aim of the institution in the following terms: 'to serve literate but isolated persons throughout the country, who wish to enlarge their knowledge and understanding of subjects of importance to national development'.[6]

Tanzania's indigenous correspondence education is not fully fledged; but an appraisal of its programmes indicates that courses are geared towards developing a socialist and self-reliant country. In accordance with the national philosophy and its objectives, there are three types of course. First, the mass-oriented courses, specially prepared for people with little or no formal education. Courses of this type are written in the national language, Swahili, and currently include National Policies and Development (Siasa) and Book-Keeping. The use of Swahili marks a 'significant development in building a national institution because until Tanzania wrote in Swahili, most correspondence courses studied in Africa were written in one of the main international languages—French or English'.[7] Swahili is also used predominantly in answers to enquires, correspondence with students, telephone interviews and information publications which will be reviewed below under the heading 'Tutorial services and experiences'.

Second, there are manpower-oriented or professional courses. These are designed to offer a variety of programmes that provide training for middle-level management and administration in the form of on-the-job training, e.g., Certificate in Law and Accounting.

Finally, there are examination-oriented courses. These were not initially given emphasis in the project because it was thought unwise to duplicate existing educational facilities. In 1971, however, Tanzania's decision to establish National Form IV and VI Examinations and to withdraw recognition of external examinations provoked the general public to demand compensatory educational opportunities for adults wishing to sit for the Tanzania National Examinations or similar academic examinations. This third category of courses is divided into three stages. Stage I is equivalent to lessons taught in Forms I and II in secondary schools. Stage II is eqivalent to subjects taught in Forms III and IV, while Stage III is equivalent to Forms V and VI. If and when a student successfully completes Stages I and II he may sit for the National Form IV Examinations without taking a qualifying test, provided he also takes Political Education and Swahili papers.

3. Course production

A fruitful discussion on course production should begin with a look at the course producers in the specific sense, and the NCI staff in general. In the early years, the NCI key positions were manned by both expatriates and Tanzanians on the counterpart system. Now in 1976, after the phasing out of expatriates, there are 80 full-time Tanzanian members of staff of whom 15 are resident tutors and 65 technical and operational staff. There are also 200 part-time tutors.

Course production is thus wholly in the hands of nationals. The actual production involves, as it may elsewhere, obtaining approved syllabi from the Ministry of National Education or institutions dealing with particular subjects, such as TANU (Political Education), and NABAA (Accountancy). The syllabus is then divided into units. The course is written by either full-time or part-time staff, individually or in a team. The full-time tutors co-ordinate the writing processes, supervise quality standards and correct or revise the scripts. Courses are designed according to demand by the students, availability of subject specialists and national or government priorities. Between 1975 and 1976 courses were produced to support the national campaigns, 'Kilimo cha Kufa na Kupona' and 'Elimu kwa Wote' (UPE).

The course manuscripts are then edited in consultation with the subject-specialist tutors and radio tutors. After printing, a course is released and the public is notified through newspapers and radio broadcasts.

The profile of course production shows that whereas in November 1972 there was only an Introductory Course in Political Education, by the end of March 1976 the NCI offered 12 subjects, namely:

1.	Political Education	Introductory
2.	Political Education	Stage I
3.	Political Education	Stage II
4.	Swahili	Stage III
5.	Mathematics	Stage I
6.	English	Introductory
7.	English	Stage I
8.	Geography	Stage I
9.	History	Stage I
10.	Book-Keeping	Introductory
11.	Kilimo cha Maharagwe (bean cultivation)	
12.	Man in Organization	

In addition to this list, many other courses for secondary and professional levels are in different stages of preparation. They will be reviewed later in the section, 'A look at the future'.

4. Tutorial services and experiences

At the end of 1972, the NCI started with an introductory course in political education, with 368 students. By December 1973 there were 4067 students, and 6997 by 1974. In July 1976, their number had risen to a total of 21 000.

Since the NCI is a service institution for the expansion and equalization of educational opportunities, students are charged incredibly low fees compared with other institutions rendering similar services. The fees for introductory courses range from 5/ = (Tsh) to 15/ = ; for Stage I the fee is 30/ =, for Stage II, 60/ = and for advanced courses, 90/ =.

The increase in student enrolment has led to the expansion of services. Recent notices in the press and radio broadcasts have helped to publicize the courses available, and those conducted under UPE have stimulated student teachers to apply also for examination-oriented courses.

Students make their enquiries by letter or telephone, or they call personally on the NCI for advisory services. At the time of writing, the advisory office takes care of an average of 150 letters daily. As already mentioned, Swahili is the language predominantly used in these contacts. Some of the enquiries are simple requests for information on certain areas, others require more serious attention. Whatever the nature of the question, every effort is made to satisfy the students' personal needs.

The organizational aspects of correspondence teaching on such a large scale can clearly not be the responsibility of one person or section. There is a variety of staff to accomplish the diverse tasks. Counsellors advise students before enrolment and during their course of studies. Accounts staff receive fees and answer queries concerning payment of fees. Registration staff check on the enrolment of students. Recorders check on the letters and assignments coming in from the students, mail them to part-time tutors for correction and marking and enter the marks on the record cards. They also remind non-active students of their studies by sending them appropriate standard form letters, or in some cases, more personal letters.

In addition to this range of services, the Resident Tutors arrange from time to time regional tours to organize contacts for distant, isolated correspondence students with the class. Furthermore, wherever possible, correspondence courses are supported by radio programmes. Evidently, successful running of correspondence education requires the continual co-operation of every staff member, reciprocated by the students themselves. Team spirit is in fact the key to efficient service.

5. A look at the future

From what has been outlined and discussed it should be evident that indigenous correspondence education is not yet fully fledged. The institution has had many plans but not all of them materialized, because the special needs and priorities of the country intervened. However that may be, the institution has both short term and long term plans for the future.

One immediate plan, for instance, is to complete all stages of the courses initially set as the first target in the 'Plan of Operation'. After their completion, there is a plan to launch a programme on technical training by correspondence. Other professional courses to be offered include teacher in-service and police officers' courses. It is further hoped that in the long run, degree courses in subjects of importance to national development will be introduced.

The NCI also has plans for employing new methods. Since until now correspondence courses have been studied individually, a need is felt to use them as a basis for group learning. This is both important and advantageous, because a group could extend the opportunity to study a course to people who may need help from more literate members of the group. These groups could further be utilized in the teaching of courses on subjects relevant to the day-to-day activities of adult learners, such as domestic science, health and agriculture, to bolster functional literacy. The organization of rigorous short-term face-to-face tutorial sessions is also envisaged, not only in academic subjects but also in practical ones.

Further, since accommodation has been limited in the IAE where correspondence education activities have been housed, they were scheduled to be moved to a special building in early 1977. The new premises were planned to be the headquarters, and the rest of correspondence education activities decentralized to prevent the ever-increasing activities from ultimately outgrowing the building. To cope with the increasing volume of work, teaching centres will be established in the regions. Students in every regional centre will be able to enrol, pay fees, and obtain tutorial services. Dar es Salaam will remain the headquarters because of its strategic location for consultancy and part-time services which are essential for advice on the preparation of correspondence courses, especially in respect of co-operation with other educational institutions such as secondary schools, colleges of varied biases and particularly the University of Dar es Salaam.

By way of conclusion there is no need to over-emphasize that, though indigenous correspondence education has begun with enthusiastic objectives, philosophy and educational programmes, its future shape undoubtedly depends on the sense of direction and management it will be given. Whilst initially, correspondence education was meant to be merely nursed by the IAE until it would be able to develop as an independent institution, the trend of events at the time of writing seems to move in a different direction. Currently the NCI is continually being reduced in complexity, volume and programmes to the level of incomparably smaller departments of the IAE. Any reference to the NCI is suppressed in preference for a newly-coined designation, Correspondence Education Department (CED). There may hopefully come a point where the general public will not condone the smothering of indigenous correspondence education. Despite growing pains and intermittent dark moments, the outlook for its development into a mature correspondence education institution seems optimistic. Once that stage is reached, the NCI will, no doubt, be more efficient in its activities, which will serve and affect not just a few thousands, but millions of people living in every part of the country and engaged in the development of a socialist and self-reliant society.

Notes

1   Kagaruki, G E and Mwakatobe, R Y 'Correspondence Education in Co-operative Training in Tanzania' in *Correspondence Education in Africa* edited by A Kabwasa and M M Kaunda. London: Routledge and Kegan Paul (1973) p. 35

2   See Erdos, R *The Role of Correspondence Education in Tanzania* Dar es Salaam: Institute of Adult Education (1974) (unpublished material.)

3 This is not suggest that all of such colleges are rendering a qualitatively inferior type of education. Some, but not all of them, are accredited within their local context. Cf. British Council for Accreditation of Correspondence Colleges. *By-Laws* London: (1970)
4 Cf. First and Second Development Plans.
5 See Nyerere, J K *Education for Self-Reliance* pp. 17–32 of this volume
6 United Republic of Tanzania *Tanzania Second Five-Year Plan for Economic and Social Development, 1st July 1969–30th June 1974, Vol. I* p. 158 Bibl. 18
7 See Note 2

Chapter 6 Research in Education

6.1 The Unproductive School

A Research report on the economic aspects of 'Education for Self-Reliance' in Tanzanian secondary schools

T L Maliyamkono

Introduction

When I proposed a study on the effectiveness of 'Education for Self-Reliance' as reflected in the productive activities in secondary schools, a friend of mine made a remark which I must quote: 'Be careful, friend, you might be treading a dangerous path'. For a minute I did not know what he meant. The argument that followed was hot and it boiled down to the difficulties envisaged in conducting a study that attempts to evaluate some parts of the whole system.

'Education for Self-Reliance' was not meant to deal with only economic issues. It is not a cement-production factory to overcome cement shortages; it is not a petroleum deposit to solve our economic problems. The primary purpose is to 'prepare people for their responsibilities as free workers in a free democratic society'. To achieve this purpose it is necessary to make use of avenues toward education which will minimize costs while maximizing returns. The latter include the inculcation of 'rightful' thinking—an awareness of social aspirations and goals. Others are more directly related to solving our immediate problems, such as the economic crisis that nations of the Third World are going to have to live with until they take their place in this world. In evaluating the policy only on

Table 6.1

Regions and their secondary schools participating in the study

(Key: U = Urban; R = Rural)

Region	Location	U/R	Boarding	Day	Boys'	Girls'	Mixed	Public	Private	Senior	Junior
Arusha	Arusha	U	–	x	–	–	x	x	–	–	x
	Karatu	R	–	x	–	–	x	x	–	–	x
	Singe	R	x	–	–	–	x	–	x	–	x
	Ilboru	U	x	–	x	–	–	x	–	x	–
	Enaboishu	U	–	x	–	–	x	–	x	–	x
	Arusha-Meru	U	x	–	–	–	x	x	–	–	x
	Makumiba	R	–	x	–	–	x	–	x	–	x
Dar es Salaam	Azania	U	–	x	x	–	–	x	–	–	x
	Porodhani	U	–	x	–	–	x	x	–	–	x
	Jangwani	U	–	x	–	x	–	x	–	x	–
	Kisutu	U	–	x	–	x	–	x	–	–	x
	Tambaza	U	–	x	–	–	x	x	–	x	–
	Zanaki	U	–	x	–	x	–	x	–	–	x
	Shaban Rob.	U	–	x	–	–	x	–	x	–	x
	Mzizima	U	–	x	–	–	x	–	x	x	–
Dodoma	Bihawana	U	x	–	x	–	–	x	–	–	x
	Dodoma	U	–	x	–	–	x	x	–	–	x
	Mazengo	U	x	–	x	–	–	x	–	x	–
	Mpwapwa	R	x	–	x	–	–	x	–	–	x
Iringa	Iringa	U	x	–	–	x	–	x	–	–	x
	Malangali	U	x	–	x	–	–	x	–	x	–
	Mkwawa	U	x	–	x	–	–	x	–	–	x
	Njombe	U	x	–	x	–	–	x	–	–	x
	Tosamaganga	R	x	–	x	–	–	x	–	x	–
	Highlands	U	–	x	–	–	x	–	x	–	x
Kigoma	Ujiji Semi	U	x	–	x	–	–	–	x	–	x
	Nary	U	x	–	–	–	x	x	–	–	x
	Kigoma	R	–	x	x	–	–	x	–	–	x
Kilimanjaro	Kibosho	R	x	–	–	x	–	–	x	–	x
	Machame	R	x	–	–	x	–	x	–	–	x
	Moshi (Techn)	U	x	–	x	–	–	x	–	–	x
	Same	U	x	–	x	–	–	x	–	–	x
	Kilimanjaro	R	–	x	x	–	–	–	x	–	x
	Siha	R	–	x	x	–	–	x	–	–	x
	Kibo	U	–	x	–	–	x	–	x	–	x

		U/R	BD	D	B	G	M	P	PR	S	J
Lindi	Lindi	U	x	–	–	–	x	x	–	–	x
	Mkonge	U	–	x	–	–	x	–	x	–	x
	Namupa	R	x	–	x	–	–	–	x	–	x
Mara	Ikuru	R	x	–	–	–	x	x	–	–	x
	Musoma	U	x	–	–	–	x	x	–	x	–
	Tarime	U	x	–	–	–	x	x	–	–	x
	Shirati	R	x	–	–	–	x	x	x	–	x
	Makoku	R	x	–	x	–	–	–	x	–	x
Mbeya	Iyunga	U	x	–	x	–	–	x	–	–	x
	Loleza	U	x	–	–	x	–	x	–	–	x
	Mbeya	U	x	–	–	–	x	x	–	–	x
	Sangu	U	–	x	–	–	x	–	x	–	x
Mtwara	Masasi	U	x	–	–	x	–	x	–	–	x
	Mtwara (Techn)	U	x	–	x	–	–	x	–	–	x
	Ndanda	R	x	–	–	–	x	x	–	x	–
Pwani	Bagamoyo	U	–	x	x	–	–	x	–	–	x
	Kibaha	R	x	–	–	–	x	–	x	x	–
Rukwa	Kantalamba	U	x	–	x	–	–	x	–	–	x
	Kaangasa	R	x	–	x	–	–	–	x	–	x
Ruvuma	Songea (Girls)	U	x	–	–	x	–	x	–	x	–
	Peramiho	R	x	–	–	x	–	x	–	x	x
	Songea (Boys)	U	x	–	x	–	–	x	–	x	–
Shinyanga	Shinyanga	R	x	–	x	–	–	x	–	x	–
	Shinyanga Comm.	U	x	–	–	–	x	x	–	x	–
	Buluba	U	–	x	–	–	x	–	x	x	–
Singida	Mwenge	U	x	–	–	–	x	x	–	–	x
	Tumaini	R	x	–	–	–	x	x	–	–	x
	Dungunyi Sem.	R	x	–	x	–	–	–	x	x	–
Tabora	Kazima	U	–	x	–	–	x	x	–	–	x
	Milambo	U	x	–	x	–	–	x	–	–	x
	Tabora (Girls)	U	x	–	–	x	–	x	–	x	–
	Tabora (Boys)	U	x	–	x	–	–	x	–	x	–
	Itaga Sem.	R	x	–	x	–	–	–	x	x	–
	Uyui	U	–	x	–	–	x	–	x	–	x
Tanga	Korogwe	R	x	–	–	x	–	x	–	–	x
	Tanga	U	–	x	x	–	–	x	–	x	–
	Usagara	U	x	–	–	–	x	x	–	x	–
	Galanos	U	x	–	x	–	–	–	x	–	x
	Popilal	U	–	x	–	–	x	–	x	–	x
West Lake	Bukoba	U	–	x	–	–	x	x	–	–	x
	Ihungo	R	x	–	x	–	–	x	–	x	–
	Kahororo	R	x	–	x	–	–	x	–	–	x
	Nyakato	R	x	–	x	–	–	–	x	–	x
	Rugambwa	R	x	–	–	x	–	x	–	x	–
	Rubya	R	x	–	x	–	–	–	x	–	x

its economic implications, it must, thus, be fully realized that the economic aspects are a sub-system within a larger system and that there are other purposes the policy is intended for. The avenues selected to evaluate the economic contribution of secondary schools in mainland Tanzania are to be seen in this light.

What has been attempted in this study is first to develop a theoretical framework which seems to fit the requirements of the policy.[1] It is argued that to emphasize academic performance at the expense of production performance or vice-versa is an undesirable course of action. The 'proper' way is to develop both objectives in such a way that they complement each other and that neither of them adversely affects the other.

Secondly, an attempt has been made to link the level of production to variables considered likely to provide some variations. Thus, comparisons have been made of the per capita income of students in boarding schools and day schools, girl' schools and boys' schools, private and public schools, junior and senior schools, as well as by regions. If anything, the results will be a starting point for future assessment. The short last chapter has been set aside for policy implications.

1. Research procedure

The study was launched in December 1975. Recording sheets were prepared by the principal researcher and a lot of details that went on the information recording sheets were drawn from related variables that were thought necessary for data gathering. That was part one of the research project, based on the school year 1974 to 1975. In May to June 1976 the second part of the study was conducted. It was intended to test student and teacher attitudes toward productive activities.[2] Altogether, 18 research assistants were involved and there were eight supervisors including the principal researcher: three members of the staff at UDSM and four practising teachers of secondary schools and teachers' colleges.

The sample: It was intended to obtain data from every secondary school on the mainland, with the exception of army schools for obvious reasons. The returns were 77 per cent. The main reasons for failing to obtain a higher return were reluctance on the part of the heads of schools to release such information and rather inconvenient timing; in some schools, teachers responsible for records of self-help activities were either on holiday or attending seminars. However, Table 6.1 showing returns by regions and different categories indicates that this may be considered a representative sample.[3]

2. Productive activities

It was found that schools have a variety of productive activities, which may be grouped as shown in Table 6.2.

At the time of gathering data there were 213 cattle on school farms, 9 sheep, 126 goats, 32406 chicken (for eggs and for meat) and 525 pigs. There were 139060 hectares of cultivated land.

Table 6.3 p. 210 shows the number of different implements used for productive activities between 1974 and 1975.

Table 6.2

Production Activities in Schools

On School Farms	Trade and Commerce	Services to the Local Community
Crop farming	**Commercial shops**	shoe repair
maize	handicraft	bookbinding
vegetables	needlework	work on village farms
beans	brick-making	maintenance of public
coffee	furniture	and other institutions
cassava	cookery	
coconuts	basket-weaving	
tea	electrical works	
pawpaws	mechanical works	
cotton	lampshade-making	
Animal husbandry		
cattle		
pigs		
goats		
poultry		
fish		

Income from self-help activities

Incomes were realized from different economic activities as Table 6.2 shows. Most of the income came from agriculture. Service and maintenance brought an income of 361 634.60 Tsh as compared to the income of 288 510.70 Tsh from trade and commerce. Table 6.4 shows the breakdown:

Table 6.4

Income from Productive Activities (in Tsh)

Source of Income	Amount
Agriculture and Animal Husbandry	1 388 490.15
Trade and Commerce	288 510.70
Services and Maintenance	361 634.60
Others	80 508.60
Total	2 119 144.05

Further categorization of income realized from self-help schemes may be made by regions, by boarding and day schools, by girls', boys' and mixed schools, urban and rural schools, public and private schools. Rather than report figures of total earnings for every one of these divisions, per capita incomes have been calculated. These are shown in Table 6.6 against per capita expenditure and the resulting per capita savings.

Table 6.3

Implements Used for Productive Activities

Region	Hoes	Rakes	Watering cans	Hoses (length in metres)	Spades	Pangas	Oxploughs	Tractors	Karais	Slashers	Others (specified)	Draft animals	Fertilizers (in kgms)	Manure (in tons)	Stores	Numbers of schools	Numbers of students
Arusha	514	39	46	800	44	144	1	2	34	176	1 Landrover 5 Wheel-barrows	4 Oxen 32 Surusa	88 546	5½	5	7	2 260
Dar es Salaam	500	138	105	2 412	56	150	—	—	33	—	—	—	600	36	4	8	5 135
Dodoma	1 900	70	64	940	84	428	3	—	80	—	2 Axes 4 Wheel-b. 11 Buckets 24 Picks 61 Sickles	6 Oxen	2 600	15	n.a.	4	2 158
Iringa	865	57	37	111	37	27	3	1	4	—		—	25 650	10	0	5	1 744
Kigoma	64	14	86	135	163	11	—	—	17	81		—	700	—	n.a.	2	564
Kilimanjaro	2 106	104	8	40	17	579	—	—	10	168	1 Coffee-pulper 18 Buckets	—	2 000	—	—	7	2 646
Lindi	537	35	20	270	25	245	1	2	24	30	6 Sprinklers	—	8 000	3	3	3	882
Mara	n.a.	45	10	770	18	168	—	—	42	90	40 Axes 15 Wheel-b. 66 Axes 10 Buckets 9 Sickles	—	1 764	1½	4	5	1 213
Mbeya	1 026	70	24	810	28	30	4	—	15	—	4 Sprinklers	2 Donkeys	5 565	2½	n.a.	4	1 802
Mtwara	718	79	92	1 240	37	67	—	—	35	159	n.a.	—	8 750	1½	0	2	977
Pwani	n.a.	n.a.	n.a.	n.a.	n.a.	—	n.a.	n.a.	n.a.	n.a.		n.a.	n.a.	n.a.	n.a.	2	822
Rukwa	280	18	8	100	0	5	4	—	15	30	—		1 599	—	2	2	542

210

Region	Hoes	Rakes	Watering cans	Hoses (length in metres)	Spades	Pangas	Oxploughs	Tractors	Karais	Slashers	Others (specified)	Draft animals	Fertilizers (in kgms)	Manure (in tons)	Stores	Numbers of schools	Numbers of students
Ruvuma	534	42	35	30	10	65	—	—	31	—	10 Axes / 5 Forks / 17 Wheel-b. / 2 Picks	—	1 850	3	n.a.	3	722
Shinyanga	365	4	85	360	8	114	—	—	25	42	—	—	3 400	10	0	3	787
Singida	808	10	15	—	10	30	—	—	5	—	12 Axes / 15 Picks / 1 Wheel-b.	—	2 000	—	3	3	928
Tabora	1 484	42	131	2 300	23	32	—	—	2	72	27 Wheel-b. / 30 Sickles / 20 Buckets	—	22 100	12	2	6	2 406
Tanga	1 750	102	20	350	88	133	—	2	102	98	—	—	7 100	7	2	5	3 201
Westlake	825	127	25	400	45	99	—	—	46	300	6 Wheel-b.	10 Oxen / 32 Surusa / 2 Donkeys	8 848	19	n.a.	6	1 325
Total	14 382	996	811	11 068	693	2 297	16	7	520	1 246		—	190 973	124	22	76	29 297 (Pwani excluded)

Items of expenditure

It was found that schools spend their incomes from self-help activities as Table 6.5 indicates:

Table 6.5

Items of Expenditure in Day Schools and Boarding Schools (in Tsh)

Items	Expenditure	Day Schools	Boarding Schools
Improved diet	167806.75	53437.70	114369.05
Recreation	57335.60	18800.00	38535.60
Repairs and maintenance	114245.45	59679.85	54565.60
Charity	15772.00	15387.00	385.00
Improved health service	62539.10	62295.00	244.10
Others	214169.15	30650.00	183519.15
Total	631868.05	240249.55	391618.50

The volume of expenditure by day schools on improved diet should be noted. Another interesting point is the difference in incomes and savings between boarding schools and day schools. Most boarding schools are in rural areas (see Table 6.1).

Table 6.6

Per Capita Income, Expenditure, and Savings from Self-Help Activities in Different Kinds of School (in Tsh)

Categories	Income	Expenditure	Savings
Boarding	84.24	18.25	66.42
Day	22.73	18.11	4.62
Girls	27.87	12.45	15.45
Boys	96.32	74.58	21.74
Mixed (boys and girls)	38.55	36.32	2.23
Public	74.28	27.05	47.23
Junior (up to Form IV)	54.38	31.85	22.53
Senior (up to Form VI)	77.12	14.90	62.22
Urban	37.84	25.46	12.84
Rural	145.13	39.27	105.86
National average per student	65.85	29.83	36.11

Table 6.7 shows incomes, expenditure and savings by regions. Among other observations it is interesting to note that Kilimanjaro with many public schools

in rural areas performs far better than Dar es Salaam region with most of the public schools in the heart of the city.

Table 6.7

Per Capita Income, Expenditure, and Savings by Regions (in Tsh)

Region	Per Capita Income	Per Capita Expenditure	Per Capita Savings
Pwani*	714.65	n.a.	—
Dodoma	158.95	n.a.	—
Lindi	108.51	100.98	7.53
Mara	81.49	55.08	26.11
Kilimanjaro	71.46	50.16	21.30
Arusha	59.92	48.53	11.39
Iringa	58.99	17.40	41.54
Mbeya	56.81	16.82	39.99
Singida	55.87	35.96	19.91
West Lake	36.13	3.15	32.98
Dar es Salaam	25.93	17.80	8.13
Kigoma	24.83	23.52	1.30
Tanga	24.51	11.17	13.34
Mtwara	19.93	11.10	8.83
Rukwa	16.95	16.50	0.45
Tabora	16.42	14.56	1.84
Shinyanga	11.78	1.25	10.53
Ruvuma	1.71	1.72	0.01

*Pwani may be influenced by Kibaha's large entry of 860.39 per capita.

In Table 6.8 productivity and academic achievement are shown in correlation to each other. Regions are ranked according to per capita income of students, and Form IV examination results have been calculated on the basis of passes and failures.[4]

3. Discussion of the data
General comments
The null hypotheses built into the study require some general comments. It is, for example, incorrect to assume that schools produce on an equal scale. The evidence provided by the data proves that rural schools produce a lot more than urban schools; that boys' schools produce more than girls' schools; that public schools have higher yields than private schools; and that the nature of an agricultural activity, e.g., perennial crops against annual crops, does not make a significant difference.

Some caution must be exercised in interpreting the results, because some findings may have been affected by the distribution. For example, the Pwani

Table 6.8

Productivity Versus Academic Achievement

Region	Rank on Productivity	Rank on Academic Achievement
Pwani	1	5
Dodoma	2	9
Lindi	3	18
Mara	4	16
Kilimanjaro	5	3
Arusha	6	13
Iringa	7	4
Mbeya	8	13
Singida	9	1
West Lake	10	6
Dar es Salaam	11	16
Kigoma	12	2
Tanga	13	8
Mtwara	14	15
Rukwa	15	7
Tabora	16	11
Shinyanga	17	9
Ruvuma	18	12

region shows higher yields than Kilimanjaro. But that may be largely due to the fact that one of the two schools in the Pwani region from which complete returns were received is Kibaha, which owing to special circumstances produces far more than any other school in the country. Compare the national average income per student of Tsh 65.85 with that of Kibaha of Tsh 860.39.

It should also be remembered that the data refer to 1974–1975 and that there will have been improvements following the 'Musoma Resolution' of November 1974 'Education and Work'. The data are, however, significant enough to provide a starting point for future research in this area.

In the discussion of the data that follows, the above comments should be borne in mind: First, there is evidently no severe shortage in schools of agricultural tools and implements which have a bearing on the production function. Table 6.3 shows that there is a hoe for almost every two students. This is not bad since students could work on the farm alternately. On the other hand, most schools, except the specialized ones, are very short of workshop equipment—saws, benches and the like.

Second, there seems to be a variety of productive activities depending on the area in which the school is situated. What is of interest is the fact that this variety provides room for experimentation. Few writers, if any, have emphasized the need for experimentation to adjust to local conditions if schools are to fulfil continuously their role as community leaders in modern productive efforts.

Third, Table 6.4 shows that over 50 per cent of the incomes accrue from agricultural activities. In general, public secondary boarding schools perform much better than day schools. From Table 6.7 it will be seen that Pwani Dodoma and Lindi students earn from 100/= (Tsh) to 700/= each per year and that in Ruvuma, Shinyanga, Tabora, Rukwa and Mtwara students earn less than 20/= each.

Fourth, Tables 6.6 and 6.7 reveal another interesting phenomenon: when schools are grouped by regions the expenditure tends to outweigh the savings, whereas the aggregate figures by kinds of school show that per capita savings are higher than per capita expenditure. Day schools at the aggregate level tend to spend over 80 per cent of their incomes, mostly on improved diet (Table 6.5) whilst boarding schools spend only 21 per cent.

Fifth, the data offer sufficient evidence that there is no correlation between a school's academic achievement and its level of production, hence the need to apply the approach used in this study.

Sixth, the average 1974 to 1975 income from production of 65.55 Tsh per student offsets only 2.5 per cent of that year's total expenditure on secondary education.[6] This is not, though, why this document has been named 'The Unproductive School'.

4. Policy implications
Research reports like the present one are pointless unless the findings are utilized. One way to do so is to develop a body of information that may be used for future research studies and also for consideration in policy decisions. In this last section possible areas for policy making will be suggested:

(a) Schools have made efforts to contribute to fulfilment of the economic requirements for self-reliance. The level they have reached may be raised through a variety of means:
Schools should have automony so that they can deal with their local situations. Cutbacks in public expenditure on secondary education should not be in real terms but rather in growth rate of public expenditure. This will make the transition from total financial dependence a little easier.
Schools should be assisted in their investment efforts. To do this no additional public funds are necessary. Boarding schools, for example, should be allowed to effect savings on items of their regular budget allocated to them by handling their own tenders for meat, beans, flour and the like.
Cutbacks on current expenditure should be directed to items considered easy for the schools to produce themselves. For instance, flour for bread is certainly cheaper than bread itself. Schools could make their own bakery goods.

(b) Schools should not be considered to be kinds of production firms, but rather as institutions developing strategies for themselves and for the larger communities. The fact that schools are a learning industry is of great significance. Is it not interesting to discover, for example, that schools have learned to produce, invest and set aside reserves for future production?

(c) Since time seems to be an influential variable affecting both academic achievement and production, severe constraints must be expected if school time is continuously controlled by individuals far removed from school localities.

(d) Regular technical assistance in agriculture, production economics and related fields is of vital importance to schools. This is not the same as saying productive efforts at the school level must be directed by specialists alone; specialists cannot unfortunately be produced cheaply. But through retraining of teachers, seminars and co-ordination, some breakthroughs are possible. This observation on shortage of technical advice has been made before.

(e) To alleviate the problem of implement and tool shortage students may be asked to bring some of their own, because it may be expected that at least by the time a student reaches Form I, he or she owns a hoe or a panga. Although this would in a sense be a private contribution to the cost of education, it would be an infinitesimal one compared to the total private or social cost of the education received.

(f) Specific cases:
The fact that private schools show less effort in productive activities than public schools needs attention if participation in productive activities is considered to be one of the means to 'test' the effectiveness of 'Education for Self-Reliance'.
That girls' schools are not at par with boys' schools in productive activities may reveal the role women play in productive work in Tanzania. It is traditionally common practice that men spend more time in the fields while women stay at home to take care of domestic affairs including looking after the children.
New means of organizing productive efforts ought to be sought for urban schools. Here is an opportunity to borrow practice from other countries. In Cuba urban school students spend certain periods in temporary homes engaging in productive activities in rural areas.

(g) A comparison of academic performance and productive effort shows no correlation between those two variables, though the expected outcome would be that the schools which produce more perform either better or worse in examinations. Assuming that examination results measure academic achievements correctly, the finding that what schools do academically is totally unrelated to what they do in their present productive efforts has many implications for curriculum development.

Conclusion
On the whole these observations may not appeal to every policy-maker, school administrator or student. They are directed to *all* who are concerned with education for the liberation of man so that he can live together with his fellow men in amity and freedom in a more amenable reality.

Notes
1   For a complete research report and a systematic description of the theoretical framework of analysis see Maliyamkono, T L *The Unproductive School. A Model for the Assessment of the Economic Aspects of the Education for Self-Reliance* Dar es Salaam: UDSM (August 1976) p. 47
2   Since the returns are not yet complete, correlations have not been run on the identified dependent variables. They will be included in the second draft of the study report.

3 There was no co-operation from Mwanza and Morogoro regions.
4 Methods used to determine examination results are described in the manuscripts.
5 See the complete research report, Note 1. Also, refer to Table 8.
6 Total expenditure of public secondary schools only, while 65.50 Tsh per capita includes students of both public and private schools.
7 See *Taarifa ya Mipango ya Ki-uchumi ya Elimu ya Taifa ya Kujitegema 1970–1973* Wizara ya Elimu ya Taifa, Dar es Salaam (January 1975) p. 54 (mimeo)

6.2 Policy and Practice in Tanzanian Adult Education—a Research Report
V M Mlekwa

The importance of adult education for national development was implied in the 'Arusha Declaration' (1967). The Second Five-Year Plan (1969 to 1974) first spelled out the content and strategies for implementing adult education in the country. In President Nyerere's Speech of December 1969, the official policy on adult education was proclaimed, to be further reflected in subsequent policies such as 'Mwongozo' (1972) and the 'Musoma Resolutions' (1974). But so far little is known about the actual programmes and how they operate in a given region, district or village.

The purpose of this study[1] is to assess the extent to which adult education policy has been implemented in Tanzania since the 'Adult Education Year' (1970), with focus on one district[2].

In this study, adult education is defined as *all educational activities planned for adults outside the formal school system*. Policy of adult education means *official statements determining the plan of action in the domain of adult education in Tanzania*. The term practice denotes *implementation* of the plan of action rather than its impact on the living habits of the target population.

In that context, the following official statements on adult education were examined:

1. The Second Five-Year Plan (1969–1974);
2. President Nyerere's 'Adult Education Year Speech' (1969);
3. The 15th and 16th TANU Biennial Conference Resolutions of 1971 and 1973 respectively;
4. The 'Prime Minister's Directive on Workers' Education in Tanzania' (1973).

From the analysis of the policy (see Figure 6.9) five variables emerged that needed empirical investigation:

1. The adult education programmes offered;
2. The agencies and personnel;
3. The adult learners and adult literacy;
4. The materials and costs;
5. The problems and constraints.

To guide the empirical investigations the following key questions were used:

1. Are the adult education programmes related to the objectives of adult education in Tanzania?
2. What agencies and personnel are involved in the dissemination of adult education in the district? To what extent are their activities co-ordinated to accord with the national philosophy of adult education?
3. Who are the adult learners and how far has the district moved in the direction of eradicating illiteracy? What problems are faced and what are their possible solutions?
4. What facilities are provided for adult education; what are the costs involved?
5. What are the general problems of adult education in the district and what are their implications?

Data were collected mainly from documents, structured and unstructured interviews and participant and non-participant observation. An interview schedule and an observation checklist were used for the structured interviews and the non-participant observation respectively.

1. Interpretation of the policy

Adult education policy, like any other policy, cannot be well implemented unless it is well understood. One of the problems of adult education is that it is so wide in its aims, objectives and methods that it can almost be equated with life itself and may be as varied. Because of its broad nature and its apparent capacity to include almost everything other than formal education of children and adolescents, there is a great deal of semantic confusion surrounding the term 'adult education'. This renders it '. . . nebulous and with no secure roots. It is about something important, but nobody is very clear what that illusive something is.'[3]

In the district studied, different categories of respondents showed that they had different interpretations of adult education, its aims and objectives and its organization. Generally speaking:

1. Professional adult educators, five of whom were interviewed, understood adult education to include literacy, functional literacy and continuing education.
2. Party leaders including affiliated bodies, government and parastatal leaders, 29 of whom were interviewed, tended to understand adult education mainly in terms of functional literacy.
3. The adult learners interviewed, including those who had been awarded certificates (ten of them altogether), considered adult education to be merely literacy.

In the last two cases the concept of adult education was thus only partially understood. One group thought of it as literacy with some function and the other, in fact the target group, perceived it as literacy without function. Such conceptions of adult education appeared to determine the way the policy was understood. Many of the Party, government and parastatal leaders who interpreted adult education as meaning mainly functional literacy tended to believe that it was the responsibility of the Ministry of National Education, rather than realizing that their respective institutions were indispensable instruments of change which adult education was all about. Indeed, the broader dimension of adult education was not vividly portrayed and the importance of co-ordinating the activities of the various adult education agencies did not seem to be an issue of much concern.

On the other hand, because the adult learners thought adult education was only literacy education, they, especially the older ones, tended to believe that it would not really benefit them. Thus, in reply to the question, 'Why do you attend adult education classes?' the general answer was, 'Because we have been told to'. Although it is true that literacy is an important element of adult education, when attention is paid to literacy alone, its significance for adults becomes difficult to justify.

Table 6.9

Indicators of Policy and Practice in Adult Education in Tanzania

Policy Document	General Aims	Specific Objectives	Programmes Specified/Implied	Specific Instructions /Recommendations
Second Five-Year Plan	Rural Development		Simple training in Agricultural techniques, craftsmanship, health education, housecraft. Simple Economics, Accounting, Political Education.	Primary Schools to become adult education centres.
President Nyerere's Adult Education Speech 1970	To shake Tanzanians out of resignation to the kind of life they have lived for centuries	To reject bad houses, bad jembes and preventable diseases and restore confidence that better houses and better health can be attained.	Simple Economics and Accounting.	All institutions to participate in war against ignorance.
	To learn how to improve their lives.	To learn how to increase productivity on the farms, and in factories and offices.	Simple agricultural training.	Organizational structure of adult education to be improved.
	To understand the national policies of Socialism and Self-Reliance.	To learn about better food, balanced diet and how to obtain it by their own efforts.	Worker's Education.	
		To learn modern methods of hygiene, furniture-making, working together to improve conditions in villages and streets.	Health Education Domestic Science. Crafts. Co-operative and Political Education.	

			...kers education.	...volved in adult education activities.
...nnial Conferences (1971 & 1973)	1973. To integrate education with work.			
Prime Minister's Directive (1973)	To raise the Workers' intellectual and professional capacities so as to raise the national income and to liberate the Workers.		Literacy education. Political education. Professional training in relevant fields. Academic Subjects.	All workplaces to give Workers' Education to *all* (from the illiterate to those with university degrees or diplomas).
				To appoint in all workplaces Workers' Education officers with full responsibilities for Workers' Education.
				To set aside a special budget (10% of the total budget) for Workers' Education.
				To conduct Workers' Education in normal working hours for not less than 1 hour daily.

2. The programmes offered

The adult education programmes offered in the district include the following: Political education, agriculture, health education, literacy, domestic science, Swahili, arithmetic, English, economics and crafts. Table 6.10 shows the number of participants per programme. There are normally three categories of adult education classes, namely literacy classes, continuing education classes (kujiendeleza) and practical projects or demonstration classes. As can be seen from Table 6.10, literacy classes have the largest enrolment, together with Swahili and arithmetic. The syllabus is derived from the primers that are being used for functional literacy. English, Swahili and domestic science are offered to those who already know how to read and write but would like to gain more knowledge.

Table 6.10

Number of Participants per Programme

Programme	Number Registered	Attendance	Attendance as percentage of registration
Political Education	24570	13225	53.8
Literacy	56078	27257	48.6
Agriculture	28876	14670	50.8
Health	11888	7146	60.7
Domestic Science	810	588	72.5
Kiswahili, Arithmetic	56078	27257	48.6
English	114	76	66.6
Economics	16387	12573	76.7
Crafts	41	16	39.0
Total	194842	102808	52.7

Source: *Monthly Report* (March 1974), available in the District Adult Education Office

The idea of integrating other subjects into the literacy campaign must be investigated further for its worthwhileness. In the district, for example, it appears that most of the focus is on literacy per se, i.e. ability to read and to write. Yet, even in the domain of literacy not all the required skills are imparted for the following reasons, among others:

1. There is no proper balance between knowledge gained in reading and ability gained in writing. Insufficient stress is put on sentence construction, and the adult learners find themselves memorizing the sentences in the primers.
2. In connection with point 1, it is noticeable that more emphasis is put on reading than on comprehension. In addition, an adult may know how to write, but since he is incapable of structuring sentences, he cannot answer questions or put them into writing.

3. Irregular attendance makes it especially difficult for the inexperienced and untrained adult education teachers to handle all students present in any particular lesson.
4. The mathematical element in some primers is too thin to benefit the learners. In centres where only such primers are used, education in literacy is therefore limited to reading and some writing; it is no longer learning the Three Rs.

The art of teaching functional literacy to adults requires that there be practical or demonstration projects enabling the adult learners to translate what they have learnt into practice, so that adult learning does not become a detached and theoretical construction of reality but a creation of reality. As far as the district is concerned, there are three such demonstration projects: (a) agriculture, (b) crafts, and (c) science. But these projects are not in operation in every ward, and even where they have been introduced, not every adult learner is participating in them. They appear to be designed only for those who have a special interest in them. For the rest, learning continues to be mainly theoretical. The projects started early enough in the district, but were initially meant only for illiterates and the facilities, i.e. materials and equipment, were inadequate, particularly for domestic science. Moreover, in January 1975, the Prime Minister's 1973 'Directive on Workers' Education' had not yet been implemented. Some subjects such as economics, accountancy and book-keeping used to be taught before the Directive was issued, but even these were discontinued, mainly owing to lack of teachers and irregular attendance by students. The main reason given by the authorities for the delay in introducing Workers' Education programmes in the district has been that, owing to the full involvement by the Party, government and parastatal officials in the re-settlement of people in the new planned villages, it was difficult to get teachers to teach in Workers' Education classes.

3. The agencies and personnel
Towards the end of his 'Adult Education Year Speech', President Nyerere emphasized that various bodies like TANU, the Ministry of Agriculture, the Ministry of Rural Development, and IAE must align their activities, which the Ministry of National Education would then co-ordinate. He also said that in 1970, more would be done to improve the organizational structure of adult education.

As far as the organizational structure is concerned, the adult education committees have been in existence since 1970, and had been operating relatively well from the district level down to the class level. However, this work was interrupted by the shifting of people to the new planned villages which began in mid-1973. By December 1974 attempts were being made to re-establish the adult education committees so that they could begin operating in January 1975.

The whole district has a total of nearly 1792 adult education teachers, the majority of whom are volunteers who are paid honoraria. Table 6.11 shows the sources from which these adult education teachers are drawn, as shown in the July to September Functional Literacy Report, 1974.

Table 6.11

Source of Adult Education Teachers, September 1974

Source	Number of Teachers
Primary School Teachers	163
TANU	6
Government Civil Servants	174
Religious institutions	14
Voluntary teachers	1 376
Others	59

The volunteer adult education teachers were supposed to be paid honoraria amounting to 30/= (Tsh) per month. This was considered to be a kind of incentive which would show the teachers that the Government did appreciate their work. But despite several attempts by the Government officials to make it clear that the 30/= were not a salary, the teachers in the district have come to believe that it is their *right* to get this amount of money. Unfortunately it is not even paid regularly. For example, the 1974 honoraria were paid only in April, May, June and July. Such irregularities tend to discourage the volunteer adult education teachers from regular and enthusiastic teaching.

Regarding the participation of the other agencies in adult education work, it still leaves much to be desired. A survey was made of the aims and objectives, the programmes, methods and organization of the major institutions in the district, such as TANU and affiliated bodies like UWT, NUTA, TYL, and TAPA; the Goverment Departments such as Health, Agriculture, Home Affairs, etc., and parastatal organizations including the Tanganyika Library Service Branch and the District Development Corporation, in order to find out how much they were involved in adult education work co-ordinated by the Ministry of National Education. The results were that only TANU, and the Department of Health, Agriculture and Prison (Home Affairs) were participating *actively* in teaching and organizing adult education classes in their places of work. TANU's role was mainly that of mobilizing the people to attend adult education classes. The other institutions seemed to be preoccupied with their own prescribed duties, as if adult education were exclusively a function of the Ministry of National Education.

4. Materials and costs

If the adult education programmes are to operate effectively, the necessary aids, such as study materials, exercise books, chalk, etc., have to be available. The country's policy is that all these materials be provided to students free of charge. The district, however, is severely short of study materials, particularly teachers' guides, exercise books, pencils, and rubbers. For example, the author visited one adult education class in which none of the 197 students had an exercise book or a pencil. Consequently there was no writing practice for the students. Furthermore, only the teacher had a copy of the Cotton Primer I that was used for the lesson. She therefore had to write sentences such as *panda pamba mapema* (grow cotton early) on the blackboard and let the students read the sentence after her in the manner of a singing group. When the authors twisted the sentence to read *mapema pamba panda* students could not identify the words, and some kept on reading *panda pamba mapema*. Almost every person who was interviewed mentioned the lack of materials as one of the main problems holding back the progress of adult education in the district.

Teaching aids such as posters and drill cards with syllables are also missing in the adult education centres and classes, and the teachers are not trained to make, if not all, at least some of the required teaching aids.

The decision of the Party and government to make adult education a priority in the country has to be accompanied by a decision to allocate sufficient funds for adult education activities. Since adult education is not the exclusive responsibility of a single institution but one shared by many agencies both statutory and non-statutory, an attempt was made to find out how much money the institutions dealing with adult education were actually allocating to adult education activities. Table 6.12 shows the results.

Table 6.12

Amount of Money Spent on Adult Education Work by Various Agencies in 1973/74 (expressed in Tsh)

Homecraft Centre	40 000/00
Health Education Division	12 640/00
TYL	700/00
Kilimo	12 000/00
Ujamaa/Ushirika	10 000/00
Prison	3 000/00
Education	217 277/00
Total	295 617/00

As against the total of 295 617 Tsh spent by various agencies on adult education, as shown in Table 6.12 the total amount spent in 1973–74 on formal (primary education) was 312 776 Tsh. Thus, formal education received 17 159 Tsh more than adult education. However, note must be taken of the fact that there are normally many hidden costs, particularly in adult education, which this study did not take into account. There may also be other agencies engaging in adult education and spending some money on it which have been left out of the analysis. Although these considerations make it difficult to draw fully valid conclusions from the comparison, it is interesting to note that the difference in money spent on adult education and on formal education is only small. This is consonant with the degree of priority that Tanzania has in fact given to adult education.

5. Problems and constraints: a summary

The problems that have held back the progress of adult education in the district may be summarized as follows:

(a) Isolated homes prior to mid-1973

Because people were living far away from one another it was difficult to enrol all adults concerned, to organize and supervise adult education classes, and to make all the required study and writing materials available. The 'Operation Vijiji' policy marks a fundamental departure from the old way of living which was individualistic, conservative and unco-ordinated. It has provided good conditions for the implementation of adult education and hence for the indispensable task of socializing and mobilizing human resources for development.

(b) Adults' lack of interest in adult education

The district has a low level of education. Indeed, it does not have a single secondary school, technical school or College of National Education. There are only 54 primary schools, 32 of which go up to Standard VII. In terms of selection for higher education, only 90 pupils out of 1 376 Standard VII candidates, or six per cent, obtained places in Form I in 1974. Generally speaking education in the district does not seem to appeal to many people, particularly not to the old ones. Even less attention is paid to adult education—in fact the very idea of being taught in a class or anywhere else by a teacher appears odd to many adults, who consider that kind of activity suitable only for children. Because of this attitude, they equate adult education with literacy, and literacy as far as they are concerned is not really for them.

(c) Lack of full participation by the other agencies

At the beginning of the campaign (1970), many government and Party leaders shared the general view that adult education meant only education in literacy for those who did not know how to read and write. On the teaching side, many primary school teachers were unwilling to accept the responsibility of teaching adult education classes because they felt that it would be too much work for them. This kind of thinking still appears to prevail. Although the Party and government leaders now interpret adult education to mean functional literacy, the tendency of the other institutions is to withdraw from adult education activities leaving the main work to the primary school teachers who feel that they are being overworked.

(d) Lack of materials

Writing materials such as exercise books, pencils, rubbers, etc., teachers' guides and teaching aids are in critically short supply. The problem is a twofold one. First, materials are not supplied in sufficient quantities from the centre to district. Second, communication within the district, necessary for transporting and distributing the materials to the respective centres, is poor. Since financial resources are also inadequate, only limited seminars for training the adult education cadres can be organized in the district.

(e) Seasonal activities

As some residents in the district are beekeepers and honey collectors, the men are

226

away for many months. In two divisions most residents are cattle herders who keep on shifting from place to place.

(f) Delay in payment of honoraria
Very often the payment of honoraria to the volunteer adult education teachers, the majority of whom are Standard VII teachers, is delayed or not made at all for several months in the year. This has tended to dishearten many of these teachers. Thus what was introduced as an incentive has produced negative results. On the other hand, its abolition would do considerable damage to the whole adult education movement.

Concluding remarks

The findings of the study show that Tanzania still faces a number of problems in the domain of adult education. However, it should not be concluded that no promising results have been achieved, nor should it be forgotten that the task which Tanzania has chosen to accomplish is so demanding that certain shortcomings in the process of implementation are virtually inevitable. Perhaps Tanzania's biggest achievement in adult education is her unreserved awareness of the fact that adult education is essential for promoting a well-integrated kind of development. She has drawn up an educational policy which spells out the strategies necessary for mobilizing the required human and other resources, and for motivating and activating the rural populace to participate in every programme at all stages of its development. The realization by the party and the government that adult education is not politically neutral, and that it therefore needs full support from political and government circles, is more than just a step towards success; it is the very foundation of success.

One important implication of the results of the study is, however, that there is a need to improve the 'information delivery system' in the country in general and in the district that has been studied in particular. Policies must be delivered from the source to the target population without losing their substance on the way. To that end it is necessary to have a wider distribution of radios and rural newspapers, to improve the services of these media and to encourage the people to develop a keener interest in reading.

The second major implication is that there are normally direct or indirect connections between policies, so much so that a change in one may necessitate a change in another. Policies may appear different whereas in the final analysis they are one and the same thing. It is necessary, therefore, to analyze policies in the context of the total system in order to find effective strategies for their implementation at minimum cost. For example, through proper planning people should be able to participate fully in the 'Life or Death' agriculture campaign without having to be absent from adult classes.

The third implication is that implementation of policies may be limited by the nature of the particular environment in which those policies are to be carried out. The administrators charged with translating the policies into practice may work diligently with all the commitment required, but they may be struggling against odds, both historical and physical, posed by the environment in which they are operating. Thus, it is necessary for the policy strategists to take into account all the major historical, economic, political and sociological factors that may act as either facilitators of change or constraints on change.

Finally, policy implementation has to be seen as a process in which all those affected by the policies are involved in the planning of the operational strategies as well as in their application. The question of who should plan for whom, and where the plans should be formulated and articulated, is an important one. Another fundamental issue is that of getting feed-back both vertically and horizontally, so that the results of implementation can be systematically recorded and adjusted. In that context, it is necessary to go beyond forming adult education committees to ensuring full participation particularly at the grassroot level. A machinery for evaluating all those efforts must not only be established but also used.

Notes

1   This research is based on an M.A. (Ed) Dissertation submitted to the University of Dar es Salaam, 1975. As Mlekwa's study was the first comprehensive research on the implementation of the national adult education programme in one specific district and describes and analyzes many of the general arguments on the problems in the development of adult education in Tanzania, we consider it a very valuable contribution to this volume.

2   The name of the district has been deliberately left out of the study in order to conform to usual research practice.

3   Coles, E T *Adult Education in Developing Countries* Oxford: Pergamon Press (1969) p. 4

6.3 Research as an Educational Tool for Development

M L Swantz

The Tanzanian policy of development primarily emphasizes development of people and not of things. In the rural sector this is accomplished through an intense programme of planned ujamaa villages with free communal services and a production system based increasingly on communal cultivation. The majority of the rural population are already living in nascent village settlements which are being formed, through a process of trial and error, by exerting some pressure on the people to move but at the same time allowing them a degree of choice in the location of their new homes.

The villages organize themselves as self-governing units and through village meetings elect their village chairmen, work leaders and members of various committees which operate under the Village Central Committee. The planning of village development is by design, if not always by practice, in the hands of the villagers.

In carrying out the villagization programme, a basic weakness in the administrative system has become evident. In spite of emphatic political statements about the development being by the people and for the people, the administrative and also District Party leadership have in practice shown little capacity to involve the villagers themselves in the planning of their own villages, either at the stage when village sites have been chosen or in developing the new village. The problem is one of inadequate communication, at least partly deriving from nascent class differences, although expediency also plays its part. In trying to achieve quick results the slower and surer way of involving the villagers in planning is by-passed. The observation that two-way communication between the administrators, district party leaders and the villagers has not been effective is based on studies made in villages at the stage of their formation and on experiences gained from student research in the Coast Region where the researchers helped to initiate village development projects and thus encountered and shared with the villagers their difficulties in efforts toward development.

In order to ensure that the larger sector of the population—the ordinary peasants—can exercise the right not only to work hard and to produce, but to influence their own development, effective ways and means are needed to facilitate their participation both in planning and implementation.

1. Research as a two-way educative communication

It is proposed here that a research approach to the task at hand can become a meaningful tool, not only in finding solutions to development problems, but in bringing together different sectors of the population and bringing about development of all those engaged in the effort. Research accompanied by participating action can become a most effective means for opening up channels of communication and for engaging administrators, researchers and villagers in a common endeavour with great educational effect on all of them.

Research as an academic exercise is an elitist concept. The prestige attached to scholarship, the status of a scientist, and the financial outlay needed for carrying it out, all tend to develop class-consciousness in those engaged in research as well as in those who become the objects of research. It can be asked, however, whether research by its design needs to have this elitist air. An intellectual exercise need not be an independent road to knowledge and discovery. Research in its goals, methods and approach can become a basic tool in the transformation process of a society. It does not need to be limited to those with higher education, trained in methods and techniques in organization of thought or formulation of problems and discursive logic. Ordinary villagers, administrators and teachers can become participants in, and not only objects of, research.

Research can become a means of communication, an educative process in which the roles of the educator and the educated are constantly reversed and the common search for solving common problems unites all those engaged in the common endeavour. Differentiating factors are likely to remain, but they do not necessarily arise from the mystifying air that a scholar creates by holding on to his scientific knowledge as if it were his private possession, nor from the design of the research.

2. Basic requirements of participatory research
Research that becomes an agent of transformation in a community must fulfil some basic requirements:

1. It needs to be planned so that at least part of it is of immediate interest to the people in the studied community and so that the community can expect to benefit from its results.
2. It should involve the people for whose benefit it is carried out in the process of research, both in formulating the immediate problems and in finding solutions to them.
3. Research should incorporate into itself as many as possible of those working locally toward the development of that community, be they village leaders, administrators, educators or extension officers.
4. The educational and motivational potential of such an engaged research method should be fully utilized for the benefit of everyone involved in it.

The principle of local participation does not mean that the total research effort should be reduced to a level comprehensible to all participants. If the researchers and the village people share the same situation of change and are involved in it, the concern of both and, on one level, the problem or parts of it are the same, although the conceptual level differs. The scientists will have to be able to operate on two levels of analysis without separating one from the other. Their task is to assist the non-professional participants to see the context and concomitants of their own problems and the direction from which the solutions can be sought. This creates awareness in people of their own situation and becomes a motivational force toward development. At the same time there remains a level of analysis that requires greater abstraction which is not shared by the villagers. However, even methods or experiments alien to villagers become an accepted part of a study if the villagers are included in the framework of larger research conducted for their own benefit.

Several research projects on questions related to women and youth, using the described approach, have been conducted under the Bureau of Resource Assessment and Land Use Planning in the University of Dar es Salaam, involving students as participants in the villages. The motivational and educational potential of the approach has been verified in relation to students, villagers and at least some of the teachers, village leaders and local officers.[1]

3. Pilot survey of 46 villages

A recent experimental pilot survey of 46 villages involved administrators, teachers and villagers of three districts in three different parts of the country. The method was based on the principle that the villagers themselves would be involved in evaluating their own level of education and skills, the extent of utilization of skills, reasons for their non-utilization, non-utilized natural resources and training needs of the villagers in view of the village development plans.

The district, divisional and ward adult education officers were involved in organizing and carrying out the survey and in training the local co-ordinators for the work. The university and the Ministry of Development planning staff in co-operation with representatives from the Ministries of Education, Agriculture and Labour, and staff from the Research Unit of the Institute of Adult Education and the Statistical Bureau prepared the plan and assisted in interpreting the approach and method to the local officers. Otherwise, the survey was carried out by villagers, with the help of adult education officers and divisional and ward secretaries.

4. Survey of skills

The survey of skills in each division was intended to cover all households. A questionnaire of 25 questions was to be answered in writing by a literate member of each household. If no one could perform the task, this fact was indicated on the form. In some villages, not one household could fill in the form itself; in others, 60 to 73 per cent of the households did not need outside assistance.

The questionnaires were administered by co-ordinators chosen by the villagers in the first village committee or village meeting where the purposes and general approach were explained. The principal co-ordinator—usually a head teacher of the primary school—supervised the work, collected the forms and with the other co-ordinators added up the statistical information on a summary sheet which was provided. The main impetus of the survey on the village level was assumed to come through the involvement of all villagers in self-evaluation, and through their meeting together to discuss their strength, needs and plans.

The 46 villages covered in the pilot survey were in Usangi in Pare District, Kilimanjaro Region, Ntebela in Kyela District, Rungwe Region and part of the Msoga division in Bagamoyo District, Coast Region. Some were traditional areas where villages had not yet been officially formed, some were new villages in formation, and some were ujamaa villages. The organization for carrying out the work was more easily accomplished in ujamaa villages than in areas where people were not yet organized in definite village units.

As could be expected, rather serious inaccuracies occurred both in filling in the forms and in summing up the statistics. If the survey is to continue, modifications will have to be made and the questionnaire simplified further.

However, the results showed that the proportionate number of literates, illiterates, educational levels and skills between various villages was correct, and the diversity of skills or their lack became evident. The percentages of those benefiting from adult education programmes were the most accurate yet provided in the country in general.

5. The educational and motivational benefits of the method
The method was used as a means whereby those participating could be both motivated to greater action and educated to greater awareness of their potential as well as to find ways of solving their developmental problems. The whole process had an educational element:

It made the leaders learn more about procedures for communicating with people and gave them a method which they could repeat in their administrative duties and thereby avoid a 'commanding' attitude in relation to villages.
It gave the leaders a way of soliciting the peoples' own ideas and of helping them to take part in the planning of their own villages.
It taught those chosen as co-ordinators some skills in handling questionnaires and processing the data from them.
It taught the village leaders and villagers the benefits of self-analysis and how to go about it.
It taught people some skills in answering questions and writing their thoughts, and at the same time revealed their weakness to those unable to respond to the challenge. This turned out to serve as a motivating force for self-improvement. In areas where villages had not yet acted as units, it created the beginning of a common thinking-process which prepared people for future planning on a village basis. This was the case particularly in Usangi.

The discussion on village resources, training needs and other Government inputs revealed that the present training schemes inadequately met specific needs, and that the extension officers spread their services too thinly without giving necessary time for teaching individual villages. The discussions also revealed that in the primary stages of their learning, the youth should be trained in the village instead of being sent elsewhere. As a result of his research the author also recommends that only after the youth have learned all there is to learn at the village level with the help of extension workers and others possessing the needed skills, and after they have shown their aptitude in an ongoing village project, should they be sent for short periods to larger training centres for more specialized training.

The survey results provide information on the following aspects of human and natural resources:

1. level of education
2. number of skills represented
3. products being made
4. obstacles to the use of particular skills
5. sources of learning.

The village reports indicate:

1. needed skills and suggestions for obtaining them
2. development plans
3. problems of development in the village
4. natural resources, especially non-utilized ones.

Despite the shortcomings of the quantitative data, the survey has given a good indication of the skills available in the villages, and yielded a great deal of useful information. Its broad results provide a good base for the further, more detailed investigations necessary or for following up the survey with practical measures to further the development of the villages. The available information is sufficiently detailed even to permit identification of individuals with particular skills. The specific recommendations made by individual villages should help the district personnel to tackle development problems at a very local level. As an example, some statistical results from the Usangi Wards are given in Tables 6.13–6.17.

Conclusion

The method described in this paper is one way in which people can become part of a larger research effort. Some aspects of research involved survey techniques which people themselves can learn. The survey under review gained another dimension by using the results of the discussions held by the villagers directly after the survey work had been accomplished. It shows that surveys can be planned so that their exploitative aspects are eliminated and they become both educational and motivational.

The survey can be the first stage for further in-depth research, as will be the case in Bagamoyo villages where a longer participatory research is planned to involve villagers in the study of various aspects of folk sciences and methods of work in the wider cultural context. The practical aim is to help the villagers use their many traditional skills for village development.

Knowledge is a continuum, not isolated facts in individual minds here and there; so too is inquiry a continuum. It is not only the scientist who is engaged in inquiry; he shares it with others and merely brings his analytical tools to the common inquiry. It is the commonality of knowledge and of inquiry that makes it possible for people from different educational levels to work together for the common good. Such a research approach becomes not only a tool for development but operates as a political levelling instrument to help minimize social and educational differences.

Note

1 Project reports are published as BRALUP Research Reports (New Series): *Youth and Development in the Coast Region of Tanzania* No. 6 (1974) and *Socio-Economic Causes of Malnutrition in Central Kilimanjaro* No. 13 (1975). See also Rudengren, Jan and Swantz, M L *Village Skills Survey, Report of the Pre-Pilot and Pilot Surveys* No. 42 (1976) and Swantz, M L and Bryceson, D F *Women Workers in Dar es Salaam. 1973/74 Survey of Female Minimum Wage Earners and Self-Employed* No. 43 (1976) Another report on the method is Swantz, M L 'The Role of Participant Research in Development'. Reprint from *Geografiska Annaler* Ser. D. (1976), 2; also BRALUP Research Report (New Series), No. 15 (1976)

Table 6.13

Main Occupation
(*Number* of people shown for villages; percentage for ward estimates).

Occupation	Agriculture	Husbandry, (Animal) Bee-keeping	Forestry, Hunting Fishing	Administration	Teaching	Trade	Medical works	Local doctors	Pottery	Handicraft	Tailoring	Shoe-making	Carpentry	Blacksmithing	Masonry	Other skilled work	Other work	Total
Kwa Koa Ward (estimated %)	65	32							3									100
Ngulu	340	92														2		434
Ruru	184	162	8			4			1									359
Kigonigoni	33	25			3					5	1					2		69
Lembeni ward (estimated %)	71	20							9									400
Kiverenge	130	96									1	1	1	1	1	1	6	238
Lembeni	463	26		1	4	6					1				2	3	11	517
Kiruru	124	79		2	1			1		4	5		3	2	4	5	13	243
Kighare ward (estimated %)	48	35							17									100
Kirongaya	137	119		1		3	3		9	6	3		5		2	7	4	299
Ngujini	158	100		2	15	11	5		3	2	3		3			12		314

Table 6.14

Secondary Occupation
(*Number* of people)

	Agriculture	Husbandry	Forestry, Hunting, Charcoal	Fishing	Carpentry	Masonry	Blacksmithing	Pottery	Handicraft	Trade	Knitting/Sewing Weaving	Tailoring	Others	Total
Kwa Koa ward														
Ngulu					6	5		19	145	1	4			180
Ruru			1	3				1	12	17	1	30		65
Kigonigoni	7	7	3	7					26	1	4		4	59
Lembeni ward														
Kiverenge			1		1			3	169		11	5	29	219
Lembeni	50	2			6	2		4	73	5	14	9	5	170
Kiruru					5	1	4	5	56		4	3		78
Kighare ward														
Kirongaya	39	21			3	11		12	5		5	7	3	106
Ngujini	53	11			4	2	2	15	2	4	17	2	3	115

Table 6.15

Skills

(x = the skill exists in the village)	Kwa Koa Ward			Lembeni Ward			Kighare Ward	
	Ngulu	Ruru	Kigonigoni	Kiverenge	Lembeni	Kiruru	Kirongaya	Ngujini
Farming	x	x	x	x	x	x	x	x
Animal husbandry	x	x	x	x	x	x	x	x
Bee-keeping	x	x		x	x	x		
Hunting		x						
Fishing		x						
Forest Work			x					x
Teaching			x		x	x		x
Trading	x	x	x		x		x	x
Medical work					x			x
Local doctors							x	x
Tailoring	x	x	x	x	x	x	x	x
Carpentry	x	x	x	x	x	x	x	x
Masonry	x		x	x	x	x	x	x
Blacksmithing				x	x	x	x	x
Construction	x			x		x	x	x
Saw-milling							x	x
Repairing bicycles/watches					x		x	x
Mechanics			x					
Injecting cattle		x						x
Administration				x	x	x	x	x
Judge, Police						x		x
Driving			x	x	x	x	x	x
Knitting	x	x	x	x	x	x		
Weaving	x					x	x	x
Pottery	x	x		x	x	x	x	x
Making shoes	x	x		x			x	x
Making mats and carpets	x	x	x	x	x	x	x	x
Making baskets	x	x	x	x	x	x	x	x
Making bags	x			x		x		
Making rope				x		x		x
Making hoehandles	x	x	x	x		x	x	
Making beehives	x			x	x	x	x	x
Making bows, arrows	x	x	x	x		x		x
Making fish traps and nets		x						
Making canoes		x						
Making spoons	x	x	x	x	x	x		

(x = the skill exists in the village)	Kwa Koa Ward			Lembeni Ward			Kighare Ward	
	Ngulu	Ruru	Kigonigoni	Kiverenge	Lembeni	Kiruru	Kirongaya	Ngujini
Making knives	x		x					
Making chairs	x	x	x	x	x	x	x	x
Making plates			x	x		x	x	x
Making clothes	x	x	x	x				x
Making sacks			x					
Making vests			x					
Making hats			x					x
Making carvings			x		x			
Making socks			x					
Making bullets			x					
Making pestles			x					
Making charcoal				x				
Making bricks						x		
Making brooms				x		x		x
Making bread							x	

Table 6.16

Means of Improving Skills

	Agriculture Officers	Veterinary Officers	Development Officers	Education Officers	TANU	Other experts	Co-operatives	Religious Organizations	Books	Magazines	Radio	Parents	Elders	Bakwata	Totals
Kwa Koa Ward	10	7	7	2	3	4	1	4	4	4	1	13			60
Ngulu	3	4	5	2	3			4	3	4		13			41
Ruru						4	1								5
Kigonigoni	7	3	2						1		1				14
Lembeni Ward	49	30	55	—	21	10	6	36	6	18	41	26	11		309
Kiverenge	6	4	11			10					4	12			47
Lembeni	31	20	34		21			32		13	27	14			192
Kiruru	12	6	10			6		4	6	5	10		11		70
Kighare Ward	28	57	80	—	22	4	2	20	12	14	46			20	305
Kirongaya	6	17	46		13	4	2		7		21			20	136
Ngujini	22	40	34		9			20	5	14	25				169
Total	87	94	142	2	46	18	9	60	22	36	88	39	11	20	674

Table 6.17

Reasons for not Using a Skill

	Lack of Equipment	Lack of Material	Lack of Capital	Lack of Market	Lack of Employment	Lack of Time	Too old	Other	Total
Kwa Koa Ward									
Ngulu	56	3							59
Ruru	8								8
Kigonigoni	15								15
Lembeni Ward									
Kiverenge	8			1	1	2	5	1	18
Lembeni	19		1			1	3	1	25
Kiruru	1	30		4	1	1	2		39
Kighare Ward									
Nigongaya			18		5	9			32
Ngujini		9	1		6		2		18
Total	107	42	20	5	13	13	12	2	214
Percent	50.0	19.6	9.4	2.3	6.1	6.1	5.6	0.9	100

Chapter 7 Education for Liberation and Development in the Perspective of Lifelong Education

A J Cropley and Hede Menke

The continuing development of education for liberation and development Tanzania is an example of how a particular society may move towards implementation of the principles of lifelong education, even though educational changes are not specifically developed with lifelong education in mind. The brief analysis which follows does not summarize the reforms that have been set under way in Tanzania, nor evaluate them. To a considerable extent this has already been done in the earlier chapters. The purpose of the present chapter is to draw readers' attention to the possibility of interpreting the Tanzanian experience from the viewpoint of lifelong education, and to give some illustrative examples. It is hoped that this will cast further light on the concept of lifelong education, especially by showing how some of its principles can be implemented in practice.

1. Aspects of lifelong education

(a) Basic principles

It is increasingly being argued that formal education concentrated into a few years during childhood, adolescence and youth is no longer appropriate in the light of the requirements of contemporary life. Schooling cannot provide all the knowledge that people will require during a lifetime. Consequently, purposeful and conscious learning in response to or even in anticipation of the successively changing requirements of life will be needed throughout each person's lifetime, and services or means to facilitate such learning should be envisaged, i.e. systems of lifelong education. Lifelong education rests upon three main principles. The first could be referred to as *vertical integration*. Learning occurs throughout life, and should be facilitated by a system in which the successive phases of learning mutually support and complement each other and are co-ordinated among themselves. The second major principle is *horizontal integration*. Learning experiences are not provided by a single, but a series of parallel agencies, many of which are part of life itself. Thus, life is a major educative force, and social experiences, cultural activities, family relationships and work have important educative functions which should be co-ordinated into a more comprehensive education system. The third major principle is that lifelong education presupposes the active involvement of the individuals concerned, who consequently should possess the necessary *personal prerequisites* including not only appropriate learning skills and abilities, but also traits such as belief in themselves as capable of changing and improving, as well as motivation for learning throughout life.

(b) Properties of a lifelong education system
An education system based on these three principles would have six main characteristics. The first is *totality*. A lifelong education system should cover the entire lifespan, include all levels of formal education such as pre-primary, primary, secondary, post-secondary and adult education, embrace all forms of education such as academic, vocational, technical or recreational and accept all delivery systems such as formal, informal and non-formal. The second characteristic is the *equality of value* of all components of the system. All educative instances have a value of their own and a value within the whole. The home, the work place, cultural and recreational activities are of no more but also of no less value than schools, universities or adult education programmes. As a logical consequence, lifelong education systems should show *flexibility*. This is manifested in the adoption of new methods, materials and media as they develop, in the introduction of alternative patterns and organizations of education, and in diversity in content, learning tools, techniques of learning, and the timing of learning.

One further characteristic of a system of lifelong education is *democratization*. The availability of formal education services to the whole of the age group concerned, and to an increasingly larger variety and number of levels of ability, would be widened to include all ages and all forms of education.

A system of lifelong education is also guided by the aim of a *better life*. Its ultimate goal is the creation of conditions that allow the self-fulfilment of each individual. It is concerned with the fulfilment of each community and society as a whole, by guaranteeing for all their members a life of respect for each other and of human dignity, so that the self-confidence and vigour of their citizens are released and they can participate to the maximum degree in political, cultural, social and economic life.

Finally, a lifelong education system is guided by the immediate purpose of developing people's *educability*. They should be able to set and pursue goals, judge their own degree of success and failure, adopt new strategies and techniques when older ones have been found wanting, learn from many different sources and in many different settings, and make use of many different kinds of information. Thus, the system would place great emphasis on self-learning and on activities fostering skill in locating information. A major learning activity would be that of inter-learning, in which students learn from each other. Finally, education which is to be linked with life requires the ability to participate in life as a learning process. Students would thus be expected to relate their school learning to the issues and problems of everyday life, and also to relate learning in life to activities carried on in school.

2. Lifelong education and the Tanzanian educational reform

Three broad themes of contemporary education in Tanzania, enunciated in the speeches of President Nyerere, appear to guide educational reform in this country. These are (1) education for liberation, (2) linking of education and life, (3) making education a lifelong process. The ways in which these principles have been employed in the design of a real-life educational system in Tanzania may be seen as a practical example of lifelong education.

(a) Education for liberation
Liberation from the colonial mentality, from passive submission to circumstances instead of changing those circumstances, and from the limitations imposed by technical ignorance is needed. Achieving such liberation requires recognition that it is possible to improve the quality of people's lives, development of the skills that will make the necessary improvements possible, fostering of co-operative attitudes, and achievement of universal participation in implementing the national policy goals. Education for liberation in Tanzania is therefore based on equality, respect for human dignity, sharing of resources and work by everyone. It may thus be understood in some of the terms mentioned above: improved quality of life, educability and democratization.

For most Tanzanians living in rural areas, an improved quality of life means largely liberation from poverty, technological ignorance and the risk of exploitation. This requires developing their rural environment and way of life towards self-reliance and co-operation. One programme which has been adopted is that of Universal Primary Education (UPE). Another is the adult literacy programme which has been under way for several years. In order to achieve independence from foreign manpower in senior positions, secondary education has been greatly expanded. In the areas of health and nutrition, major public education campaigns have been launched, while the socio-economic development of villages has been fostered through the initiation of a large number of local projects emphasizing self-reliance, such as clearing of land for vegetable-growing, opening of poultry-keeping facilities, and similar plans.

Within the context of Tanzania, education involves the process of learners recognizing their own capacities and developing confidence in them. It also involves the further development of their capacities as a result of using them, the collective process of working together to improve their lives, and their understanding of the concept of self-reliance. In this sense, it is concerned with educability. This goal has been pursued by the encouragement of self-help activities, by local participation in the development of the school curriculum, by recognition of the importance of Tanzanian history and culture, and by the acknowledgement of Swahili as the official language. It has also involved activities such as school farms to encourage the pupils to recognize their own working capacities and to gain self-confidence in their exercise. Finally, opportunities have been created to develop learning abilities through programmes such as radio study groups, adult literacy projects and similar activities.

Democratization, or equality in education for all people, has been pursued through the establishment of UPE for all Tanzanians, regardless of religious, racial or economic origin. School fees have been abolished. The school curriculum has been adapted to local conditions. Formal entrance examinations are no longer the only criterion for entrance to higher education. Opportunities for education have been extended to include workers as well as students, through various institutions and through expedients like correspondence courses and radio study groups. Another relatively underprivileged group, women, has also been encouraged to participate in higher education.

Finally, democratization has been implemented through the sharing of decision-making and co-operation among people of different status in the educational process, at all levels of the system. Enterprises employing more than ten people have to establish workers' councils which participate in the planning of worker training programmes. Pupils participate in decision-making in schools through students' councils. Pupils are also involved in the planning of self-help activities, while for their part, villagers participate in decisions about schools. Even at the level of designing educational research projects, villagers who would be affected by the findings have shared with researchers in the planning.

(b) Linking education and life

A second major characteristic of the Tanzanian educational system is the integration of education with life. A number of measures have been undertaken which may be considered as administrative pre-conditions facilitating local input into this integration, such as the appointment of local education officers responsible for co-ordinating educational programmes in their areas, formation of adult education committees at national, regional and local levels to foster co-ordination between different formal and non-formal educational activities, and establishment of workers' educational committees at all levels, in order to provide work-oriented control of programmes and mobilize workers for enrolment.

Learning facilities are also integrated in the sense, for example, that formal educational institutions, particularly primary schools, function simultaneously as institutions for non-formal and adult education. In community centres, folk development colleges and similar institutions, this co-ordination permits the introduction into the formal classroom conditions of such activities as library work, handicraft and workshops, and the articulation of a variety of formal and non-formal programmes such as UPE, literacy courses, women's education, nutrition and health projects, self-help activities, and so on. This reduces the barriers between school and non-school learning.

Work is an important aspect of life. In Tanzania, education and work have been combined according to the needs of the local communities and the national policy of self-reliance. At primary and secondary school level, for example, work has become an integral part of the curriculum, so that schools also function as farms, workshops or other work places. On the other hand, factories, community centres and villages have also become places of education. In universities too, practical and professional work is part of the curriculum, while at least two years' work experience is required before entering university. Former bursary holders are required to work in government service as a way of repaying the support they have received from society. These aspects of Tanzanian education are aimed at permitting learners to contribute to the cost of their studies, discouraging intellectual arrogance among the highly educated, and, through work activities, integrating the students' learning with the workers' mode of living. Amalgamation of educational programmes and the contents of learning with the lives of local communities and with their developmental needs is a focal principle of all Tanzanian education.

(c) Making education lifelong

The third major theme identified in the Tanzanian reform is education as a lifelong process. Basically this has been achieved in Tanzania in three ways. The first involves the integration of formal and non-formal education, for example, through the development of a common administrative structure, through the imposition on all primary schools of the requirement that they become centres for adult education classes, and through the requirement that all school teachers assume responsibility for teaching adults as well as children. In this way, among other things, an attempt has been made to upgrade the status of adult education and to give it official legitimacy. The second step involves the development of facilities for adult education. This has been attempted by the training of specialist adult education teachers and the development of community centres or folk development colleges. Educative experiences have also been brought to adults who cannot attend schools in the conventional sense, through the use of the media, and especially radio. Finally, the knowledge of non-professional teachers has been mobilized through a system of volunteer teachers.

The first two of these steps are largely concerned with providing the opportunity for lifelong eduation. The third is more concerned with fostering the skills of lifelong learning in conventional classrooms. This has been attempted through such expedients as concentration on educability as it has already been defined, changes in evaluation processes to encourage self-directed learning, self-evaluation, student-setting of goals, and similar activities. Attempts have also been made to change teaching and learning procedures and techniques, in order to foster attitudes and motives conducive to lifelong learning.

3. Studying the Tanzanian experiences from the point of view of lifelong education

The discussion of Tanzanian educational reform in this chapter has not been exhaustive. It has merely attempted to make some of the more obvious linkages between the principles of lifelong education and the theory and practice of education for liberation and development. Even this preliminary analysis, however, shows that both the theoretical basis of the reforms, as stated in the speeches of President Nyerere, and the practices adopted in implementing the theory, are highly consistent with the ideas of lifelong education. For this reason, although the reforms were not specifically developed in the light of lifelong education, they provide valuable insights into the problem of how to give it concrete expression.

Although they need not necessarily be studied in this way, the earlier chapters can be treated as a case study in lifelong education. It then becomes apparent that they provide many insights into how to give reality to the ideas of lifelong education, some of the problems to be expected, conditions which help or hinder the process, and similar information. Readers who wish to extend the present illustrative review will be assisted by the subject index to be found at the end of the book. This index may be treated as a kind of content analysis of the earlier chapters in terms of lifelong education, and will facilitate using the book as a study of the practical application of its principles. In this way it is hoped that the present report will increase understanding of lifelong education, at the same time as it increases knowledge of education for liberation and development.

List of Translated Swahili/English Words and Phrases appearing in the Text

Akida	German-trained Arab and Swahili administrators and tax-collectors in the early 19th century
Chakula ni Uhai	Food is Life (Slogan of nutrition education mass campaign)
Kilimo cha Kufa na Kupona	Agriculture as a Matter of Life or Death (Slogan of agricultural campaign)
Kiswahili	The Swahili language (in differentiation from other uses of the word 'Swahili')
Liwali	Local rulers set up by the German colonial administration
Mtu ni Afya	Man is Health (Slogan of health education mass campaign)
Mwalimu	Teacher
Operation Vijiji	Villagization Programme (settling of scattered population in Ujamaa villages)
Panga	Machete, broad heavy knife
Pwani	Coast (Region)
Shamba	Field, garden
Uhuru	Freedom
Ujamaa	Familyhood and Socialism (Planned self-contained villages)
Ushirika	Co-operative

Bibliography

A Selected and Structured Bibliography on Tanzanian Education Within Overall National Development
H Hinzen and V H Hundsdörfer

Some of the literature on education and development in Tanzania is not easily obtainable. Requests for most of the books and papers listed in this bibliography could be made to one of the following addresses as applicable:

Tanzania Publishing House
P.O. Box 2138, Dar es Salaam, Tanzania

East African Literature Bureau
P.O. Box 1408, Dar es Salaam, Tanzania

East African Publishing House
P.O. Box 30571, Nairobi, Kenya

Oxford University Press
P.O. Box 5299, Dar es Salaam, Tanzania

Institute of Education
P.O. Box 35094, Dar es Salaam, Tanzania

Institute of Adult Education
P.O. Box 20679, Dar es Salaam, Tanzania

Department of Education, University of Dar es Salaam
P.O. Box 35048, Dar es Salaam, Tanzania

Bureau of Resource Assessment and Land Use Planning
University of Dar es Salaam
P.O. Box 35097, Dar es Salaam, Tanzania

Economic Research Bureau, University of Dar es Salaam
P.O. Box 35097, Dar es Salaam, Tanzania

The Tanzania Education Journal
P.O. Box 9121, Dar es Salaam, Tanzania

Mbioni. The Journal of Kivukoni College
P.O. Box 9193, Dar es Salaam, Tanzania

Unesco: International Bureau of Education
Palais Wilson, CH-1211 Geneva 14, Switzerland

International Council for Adult Education
29 Prince Arthur Avenue, Toronto, Canda, M5R 1B2

A Bibliographies

1. Auger, George A (ed.) *Tanzania Education since Uhuru. Bibliography 1961–1971* Dar es Salaam: Institute of Education (1971) 269 pp. (mimeo.)
2. Hundsdörfer, Volkhard and Küper, Wolfgang *Bibliographie zur sozial-wissenschaftlichen Erforschung Tanzanias/Bibliography for Social Science Research on Tanzania* München: Weltforum (1974) X, 231 S. (Arnold-Bergstraesser-Institut: Materialien zu Entwicklung und Politik, Bd 6)
3. Institute of Adult Education, University of Dar es Salaam *A Source Book of Adult Education in Tanzania. A structured bibliography of books, papers and speeches on adult education* Dar es Salaam: Institute of Adult Education (June 1974) 63 pp. (Studies in Adult Education, No. 13)
4. Rweyemamu, A H *Government and Politics in Tanzania. A bibliography* Nairobi: The East African Academy (1972) 39 pp. (mimeo.) (Information Circular, No. 6, January 1972)

B General and collections

5. Cliffe, Lionel and Saul, John S (eds.) *Socialism in Tanzania* Dar es Salaam: East African Publishing House EAPH (1972 and 1973) (Political Studies 14)
   Vol. I: *Politics* (1972) 346 pp.
   Vol. II: *Policies* (1973) 358 pp.
6. Egero, E and Henin, R A *The Population of Tanzania. An analysis of the 1967 population census* Dar es Salaam: BRALUP and Bureau of Statistics (1973) 292 pp.
7. Kokuhirwa, H 'Towards Social and Economic Promotion of Rural Women in Tanzania'. In *Rikara* (Dar es Salaam: IAE) No. 1, (May 1975) 14 pp. and 2 app.
8. Mbughuni, L A *The Cultural Policy of the United Republic of Tanzania* Paris: The Unesco Press (1974)
9. Mushi, S S 'African Traditional Culture and the Problems of Rural Modernization'. *Taamuli* 2 (July 1972) No. 2, pp. 3–16
10. Nyerere, J K *Freedom and Unity/Uhuru na Umoja. A selection from writings and speeches 1952–1965* Dar es Salaam etc.: OUP (1966)
11. Nyerere J K *Freedom and Socialism/Uhuru na Ujamaa. A selection from writings and speeches 1965–1967* Dar es Salaam etc.: OUP (1968)
12. Nyerere, J K *Freedom and Development/Uhuru na Maendeleo. A selection from writings and speeches 1968–1973* Dar es Salaam etc.: OUP (1973)
13. Nyerere, J K *Speech in Parliament, 18th July, 1975* Dar es Salaam: The Government Printer (1975)
14. Ruhumbika, Gabriel (ed.) *Towards Ujamaa. Twenty years of TANU leadership* Dar es Salaam etc.: EALB (1974)
15. Rweyemamu, A H (ed.) *Nation Building in Tanzania. Problems and issues* Nairobi etc.: EAPH (1970)
16. Svendsen, K E and Teisen, M (eds.) *Self-Reliant Tanzania. A series of articles* Dar es Salaam: TPH (1969)
17. Tanganyika and Zanzibar, The United Republic of, *Tanganyika Five Year*

Plan for Economic and Social Development, 1st July, 1964–30th June, 1969 Dar
es Salaam: The Government Printer 1964
Vol. I: *General Analysis* p. 114
Vol. II: *The Programmes* p. 151

18. Tanzania, The United Republic of, *Tanzania Second Five-Year Plan for
Economic and Social Development, 1st July, 1969–30th June, 1974* Dar es
Salaam: The Government Printer (1969 and 1970)
Vol. I: *General Analysis* (1969) p. 227
Vol. II: *The Programmes* (1969) p. 115
Vol. III: *Regional Perspectives* (1970) p. 327
Vol. IV: *Survey of the High and Middle Level Manpower Requirements and
Resources* (1969) v. p. 18

19. Tanzania, The United Republic of, *Ten Years of National Service 1963–1973*
Dar es Salaam: TPH, n.d.

20. Tschannerl, G 'Employment and Population Growth in Tanzania' *Maji
Maji* (August 1975) No. 23, pp. 9–17

C History

21. Alpers, E A *The East African Slave Trade* Nairobi: EAPH (1967) (Historical
Association of Tanzania, Paper No. 3)

22. Iliffe, J *Tanganyika under German Rule 1905–1912* Nairobi: EAPH; London:
Oxford University Press (1969)

23. Kimambo, I N and Temu, A J (eds.) *A History of Tanzania* Published for
the Historical Association of Tanzania, Nairobi: EAPH (1969)

24. Listowel, Judith *The Making of Tanganyika* London: Chatto and Windus
(1965) p. 451

25. Ogot, B K and Kierch, J A (eds.) *Zamani. A survey of East African history*
Published for the Historical Association of Kenya, Nairobi: EAPH and
Longmans of Kenya (1965) p. 407

26. Omer-Cooper, J D *Tanzania before 1900* Published for the Historical
Association of Tanzania, Nairobi: EAPH (1968)

27. Ranger, T O *The Recovery of African Initiative in Tanzanian History* Dar es
Salaam: The University College (March 1969) p. 14 (Inaugural Lecture
Series, No. 2)

D Government and politics

28. Election Study Committee, The University of Dar es Salaam *Socialism and
Participation. Tanzania's 1970 national election* Dar es Salaam: (1974) p. 464

29. Harris, Belle 'Tanzania Elections 1965' *Mbioni* II (1965) No. 5, pp. 14–56

30. Martin, R *Personal Freedom and the Law in Tanzania. A study of socialist state
administration* Nairobi etc.: OUP (1974)

31. Mwansasu, Bismarck U 'Commentary on Mwongozo wa TANU, 1971
(= TANU Guidelines)' *The African Review* 1 (April 1972), No. 4, pp. 9–24

32. Mytton, Graham 'Mass Media and TANU. Information flow in Tanzania
and its relevance to development' In: *Provisional Council for the Social Sciences
in East Africa* 1st Annual Conference, University of Dar es Salaam
(December 1970) pp. 258–284 (Proceedings, Vol. 4)

33. Proctor, J H (ed.) *The Cell System of the Tanganyika African National Union* Dar es Salaam: TPH (1971) 6 pp. (University of Dar es Salaam: Studies in Political Science, No 1)

34. Rweyemamu, P 'From "Fear Discipline" to Socialist Self-Discipline: Problems of Organization and Democracy in Tanzania' *Taamuli* 3 (1973), No. 2, pp. 14–21

35. TANU 'TANU Guidelines on Guarding, Consolidating and Advancing the Revolution of Tanzania, and of Africa' *The African Review* 1 (April 1972), No. 4, pp. 1–8

36. Tanzania, The Prime Minister's Office *The Policy of Decentralization* 'Adult Education for Development', Conference and Study Tour on the Tanzanian Experiences in Functional Adult Education (July 29–August 7, 1974) in Dar es Salaam/Mwanza, Tanzania. p. 8 (mimeo.)

37. Tordoff, W *Government and Politics in Tanzania. Collection of essays covering the period from September 1960 to July 1966* Nairobi: EAPH (1967)

E Economy and rural development

38. Bienefeld, M 'The Informal Sector and Peripheral Capitalism: The Case of Tanzania' *Institute of Development Studies (Brighton) Bulletin*, 6 February 1975), No. 3, pp. 53–73

39. Clark, E 'Socialist Development in an Underdeveloped Country: The Case of Tanzania' *World Development* 3 (April 1975), No. 4, pp. 223–228

40. Coulson, A C *A Simplified Political Economy of Tanzania* Dar es Salaam: University of Dar es Salaam (November 1974) (ERB Paper 74.9)

41. Finucane, James R *Rural Development and Bureaucracy in Tanzania. The case of Mwanza region* Uppsala: Scandinavian Institute of African Studies (1974) p. 192

42. Freyhold, Michaela v. *The Workers and the Nizers. A study in class relations* Dar es Salaam: Institute of Finance Management (1975) 146 pp. and 51 tables (mimeo.) London: Monthly Review Press 1977 (revised edition)

43. Gitelson, S A *Multilateral Aid for National Development and Self-Reliance. A case study of the UNDP in Uganda and Tanzania* Kampala etc.: EALB (1975)

44. Hänsel, H; Vries, J de; Ndedya, P C (eds.) *Agricultural Extension in Ujamaa Village Development* Papers and Proceedings of a Workshop, Morogoro (September 22–27, 1975)

45. Hyden, Goran (ed.) *Co-operatives in Tanzania. Problems of organisation* Dar es Salaam: TPH 1976, 93 pp. (University of Dar es Salaam: Studies in Political Science, No. 4)

46. Kahama, C G 'Participation in Tanzania: The Role of National Development Corporation' *Mbioni* VI (1972), No. 11

47. Kahama, C G 'Promotion of Small Scale Industries in Ujamaa Villages' *Mbioni* VII (1973), No. 2, pp. 5–26

48. Loxley, J and Saul, J S 'Multinationals, Workers and Parastatals in Tanzania' *Review of African Political Economy* (January to April 1975), No. 2, pp. 54–88

49. Macpherson, G A *First Steps in Village Mechanization* Dar es Salaam: TPH (1975)

50. Mapolu, H (ed.) *Workers and Management* Dar es Salaam: TPH (1976) (Tanzania Studies Series, No. 4)
51. Mbilinyi, S M (ed.) *Agricultural Research for Rural Development. How do we use what we know?* Nairobi etc.: EALB (1973) (Proceedings of the 6th Annual Symposium of the East African Academy, Vol. 6 (1968)
52. Msuya, C D 'Foreign Aid and Tanzania Development' *Mbioni* VII (1974) No. 4, pp. 24–45
53. Mwapachu, J V 'Operation Planned Villages in Rural Tanzania. A revolutionary strategy for development' *Mbioni* VII (1975), No. 11, pp. 5–39
54. Nyalali, F L *Aspects of Industrial Conflicts. A case study of trade disputes in Tanzania 1967–1973* Dar es Salaam, Kampala, Nairobi: EALB (1975) p. 219
55. Nyerere, J K *The Third World and the International Economic Structure* Address given in Bonn, FRG, in the Headquarters of the Friedrich-Ebert-Stiftung and the Institute for International Relations (May 4, 1976)
56. Proctor, J H (ed.) *Building Ujamaa Villages in Tanzania* Dar es Salaam: TPH (1971) 69 pp. (University of Dar es Salaam: Studies in Political Science, No. 2)
57. Rural Development Research Committee, University of Dar es Salaam (ed.) *Rural Co-operation in Tanzania* Edited by Lionel Cliffe, Peter Lawrence, William Luttreell, Shem Migot-Auhoska and John S Saul. Dar es Salaam: Tanzania Publishing House (1975) p. 554
58. Saul, John S 'African Socialism in One Country: Tanzania'. In Arrighi, Giovanni and Saul, John S *Essays on the Political Economy of Africa* London/New York: Monthly Review Press (1973) pp. 237–335
59. Shivji, Issa G *Class Struggles in Tanzania* Dar es Salaam: TPH (1975) p. 182
60. Shivji, Issa G; Guruli, Kassim; Rodney, Walter; Rweyemamu, J F; Saul, John S; Szentes, Thomas *The Silent Class Struggle* Dar es Salaam: TPH (1973) p. 138 (Tanzanian Studies, No. 2)
61. Tanzania, The United Republic of, 'An Act to Provide for the Registration of Villages, the Administration of Registered Villages and Designation of Ujamaa Villages' *Acts Supplement to the Gazette of the United Republic of Tanzania* LVI (August 8 1975), No. 33, pp. 305–312
62. Tanzania, The United Republic of, *The Economic Survey 1973–1974* Dar es Salaam: The Government Printer 1975

F Education
F.1 History and development

63. Cameron, John 'The Integration of Education in Tanganyika' *Comparative Education Review* XI (February 1967), No. 1, pp. 38–56
64. Cameron, J and Dodd, W A *Society, Schools and Progress in Tanzania* Oxford, New York: Pergamon Press; Braunschschweig: Vieweg und Sohn (1970) XVI, p. 256
65. Lawuo, Z B 'Education and Training in Pre-Colonial Tanzania' In *Seminar on Teacher Education* Preliminary Report on the Teacher Education

Seminar held at the Institute of Education, Dar es Salaam (June 4–16) 1973) Dar es Salaam: University of Dar es Salaam, Institute of Education 1973

66. Mbilinyi, M J *African Education in the British Colonial Period (1919–1961)* Dar es Salaam: University of Dar es Salaam, Education Department (1975) (mimeo.)

67. Saul, P *Agricultural Education in Tanganyika 1925–1955. The policy programmes and practices* Paper read at the 5th Annual Symposium of the East African Academy, Dar es Salaam (September 15–16 1968) p. 17 (mimeo.)

68. Sifuna, D N *Vocational Education in Schools. A historical survey of Kenya and Tanzania* Dar es Salaam, Kampala, Nairobi: EALB (1976) p. 200

69. Tanganyika *The Education Ordinance, 1961 (No. 37 of 1961), Regulations* Dar es Salaam: The Government Printer (1962) p. 9

70. Tanzania, The United Republic of, 'The Education Act, 1969. (No. 13 of 1969)' *Bill Supplement to the Gazette of the United Republic of Tanzania* L (November 28 1969), No. 51. Dar es Salaam: the Government Printer (1969)

F.2 General conception, planning and research

71. Besha, M R *Education for Self-Reliance and Rural Development* Based on 'Study of Some Schools and Villages in Bagamoyo and Rufiji Districts'. First draft for private circulation. Dar es Salaam: University of Dar es Salaam, Institute of Education (1973) p. 41 (mimeo.)

72. Chamungwana, W M *Socialization Problems in Tanzania: An Appraisal of Education for Self-Reliance as a Strategy of Cultural Transformation* Dar es Salaam: University of Dar es Salaam, Institute of Education (July 1975) pp. 51–67 (Studies in Curriculum Development, No. 5)

73. Heijnen, J D *Development and Education in the Mwanza District (Tanzania): A Case Study of Migration and Peasant Farming* (Report). Rotterdam: Bronder Offset for CESC (Center for the Study of Education in Changing Societies) (1968) p. 171

74. Ishumi, A`G M *Education. A review of concepts, ideas and practices* Dar es Salaam: University of Dar es Salaam, Institute of Education 1974

75. Ishumi, A G M 'Some Significant Factors Influencing Community Access to Education and Modernization: A Case of Rural and Suburban Tanzania in *Annual Social Science Conference of the East African Universities* Dar es Salaam (1973) (Collected Papers, edited by E O Okumu) Dar es Salaam: University of Dar es Salaam (September 1974) pp. 507–606

76. Jengo, E 'Educational Technology: Its Place in the Process of Lifelong Education in Tanzania' *Programmed Learning and Educational Technology* (London), 12 (September 1975) No. 5, pp. 270–273

77. Kassam, Y O *The Relationship Between Formal and Non-Formal Education: A Case Study—Tanzania* Dar es Salaam: University of Dar es Salaam, Department of Education, n.y. (typescr.)

78. Kinunda, M J *The Place of Evaluation in the Tanzanian System of Education* Paris: IIEP (September 16 1974) p. 34

79. Knight, J B 'The Costing and Financing of Educational Development in Tanzania' in: *Costing and Financing* Paris: Unesco (1969) pp. 9–83

(Unesco: IIEP African Research Studies *Educational Development in Africa* II

80. Lema, A A *Education for Self-Reliance. A brief survey of self-reliance activities in some Tanzanian schools and colleges* Dar es Salaam: Institute of Education, University of Dar es Salaam (1973) p. 110 (mimeo.)

81. Mbilinyi, M J *The Education of Girls in Tanzania. A study of attitudes of Tanzanian girls and their fathers towards education* Dar es Salaam: Institute of Education, University College (1969) p. 62

82. Mbilinyi, M J 'Education for Rural Life or Education for Socialist Transformation' in: *Collected Papers of the Ninth Science Conference of the East African Universities* (December 18–20, 1973) at the University of Dar es Salaam (Edited by E O Okumu) Dar es Salaam: University of Dar es Salaam (September 1974) pp. 437–464

83. Mbilinyi, M J 'Education, Stratification and Sexism in Tanzania: Policy Implications' *The African Review* 3 (June 1973), No. 2, pp. 327–340

84. Mbilinyi, M J *Educational Innovations in Tanzania* Paper presented to ICI Conference on Education, University of Ottawa (April 7–12, 1975) p. 32 (mimeo.)

85. Ministry of National Education *Community Education Centres. Proposals for improvement of international efficiency in the primary education system* Dar es Salaam: Ministry of National Education, Directory of Planning and Development (November 9, 1973) p. 19 (mimeo.)

86. Morrisson, D R *Education and Politics in Africa. The Tanzanian case* London: Murst & Company (1976)

87. Mwingira, A C and Pratt, Simon 'The Process of Educational Planning in Tanzania' in: *The Planning Process* Paris: Unesco (1969) pp. 103 199 (Unesco: IIEP African Research Studies *Educational Development in Africa*, I)

88. Mwobahe, B L and Mbilinyi, M J (eds.) *Challenge of Education for Self-Reliance in Tanzania* A Report based on the Workshop on Education (March 22–23, 1974) organized by the Institute of Education in conjunction with the Department of Education. Dar es Salaam: Institute of Education (1975)

89. Overseas Liaison Committee, American Council of Education *Tanzania: A Nation-Wide Learning System* Submitted to the Education Projects Department, International Bank of Reconstruction and Development, International Development Association and to the Government of Tanzania (November 15, 1971)

90. Prewitt, Kenneth (ed.) *Education and Political Values. An East African case study* Nairobi: EAPH (1971) p. 249

91. Resnick, Idrian (ed.) *Tanzania: Revolution by Education* Arusha: Longmans of Tanzania (1968) p. 252

92. Sabot, R H *Education, Income Distribution, and Rates of Urban Migration in Tanzania* Dar es Salaam: University of Dar es Salaam (September 1972) p. 40 (ERB Paper 72.6)

93. Skorov, George 'Integration of Educational and Economic Planning in Tanzania' in *Integration and Administration* Paris: Unesco (1969) pp. 9-82 (Unesco: IIEP African Research Studies *Educational Development in Africa*, III)

94. Tanzania, The United Republic of, 'The Institute of Education Act, 1975' *Acts Supplement to the Gazette of the United Republic of Tanzania* (August 12, 1975), No. 5, pp. 115–126

95. Toroka, S 'Education for Self-Reliance: The Litowa Experiment' *Mbioni* IV (May 1968), No. XI, pp. 2–25

96. Varkevisser, C M *Socialization in a Changing Society. Sukuma childhood in rural and urban Mwanza, Tanzania* Dar es Salaam: Centre for the Study of Education in Changing Societies (CESC) (1973) p. 334

97. Wood, A W 'The Community School Tanzania—The Experience at Litowa's *Teacher Education in New Countries* X (1969) No. 1, pp. 4–12

98. Zanolli, Noa Vera *Education toward Development in Tanzania. A study of the educative process in a rural area (Ulanga district)* Basel: Pharos-Verlag Hansrudolf Schwabe (1971) p. 368 (Baseler Beiträge zur Ethnologie, Bd 8)

F.3 Formal schooling

99. Court, D 'The Social Functions of Formal Schooling in Tanzania' *The African Review* 3 (1974) No. 4, pp. 577–593

100. Hirji, K F 'School Education and Underdevelopment in Tanzania' *Maji Maji* (September 1973) No. 12, pp. 1–22

101. Kibodya, G *The Teaching of African History* Dar es Salaam: University of Dar es Salaam, Institute of Education, n.y. p. 53 and p. 4 bibliography

102. Mmari, G R V 'The Role of Formal Education in Developing Countries: The Tanzanian Case' in *Policy and Practice in Tanzanian Education* Dar es Salaam: University of Dar es Salaam, Department of Education (July 1975) pp. 1–21 (Papers in Education and Development, No. 1)

F.3.1 Primary education

103. Auger, G A *Absenteeism in Primary Schools in Tanzania* Dar es Salaam: Institute of Education (March 1970) (Studies in Tanzanian Education, No. 2)

104. Center for the Study of Education in Changing Societies (CESC) *Primary Education in Sukumaland, Tanzania* A Summary Report of a study made by the Center for the Study of Education in Changing Societies, The Hague. Groningen: Wolters-Noordhoff (for CESC) (1969) p. 147

105. Dubbledam, L F B *The Primary School and the Community in Mwanza District, Tanzania* Groningen: Wolters-Noordhoff (for CESC) (1970) p. 199

106. Institute of Education *The Tanzania UNICEF/Unesco Primary Education Reform Project. Evaluation report no. 1* Dar es Salaam: University of Dar es Salaam, Institute of Education (December 1973) p. 108

107. Institute of Education *The Tanzania UNICEF/Unesco Primary Education Reform Project. Evaluation report no. 2* Dar es Salaam: University of Dar es Salaam, Institute of Education (December 1974) p. 95

108. Mbilinyi, M J *The Problem of Unequal Access to Primary Education in Tanzania* Paper No. 21 for Annual Social Science Conference of the East African Universities, December 18–20 (1973) at the University of Dar es Salaam. Dar es Salaam: University of Dar es Salaam 1974, p. 22

109. Mbunda, D *U P E by 1977* Dar es Salaam: IAE, n.y. p. 7 and App. (mimeo.)

110. Meer, F W van 'Art and Craft Education in Primary School. Choice and emphasis' *The Tanzania Education Journal* 3 (1974) No. 7, pp. 32–34
111. Mvungi, M V *When to Introduce English in Tanzania Primary Schools* Dar es Salaam: Institute of Education (December 1974) pp. 12–23 (Studies in Tanzanian Education, No. 4)
112. Omari, I O *The Credibility of Primary 7 School Leaving and Selection Examination* Dar es Salaam: Institute of Education (December 1974) pp. 3–11 (Studies in Tanzanian Education, No. 4)

F.3.2 Secondary education
113. Brumfit, C J *English Language in the Secondary School* Dar es Salaam: University of Dar es Salaam, Institute of Education (1972) pp. 77–85 (Studies in Curriculum Development, No. 1)
114. Evans, J F *The School Science Project in Physics for the Secondary School* Dar es Salaam: UDSM, IE (1972) pp. 112–116 (Studies in Curriculum Development, No. 1)
115. Hyslop, G *The Study of African Music in Secondary Schools* Dar es Salaam: UDSM, IE (1972) pp. 8–20 (Studies in Curriculum Development, No. 2)
116. Kanyili, A *Introducing the New Curricula for Technical Schools in Diversified Secondary Education* Dar es Salaam: UDSM, IE (July 1975) (Studies in Curriculum Development, No. 5)
117. Meena, A S 'Biology Examinations in Secondary Schools' *The Tanzania Education Journal* 2 (1973) No. 4, pp. 26–28
118. Meena, A S 'New Change in Biology Curriculum for Secondary Schools in Tanzania' *The Tanzanian Education Journal* 1 (1972) No. 2, pp. 16–21
119. Ministry of National Education, Directorate of Planning 'Diversification of Secondary Education' *The Tanzania Education Journal* 2 (1973) No. 5, pp. 11–16
120. Mmari, E E *A Study of the Understanding of Mathematical Ideas and Concepts among Tanzanian Secondary School Pupils. (A summary report)* Dar es Salaam: University of Dar es Salaam, Institute of Education (December 1974) pp. 26–30 (Studies in Tanzanian Education, No. 4)
121. Pendaeli, J *The School Science Project in Chemistry for the Secondary School* Dar es Salaam: UDSM, IE (1972) pp. 101–111 (Studies in Curriculum Development, No. 1)
122. Pochard, J C *Guidelines for French Teaching in Secondary Schools Form I to Form IV* Dar es Salaam: UDSM, IE (1973) pp. 1–8 (Studies in Curriculum Development, No. 3)
123. Vella, J *Developing a Revised Syllabus in Literature for Tanzania Secondary Schools* Dar es Salaam: UDSM, IE (1973) pp. 15–28 (Studies in Curriculum Development, No. 3)

F.4 Teacher training
124. Jiboku, S O 'Some Aspects of Leadership Behaviour of Tanzania Headmasters' *Education in Eastern Africa* 4 (1974) No. 1, pp. 155–162
125. Michongwe, E M P 'The Teacher's Role in School and Society' *The Tanzania Education Journal* 3 (1974) No. 6, pp. 34–35

126. Ministry of National Education *Programme Grade 'A' Teacher Education* Dar es Salaam: Issued by the Ministry of Education (Printtak Tanzania) (1969) p. 39 and App. (photos)

127. Mmari, G R V *The Role of the Teacher in the Development Process* Paper presented to a Regional Workshop on Unsolved Problems in Preparing Teachers for Basic Education (December 1–5, 1975) Dar es Salaam p. 24 (mimeo.)

128. Moshi, E E *Professional Training of the Primary School Teaching Force* Dar es Salaam: University of Dar es Salaam, Institute of Education (1973) pp. 11–23 (Studies in Curriculum Development, No. 4)

129. Nwagwu, N A *Teachers and Curriculum Development* Dar es Salaam: UDSM, IE (1973) pp. 26–34 (Studies in Curriculum Development, No. 4)

130. Rones, P S *Teacher Training at Batimba. A case study in Tanzania* Groningen: Wolters-Noordhoff (for CESC, The Hague) 1970, p. 197

131. Tunginie, S *Teacher Education in Tanzania* Paper presented to a Regional Workshop on Unsolved Problems in Preparing Teachers for Basic Education (December 1–5, 1975) Dar es Salaam. p. 5 (mimeo)

132. White, M J *The Education of Teachers for the People of Tanzania* Dar es Salaam: UDSM, IE (1972) pp. 36–54 (Studies in Curriculum Development, No. 1)

F.5 Adult education in general

133. Hall, B L *Adult Education and the Development of Socialism in Tanzania* Dar es Salaam: EALB (1975)

134. Hall, B L and Mhaiki, P J *The Integration of Adult Education in Tanzania* Dar es Salaam: University of Dar es Salaam, Institute of Education (1975)

135. Institute of Adult Education *Adult Education Directory 1975. A guide to agencies, courses and facilities in Tanzania* Dar es Salaam: University of Dar es Salaam, Institute of Adult Education 1975

136. Kassam, Y O (ed.) *Adult Education and Development. A Tanzanian case study* Prepared for the International Conference of Adult Education and Development/Elimu ya Watu Wazima na Maendeleo, Dar es Salaam (June 21–26, 1976)

137. Kibira, E 'Adult Education in Tanzania' *Kenya Journal of Adult Education* (March 1975) No. 1, pp. 8–12

138. Kubanga, N A *Organization and Administration of Adult Education in Tanzania* Dar es Salaam: Institute of Adult Education (1975) p. 21 (mimeo.)

139. London, J 'A Model of a Comprehensive Programme of Adult Education in the Third World. A case study of Tanzania' *Literacy Discussion* IV (1973) No. 3, pp. 285–322

140. Mayani, Y H *The TANU Educational Concept in the Context of Adult Education* 'Adult Education for Development', Conference and Study Tour on the Tanzanian Experiences in Functional Adult Education (July 29–August 7) in Dar es Salaam/Mwanza, Tanzania p. 26 (mimeo.)

141. Mbunda, D *Adult Education in Tanzania. Lifelong process for national development* Study for the Interdisciplinary Symposium on Lifelong Education, organized by Unesco in Paris (September 25–October 2 1972) p. 11 Paris: Unesco (1972)

142. Mbunda, D 'The Institute of Adult Education and it's Obligation to Tanzania' *The Tanzania Education Journal* 3 (1974) No. 7, pp. 17–20

143. Mhaiki, P J 'Political Education and Adult Education' *Convergence* VI (1973) No. 1, pp. 15–21

144. Müller, J *International Symposium on Adult Education for Development* Conference and Study Tour on the Tanzanian Experiences in Functional Adult Education (July 29–August 7 1974) in Dar es Salaam/Mwanza, Tanzania. Summary Report, Bonn: German Foundation for International Development (DSE); Ministry of National Education of the United Republic of Tanzania and the Institute of Adult Education, Dar es Salaam (1974) p. 49

145. National Adult Education Association of Tanzania (ed.) *Adult Education and Development in Tanzania* Vol. I Dar es Salaam: NAEAT (1975) p. 151

146. Nyerere, J K *Adult Education and Development* Speech given at the International Conference on Adult Education and Development and Elimu ya Watu Wazima na Maendeleo, Dar es Salaam (June 21–26 1976) organized by Tanzanian National Conference Committee and International Council for Adult Education.

147. Sallnäs, I *Comparative Adult Education. Tanzania, United States, Sweden, Soviet Union, China, Cuba, Mozambique, Somalia. A handbook* Dar es Salaam: Institute of Adult Education (1975) p. 350

148. Tanzania, The United Republic of, 'The Institute of Adult Education Act, 1975' *Acts Supplement to the Gazette of the United Republic of Tanzania* (August 12 1975) No. 4, pp. 103–114

F.5.1 Basic education for adults

149. Evaluation Unit Mwanza, The, *UNDP/Unesco Work-Oriented Adult Literacy. Pilot Project Lake Regions Tanzania: Final evaluation report, 1968–1972* Mwanza: WCALPP (May 1973) p. 136

150. Grenholm, L H *Radio Study Group Campaigns in the United Republic of Tanzania* Paris: The Unesco Press (1975) (International Bureau of Education: Experiments and innovations in education No. 15)

151. Hall, Budd L; Maganga, C K; Malya, Simon; Mhaiki, Paul J *The 1971 Literacy Campaign Study* Dar es Salaam: Institute of Adult Education (April 1972) p. 72 (Monograph). (mimeo.)

152. Hall, B L and Zikambona, C *Mtu ni Afya. An evaluation of the 1973 mass health education campaign* Dar es Salaam: Institute of Adult Education (1973) p. 174 (Studies in Adult Education No. 12)

153. Kassam, Y O 'Towards Mass Adult Education in Tanzania: The Rationale for Radio Study Group Campaigns' *Literacy Discussion* VI (Spring 1975) No. 1, pp. 79–94

154. Kaungamno, E E *After Literacy What? The role of libraries in post-literacy adult education* A paper presented at NAEAT seminar (November 17–18 1972) Dar es Salaam: Institute of Adult Education (1972)

155. Mahai, B A P; Haule, G S; Timotheo, E K; Joachim, A K *Chakula ni Uhai. A guide to evaluation of the Food is Life Campaign—1975* Dar es Salaam: Institute of Adult Education (1975) p. 38 (mimeo.)

156. Malya, S *Traditional Oral Literature Procuring Post-Literacy Reading Material*

and Capturing Culture Dar es Salaam: Institute of Adult Education (1974) p. 16 (Studies in Adult Education No. 10)

157. Mbakile, E P R *The Evaluation of the UNDP/Unesco Functional Literacy Project in Tanzania* Mwanza: UNDP/Unesco Functional Literacy Curriculum Programmes and Materials Development Project, Tanzania (1974) p. 14 (mimeo.)

158. Mbakile, E P R *The National Literacy Campaign: A Summary of Results of the Nation-Wide Literacy Tests* Mwanza: The Ministry of National Education, Tanzania, UNDP/Unesco Functional Literacy Curriculum, Programmes and Materials Development Project (February 1976) (mimeo.)

159. Mbakile, E P R *Radio Education Programmes as a Support to Literacy Methods: The Experiences in Tanzania* Mwanza: Literacy Project (February 1976) (mimeo.)

160. Mlekwa, V M *Mass Education and Functional Literacy Programmes in Tanzania. Searching for a model* Dar es Salaam: Institute of Adult Education (1975) (Studies in Adult Education No. 21)

161. Mpogolo, Z J *Implementation of Functional Literacy in Tanzania by the UNDP/Unesco Work-Oriented Adult Literacy Pilot Project in the Lake Regions* Prepared by the National Deputy Director of the Project, Mwanza, Tanzania. 'Adult Education for Development', Conference and Study Tour on the Tanzanian Experiences in Functional Adult Education, (July 29–August 7 1974) in Dar es Salaam/Mwanza, Tanzania. p. 19 (mimeo.)

162. Österling, O *The Literacy Campaign. A short introduction* Produced within the Directorate of Adult Education, Ministry of National Education, Tanzania. n.p.: SIDA (1974) p. 24

F.5.2 Manpower-oriented training and education

163. Barkan, Joel D *An African Dilemma. University students, development and politics in Ghana, Tanzania and Uganda* Nairobi, London, New York: OUP (1975) p. 259

164. Chale, E M *Towards Effective Teaching of Adults by Correspondence Education Method in Tanzania* Dar es Salaam: University of Dar es Salaam (1975) p. 59 (M.A. Diss.)

165. Erdos, R F *Establishing an Institution by Correspondence* Paris: The Unesco Press (1975) p. 59 (International Bureau of Education: Experiments and Innovations in Education No. 17)

166. Grabe, S 'Tanzania: An Educational Program for Co-operatives' in: Ahmed, M and Coombs, P H (eds.) *Education for Rural Development. Case studies for planners* New York etc.: Praeger (1975) pp. 589–616

167. Hall, B L *Who Participates in University Adult Education?* Dar es Salaam: Institute of Adult Education (1973) p. 17 (Studies in Adult Education No. 5)

168. Kassam, Y O *The Diploma Course in Adult Education. An Evaluation of the Diploma Course in Adult Education in Relation to the Functions of Professional Adult Educators in Tanzania* Dar es Salaam: Institute of Adult Education (1974) p. 26 (Studies in Adult Education No. 11)

169. Maliyamkono, T L *Higher Education for Economic Development. Training of middle level manpower* A paper presented at the Eastern African Universities

Conference at the National University of Lesotho (June 28–July 2, 1976) p. 21 and tables (mimeo.)

170. Mbunda, D *Manpower Training for Increased Productivity in Tanzania* Paper for Regional Seminar on University-Level Continuing Education for Manpower Development in Africa. Conjoined with the Fourth Conference of the African Adult Education Association, Addis Ababa (September 3–14, 1973) p. 32 and App. I–III

171. Ministry of Economic Affairs and Development Planning, Manpower Planning Division *Annual Manpower Report to the President 1973* Dar es Salaam: Ministry of Economic Affairs and Development Planning (November 1974) p. 109 and App. No. 1–4

172. Ministry of Manpower Development, Manpower Planning Division *Annual Manpower Report to the President 1974* Dar es Salaam: Ministry of Manpower Development (1975) p. 134 and App. p. 100

173. Mkunduge, G (ed.) *Tanzania and Somalia* Dar es Salaam: Institute of Adult Education (1975) p. 97

174. Mwambene, N K M The National Institute for Productivity, Ministry of Labour and Social Welfare *Adult Education in the Context of Industrial Productivity and Manpower Development* 'Adult Education for Development', Conference and Study Tour on the Tanzanian Experiences in Functional Adult Education (July 29–August 7 1974) in Dar es Salaam/Mwanza, Tanzania. p. 31 (mimeo.)

175. National Institute for Productivity (ed.) *Guide to Workers' Education. Manual in workers' education for workers' education officers, organizers, instructors and teachers* Dar es Salaam: NIP (1973) p. 103

176. 'New Terms and Conditions for Application to Civil Servants Attending Courses of Higher Education' *The Tanzania Education Journal* (1976) No. 11, pp. 20–25

177. Rwegasira, D 'Career Guidance, Career Policy and High-Level Manpower Efficiency in Tanzania' *The African Review* 4 (1974) No. 1, pp. 111–126

178. Southall, Roger *Federalism and Higher Education in East Africa* Nairobi: EPH (1974) p. 160 (East African Specials, 16)

179. Tanzania, The United Republic of 'The University of Dar es Salaam Act, 1970' *Bill Supplement (No. 4) to the Gazette of the United Republic of Tanzania* LI (June 5 1970) No. 23, p. 39 Dar es Salaam: Government Printer 1970

180. Working Party on Ujamaa and Co-operative Training *Ujamaa and Co-operative Education Plan, Tanzania, 1973–1979* n.p.: (1973) p. 29 (mimeo.)

G Late additions

181. Ergas Z *La 3ᵉ Métamorphose de l'Afrique noire: Essai sur l'économie politique de l'éducation et le développement rural* with a case study on Tanzania. Genève: Editions Médicine et Hygiène (1977)

182. Gillette, A 'L'Education en Tanzanie: Une réforme de plus ou une révolution éducationnelle?' *Tiers Monde* Paris. (octobre–décembre 1975)

183. Gillette, A *Beyond the Non-Formal Fashion: Towards Educational Revolution in*

Tanzania Amherst, Massachusetts: University of Massachusetts, Centre for International Education (1977) p. 321

184. Hall, Budd 'The United Republic of Tanzania: A National Priority to Adult Education' *Prospects* (1974) No. 4

185. Mmari, G R V 'Attempts to Link School with Work: The Tanzanian Experience' *Prospects* (1977) No. 3

186. Swantz, N L 'Research as an Educational Tool for Development', a case study on adult education in Tanzania. *Convergence* (English with summaries in French, Spanish and Russian) Toronto: ICAE. (1975) No. 2

187. 'Tanzania, a case study on literacy' in *The Experimental World Literacy Programme: A Critical Assessment* Paris: Unesco Press/UNDP (1976)

188. Vacchi, L 'La politica educativa della Tanzania: l'educazione per "l'autofiducia"' *Terzo Mondo* Milano (December 1973)

Subject Index